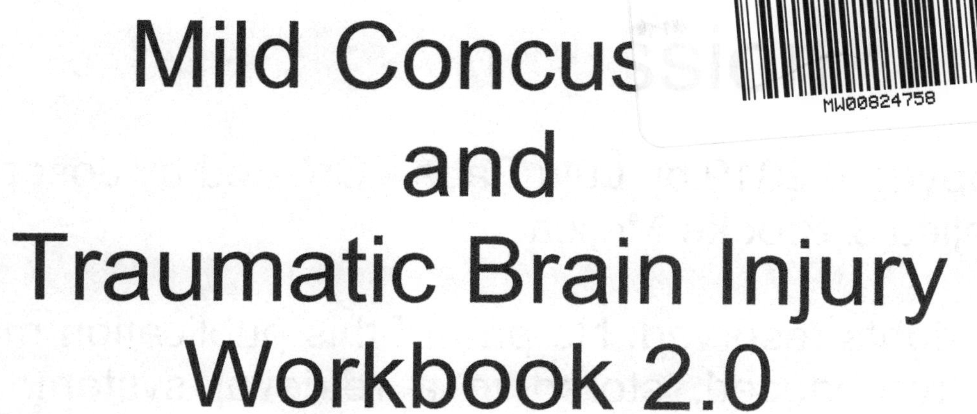

Mild Concussion and Traumatic Brain Injury Workbook 2.0

MW00824758

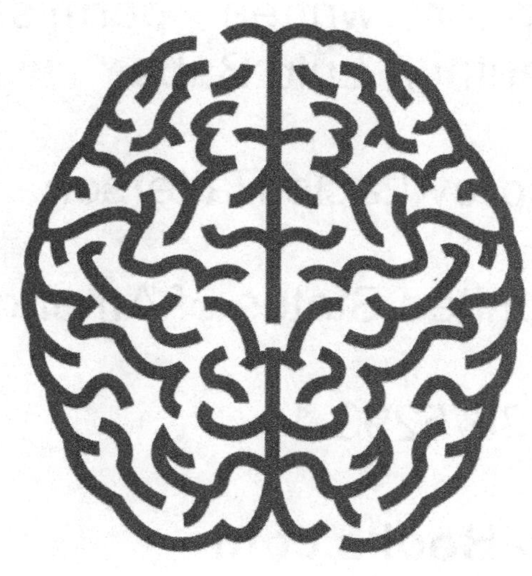

A Method to Help

Track your Recovery Process

Lulu Baba

Copyright 2019 by Lulu Baba - Created by Joseph Mejica & Brooke Mejica

All rights reserved. No part of this publication may be reproduced, stored in a retrieval system, or transmitted, in any form or by any means, electronic, photocopying, recording, or otherwise, without the prior written permission of the publisher and author, Lulu Baba.

Cover illustrated by Lacie Patterson

Printed in the United States of America

ISBN 978-1-5136-5293-1

www.LuluBabaBooks.com

Follow us on Facebook:
www.facebook.com/lulubababooks

Follow us on Twitter:
@lulubababooks

Follow us on instagram:
@lulubababooks

DEDICATION

To all who wish to be healed, whole and free
We wish you may
We wish you might
Have the wish you wish tonight.

—Lulu Baba

No matter what the issue is and no matter how long you have struggled with it, the possibility exists for you to become absolutely FREE, WHOLE and HEALED.

—Brandon Bays

CONTENTS

2.0 UPGRADE

The *Mild Concussion and Traumatic Brain Injury Workbook 2.0* now comes in LARGE font for a clear and simple reading experience. This book also features larger pages, 8x10, in comparison to the 6x8 travel-sized format of the first book. The maze passageways have grown in size which makes for easier navigation with your pen. The principal upgrade includes the ability to record your completion time of each maze so you can track your progress. The maze count has also more than doubled from the previous book. There are now 255 mazes.

Track your recovery by timing the completion of the same maze three times. There are 85 unique and thoughtfully designed mazes to help aid in your recovery. The mazes get gradually harder, and every maze comes in triplicate with a place to record your time. If you're consistently achieving better times, your memory, cognitive function and executive skills should also be improving.

If your time stays the same or gets worse, don't be discouraged, you can show your health care provider valuable data regarding where you are on your path to recovery. If your time is getting faster, you can share evidence of some of the positive results you are experiencing on your road to recovery.

It is always prudent to inform your physician about the

exercises you are pursuing. Your professional healthcare team can help you incorporate supportive and complementary activities, in accordance with this book, that can aid in your rehabilitation goals.

To ensure this book is appropriate for where you are in your recovery process, we highly recommend consulting your physician before adding any new therapies to your rehabilitation regimen.

Good tidings on your journey.

Preface

In addition to working with professionals (e.g., medical doctor, neuropsychologist, occupational therapists, etc.), honing your puzzle skills can improve memory and cognitive function.

Activities designed to assist individuals recover from traumatic brain injuries often include puzzles such as mazes. Individuals that have used mazes in their cognitive rehabilitation therapies have reported improved memory and cognitive function.

Additionally, a positive outlook can help greatly on your road to recovery. Accordingly, encouraging quotes are used throughout this workbook to maintain optimism.

The exercises in this workbook are not intended to replace therapy with professionals. We encourage you to consult your doctor or therapist before making any changes to your rehabilitation program.

Coping

Coping is a way to adjust to circumstances that fall outside of our comfort zones. When we are physically injured, we may have to cope with the rehabilitation process. This may involve using a cane or assistive device to help perform and complete activities of daily life.

A cognitive injury requires coping as well. There are internal and external ways to adjust and adapt. A good internal adaptation for a cognitive injury could be using visual images to stimulate memory. Likewise, a great external adaptation might be keeping a journal to help recall experiences and track improvements in recovery.

People with brain injuries seek to improve memory, concentration and executive function skills while managing fatigue, frustration and anger.

Solving a maze requires memory, focus and executive function skills to complete. Instead of being angry at what caused the injury, or being anxious about the future, mazes can compel a person to be in the moment, helping the person to operate and interact in a real-time experience that may aid in the persons recovery.

Awareness and Insight

Even at our best it may be difficult to be objective about ourselves. This becomes more apparent after a brain injury. After a brain injury, lack of awareness and insight can be a persistent obstacle.

It is important to remember that recovering from a brain injury can be a very slow and gradual process. You may casually realize the difficulties you will need to cope with. This process can be described as a fog slowly lifting.

Slowly, mazes can help to clear the fog and give you an improved understanding of your cognitive ability. Accepting and understanding where you are in the rehabilitation process will assist you in integrating the methods best suited for your recovery.

There are many stages in recovering from a brain injury. Depending on the type of brain injury and where you are at in your recovery, this book may or may not help you. You may require a rehabilitation activity more suited for your stage in the healing process.

If this book seems too difficult or frustrating, put it away and come back to it again later.

We wish you a blessed and insightful recovery.

Chapter 1.

35 SIMPLE PUZZLES (in Triplicate to Track your Progress)

Wounds don't heal the way you want them to, they heal the way they need to. It takes time for wounds to fade into scars. It takes time for the process of healing to take place. Give yourself that time. Give yourself that grace. Be gentle with your wounds. Be Gentle with your heart.

You deserve to heal.

—*Dele Olanubi*

The natural healing force in each one of us
is the greatest force in getting well.

—*Hippocrates*

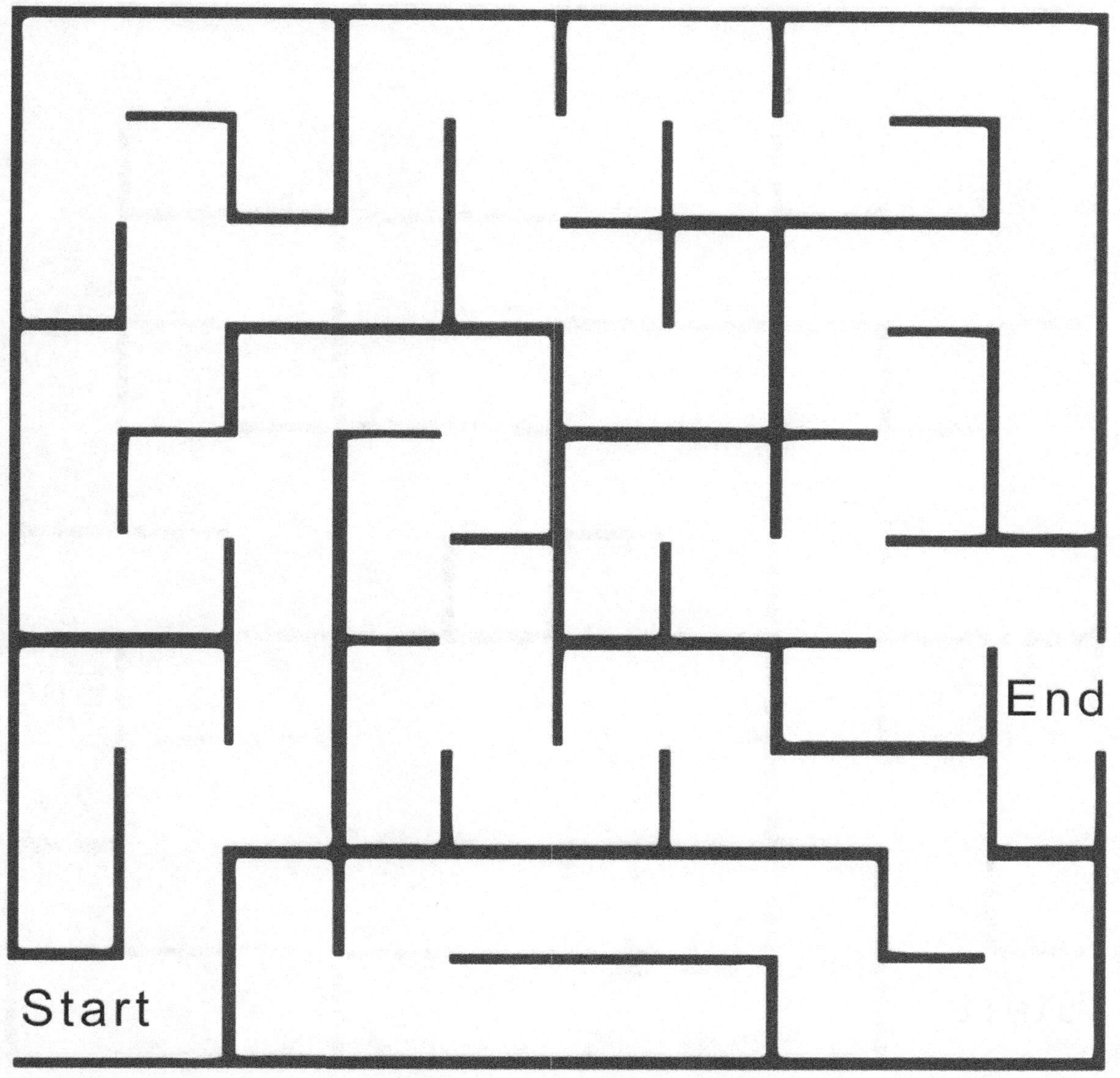

Start time: __________ End time: __________

Total time, maze 1: __________

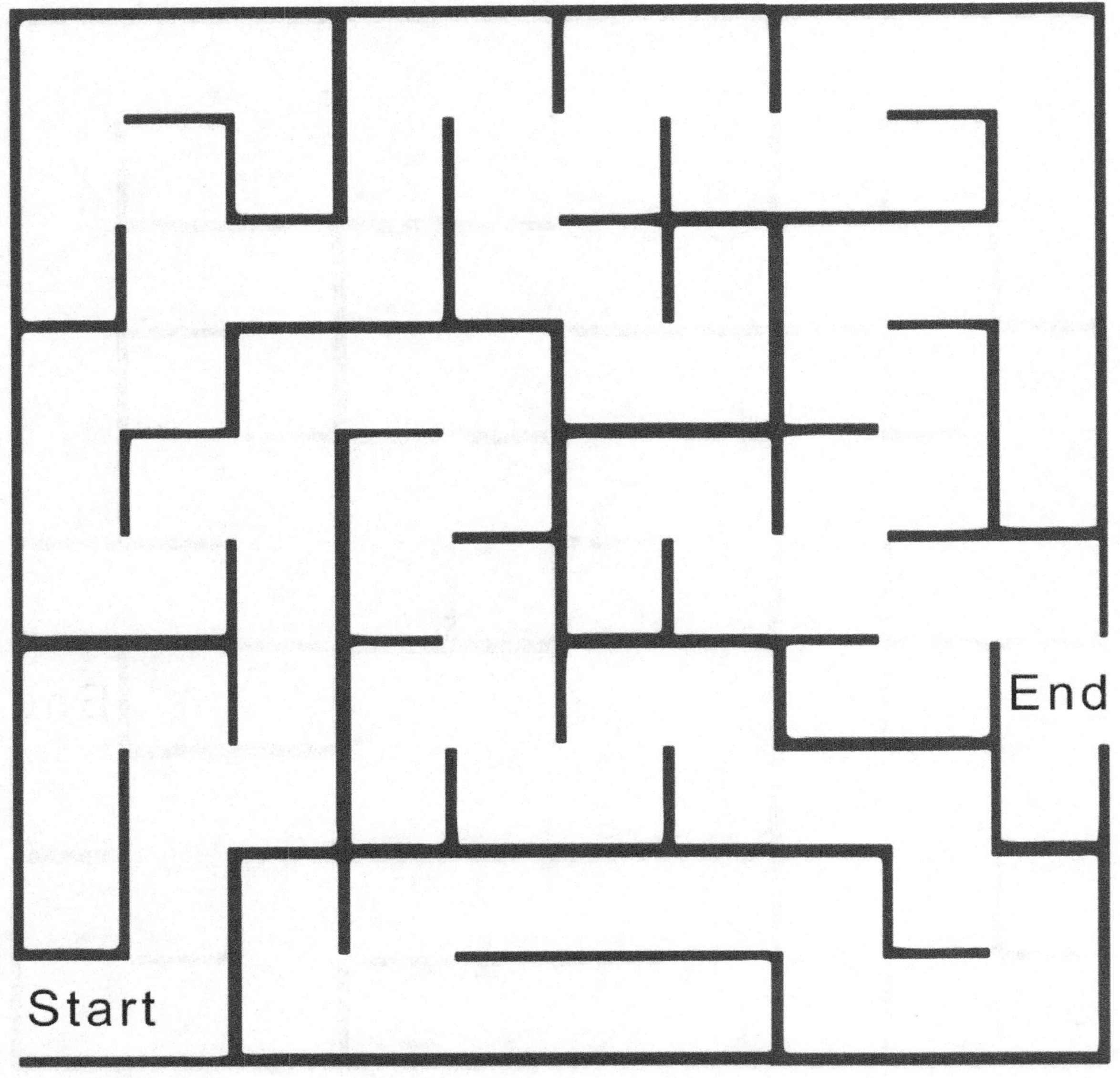

Start time: __________ End time: __________

Total time, maze 2: __________

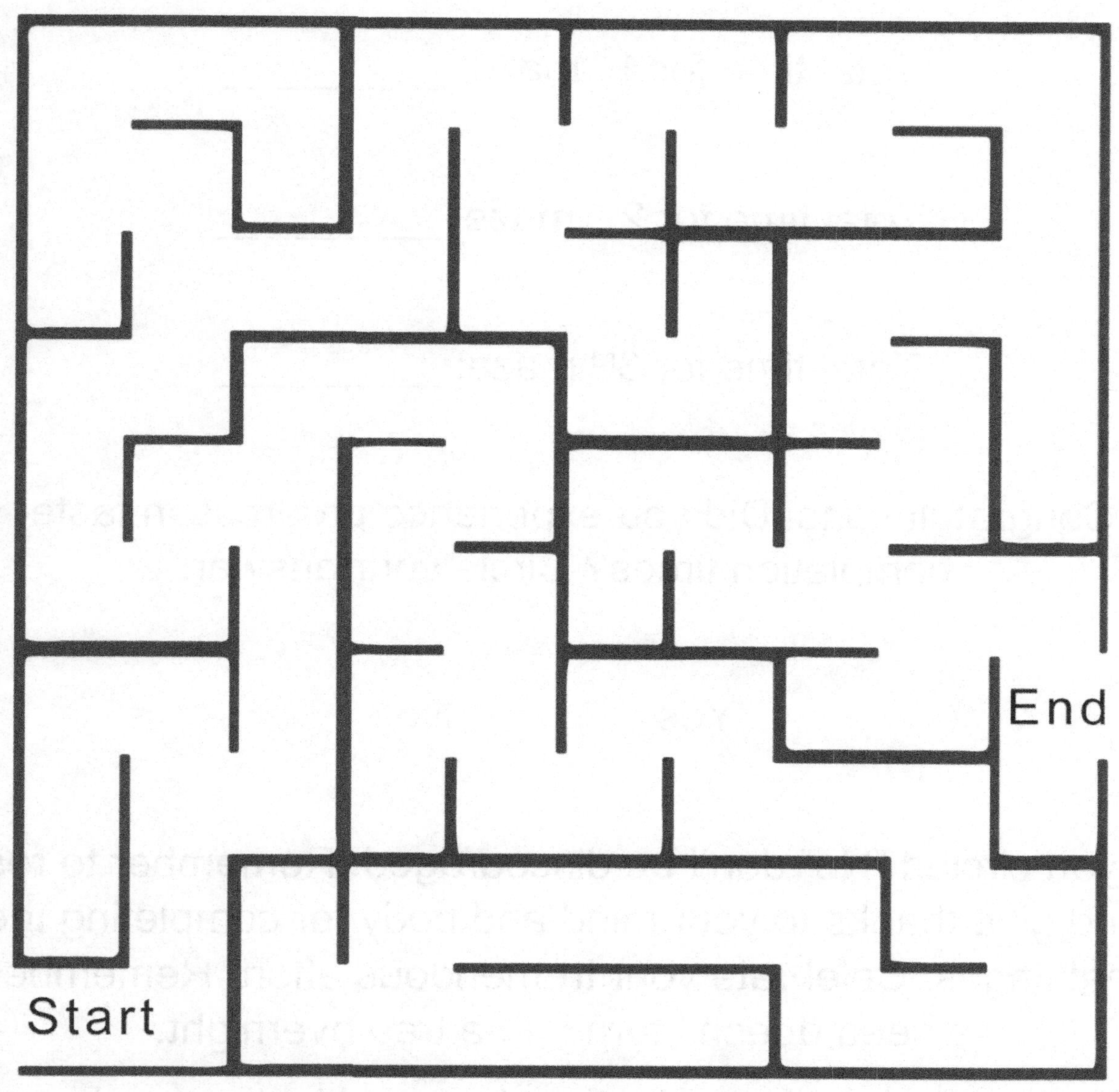

Start time: __________ End time: __________

Total time, maze 3: __________

Total time for 1st maze: __________

Total time for 2nd maze: __________

Total time for 3rd maze: __________

Congratulations! Did you experience progress in faster completion times? Circle your answer.

Yes No

If you circled "No" don't be discouraged. Remember to rest and give thanks to your mind and body for completing the challenges. Celebrate your tremendous effort. Remember, a seed doesn't turn into a tree overnight.

Keep watering, keep planting, keep cultivating, and one day your garden will bloom.

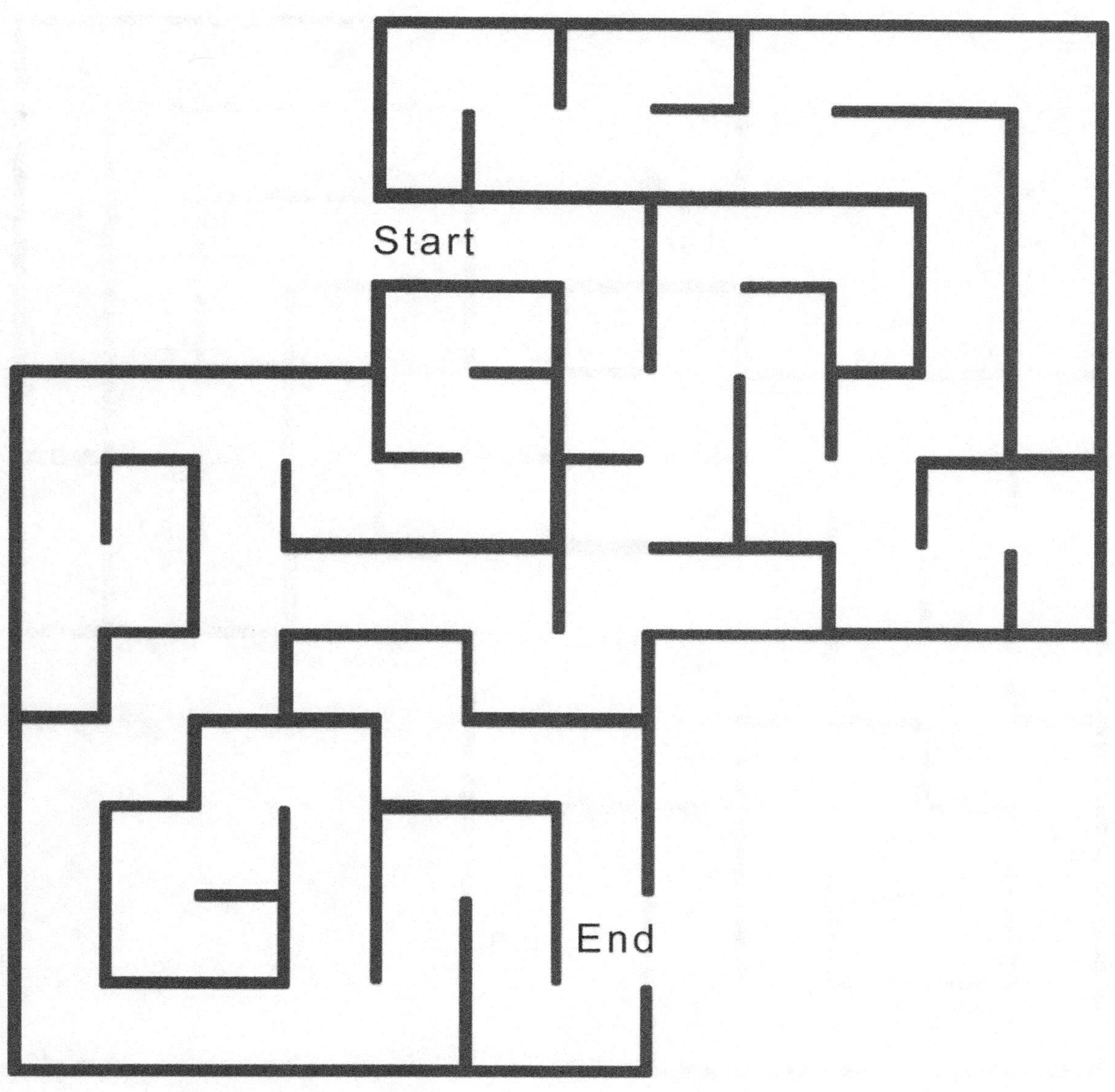

Start time: __________ End time: __________

Total time, maze 1: __________

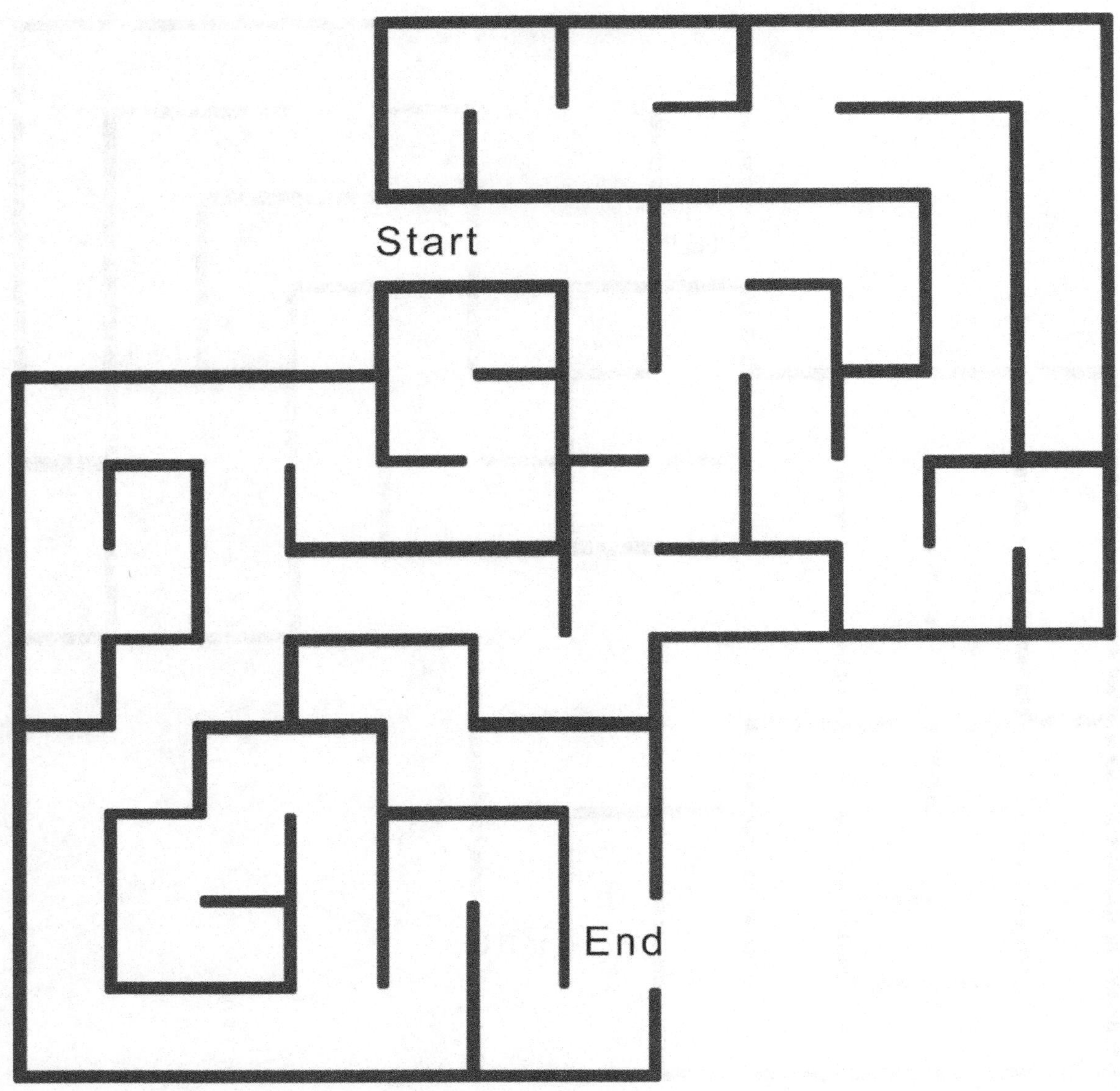

Start time: __________ End time: __________

Total time, maze 2: __________

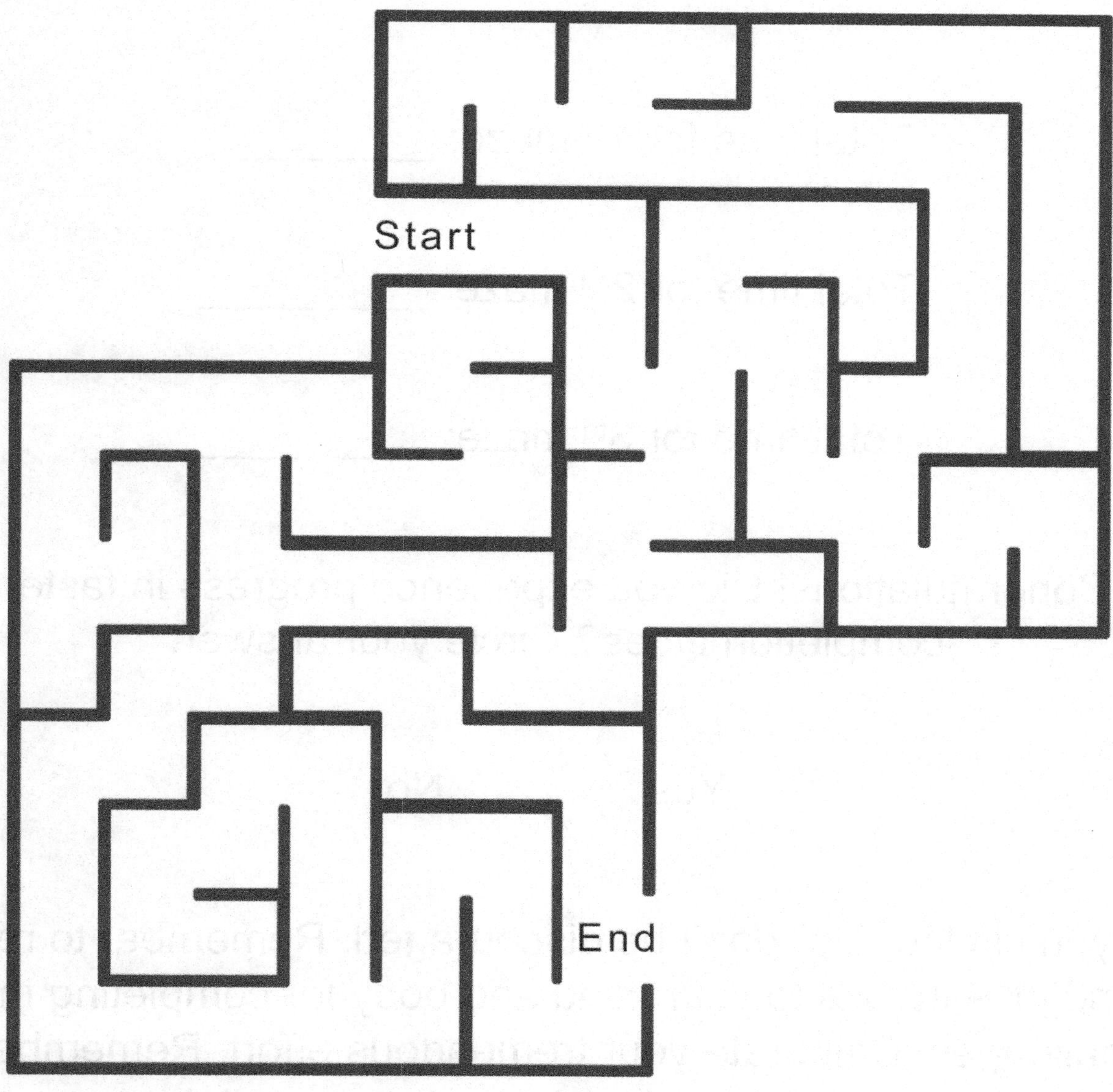

Start time: __________ End time: __________

Total time, maze 3: __________

Total time for 1st maze: __________

Total time for 2nd maze: __________

Total time for 3rd maze: __________

Congratulations! Did you experience progress in faster completion times? Circle your answer.

Yes No

If you circled "No" don't be discouraged. Remember to rest and give thanks to your mind and body for completing the challenges. Celebrate your tremendous effort. Remember, a seed doesn't turn into a tree overnight.

One of the things I learned the hard way was that it doesn't pay to get discouraged. Keeping busy and making optimism a way of life can restore your faith in yourself.

—Lucille Ball

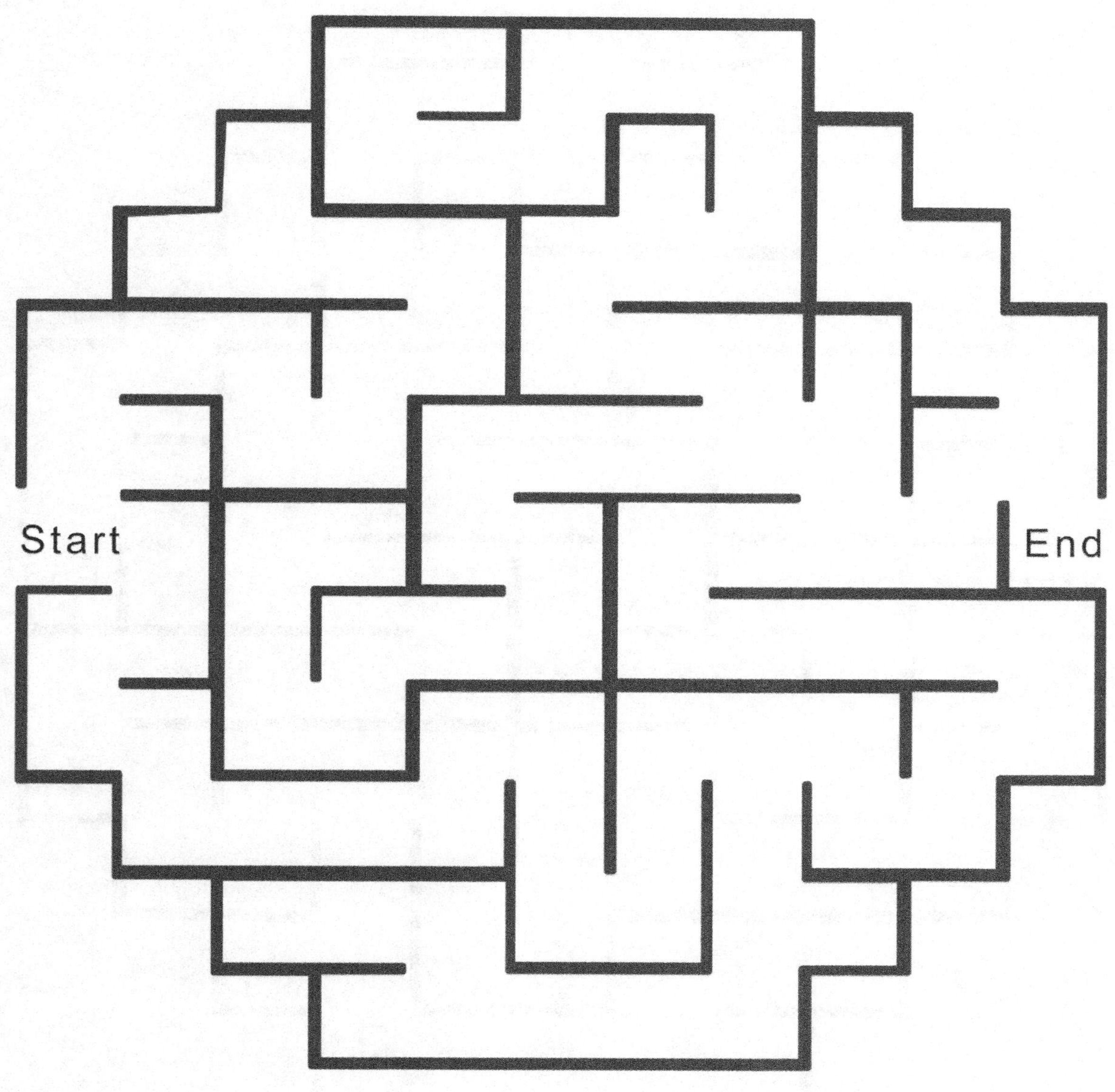

Start time: __________ End time: __________

Total time, maze 1: __________

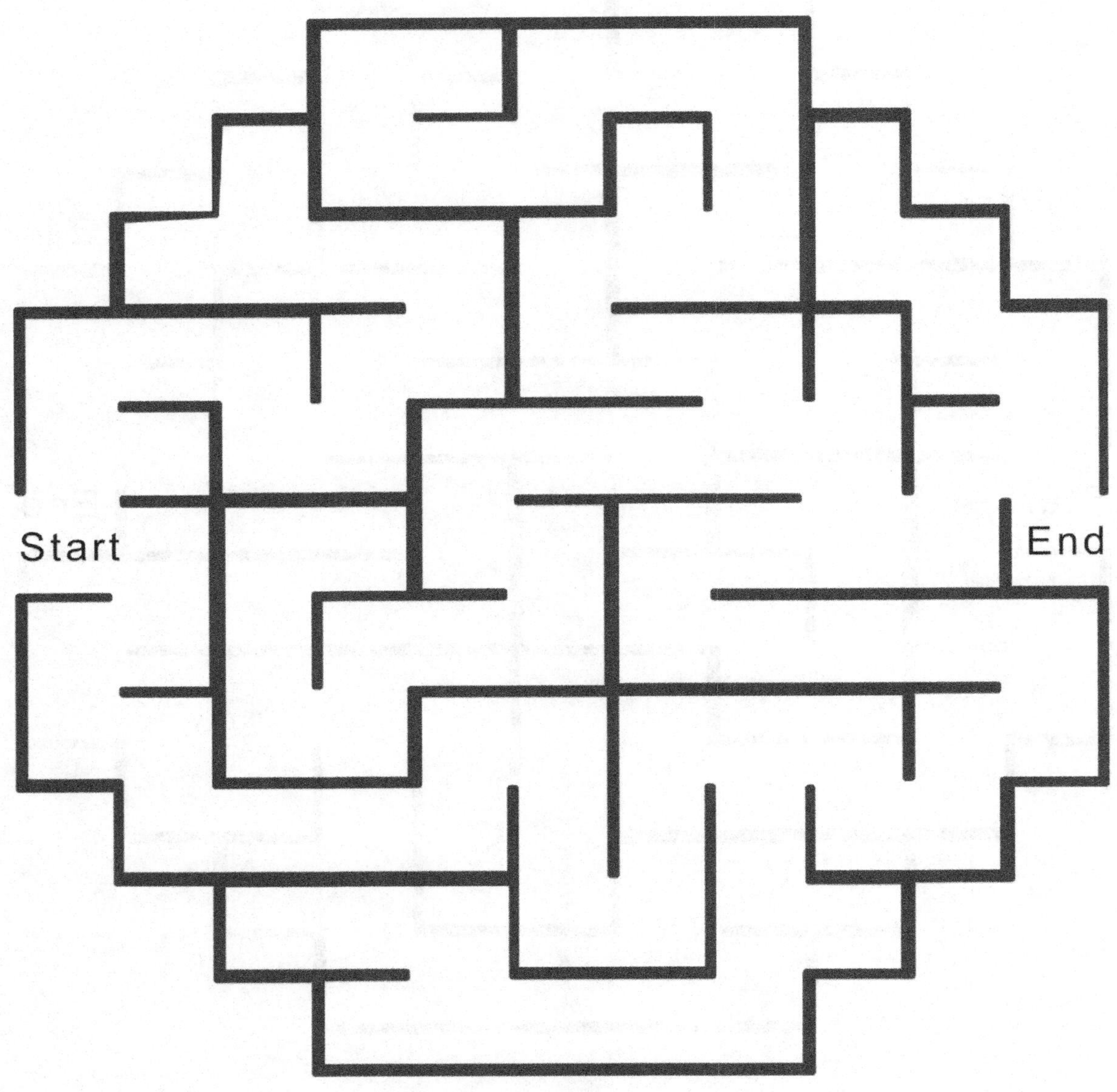

Start time: __________ End time: __________

Total time, maze 2: __________

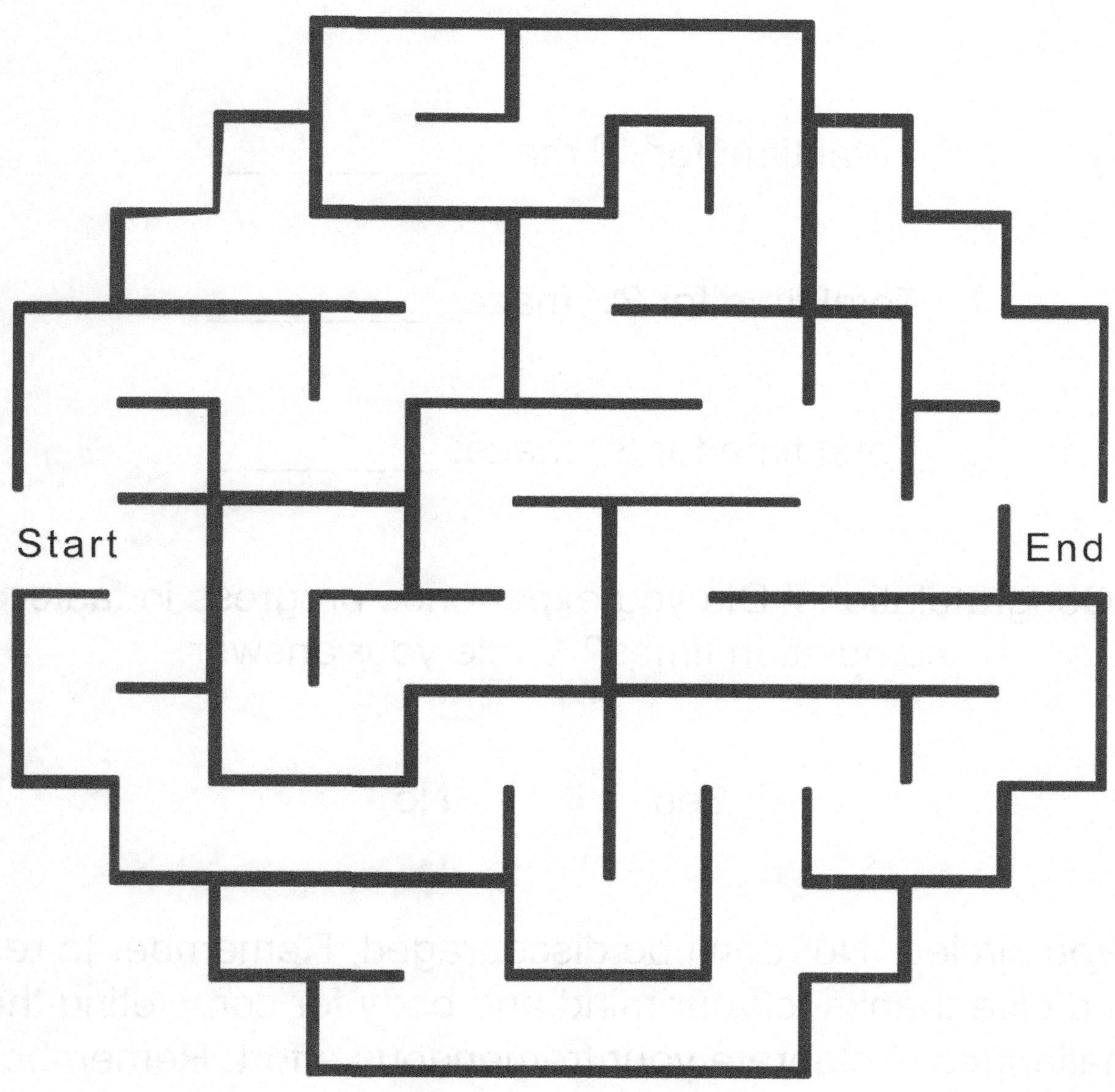

Start time: __________ End time: __________

Total time, maze 3: __________

Total time for 1st maze: __________

Total time for 2nd maze: __________

Total time for 3rd maze: __________

Congratulations! Did you experience progress in faster completion times? Circle your answer.

Yes No

If you circled "No" don't be discouraged. Remember to rest and give thanks to your mind and body for completing the challenges. Celebrate your tremendous effort. Remember, a seed doesn't turn into a tree overnight.

Edison failed 10,000 times before he made the electric light. Do not be discouraged if you fail a few times.

—*Napoleon Hill*

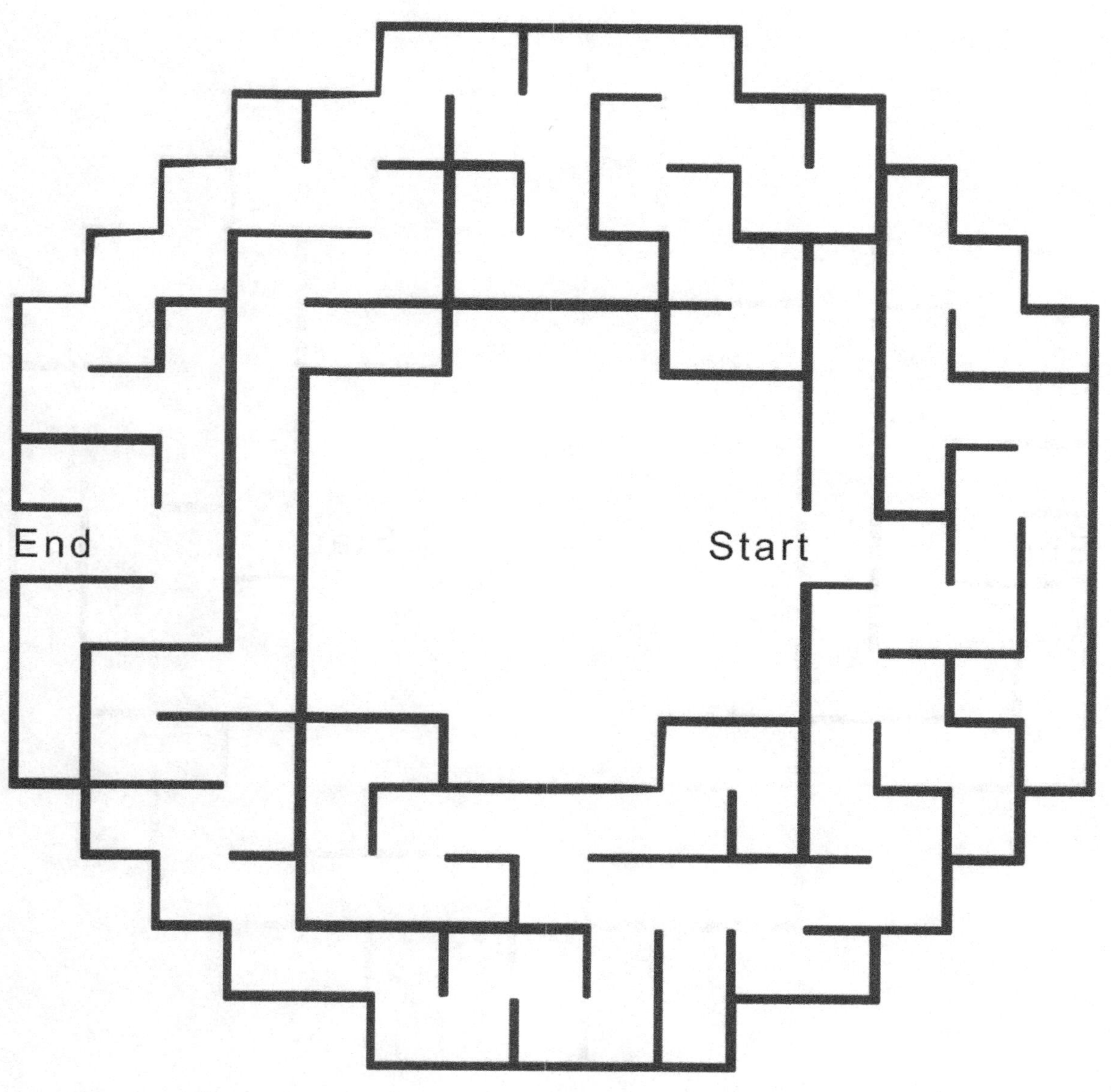

Start time: __________ End time: __________

Total time, maze 1: __________

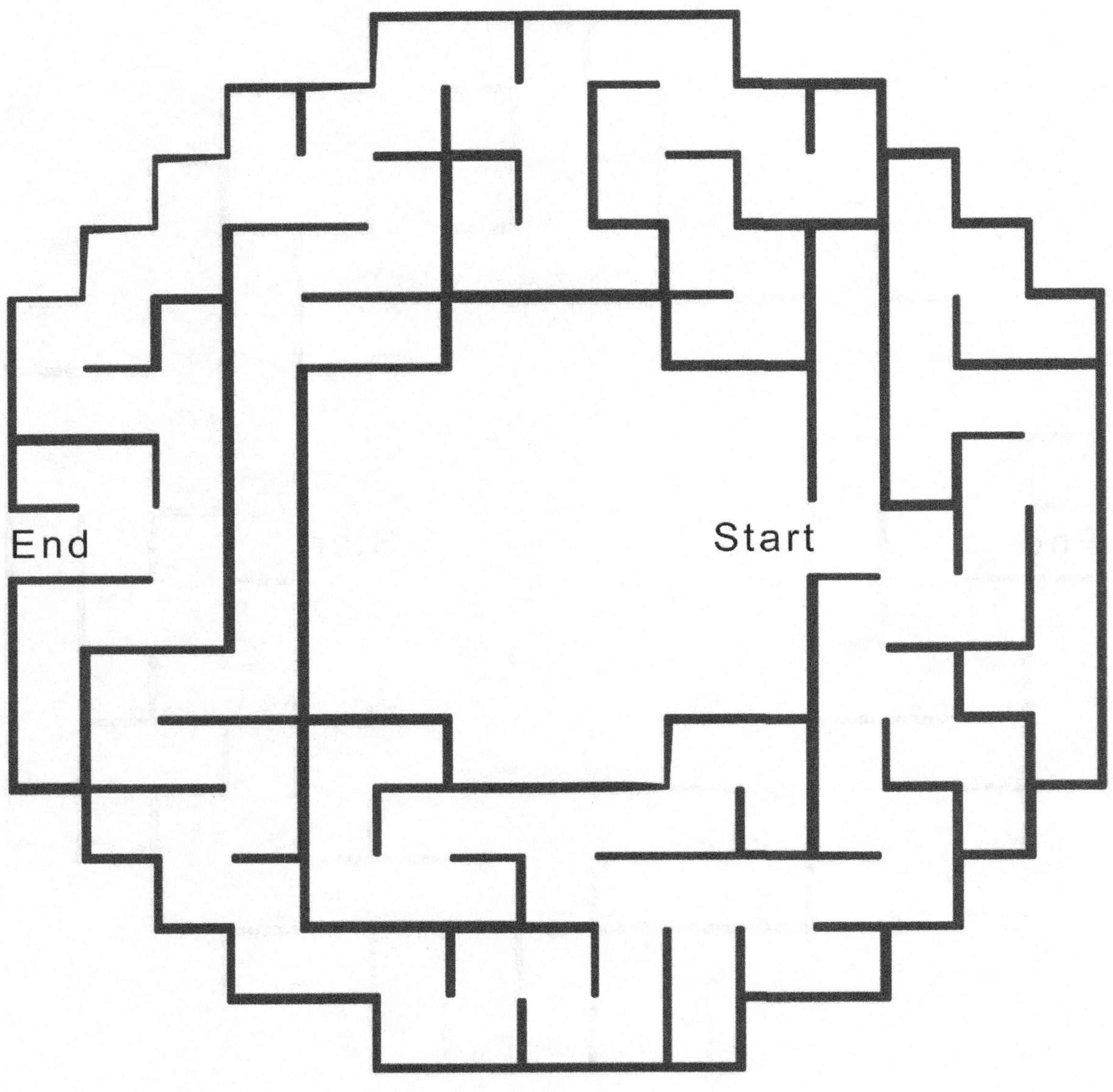

Start time: __________ End time: __________

Total time, maze 2: __________

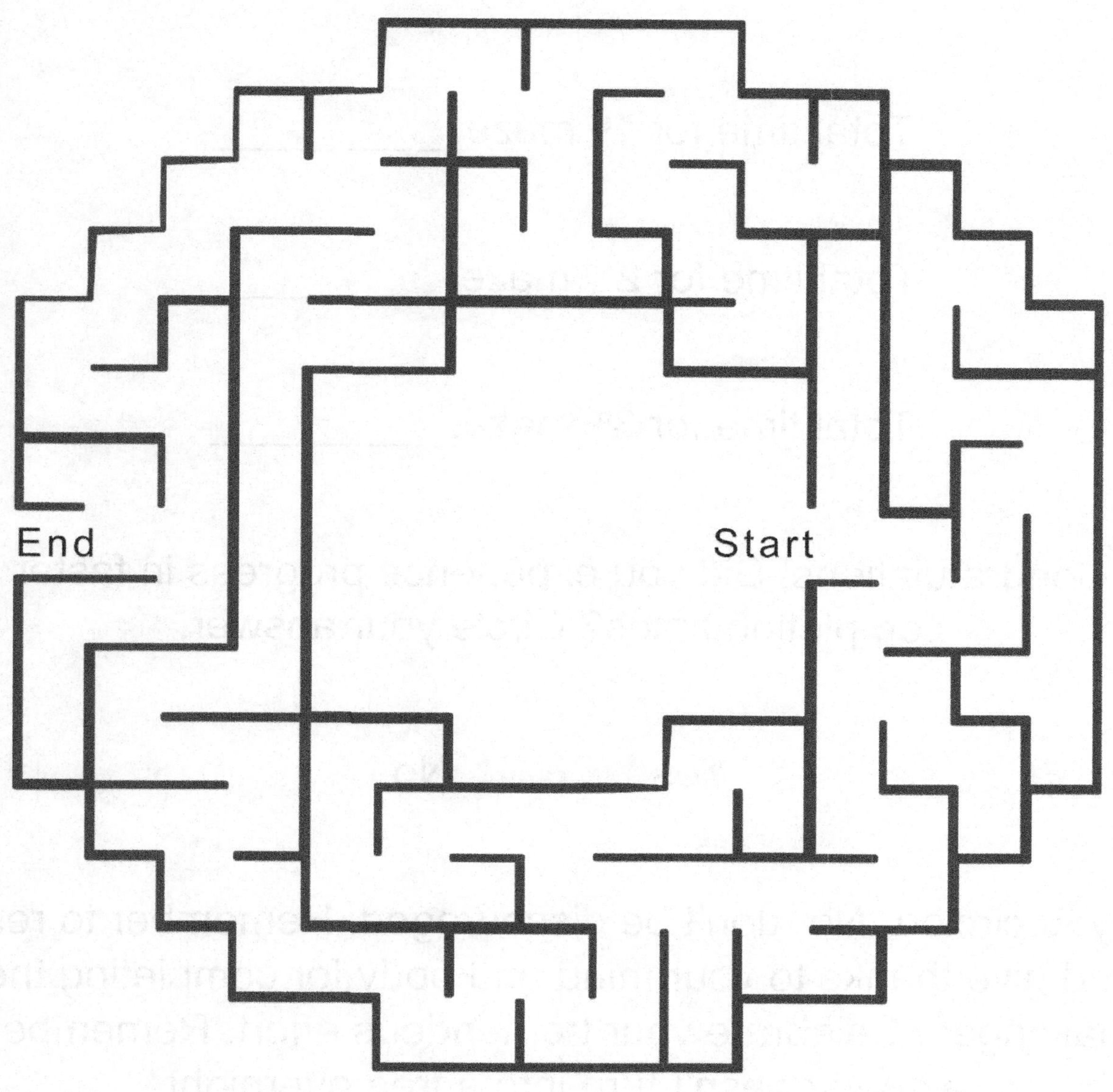

Start time: __________ End time: __________

Total time, maze 3: __________

Total time for 1st maze: __________

Total time for 2nd maze: __________

Total time for 3rd maze: __________

Congratulations! Did you experience progress in faster completion times? Circle your answer.

Yes No

If you circled “No” don’t be discouraged. Remember to rest and give thanks to your mind and body for completing the challenges. Celebrate your tremendous effort. Remember, a seed doesn’t turn into a tree overnight.

A man can get discouraged many times but he is not a failure until he begins to blame somebody else and stops trying.

—*John Burroughs*

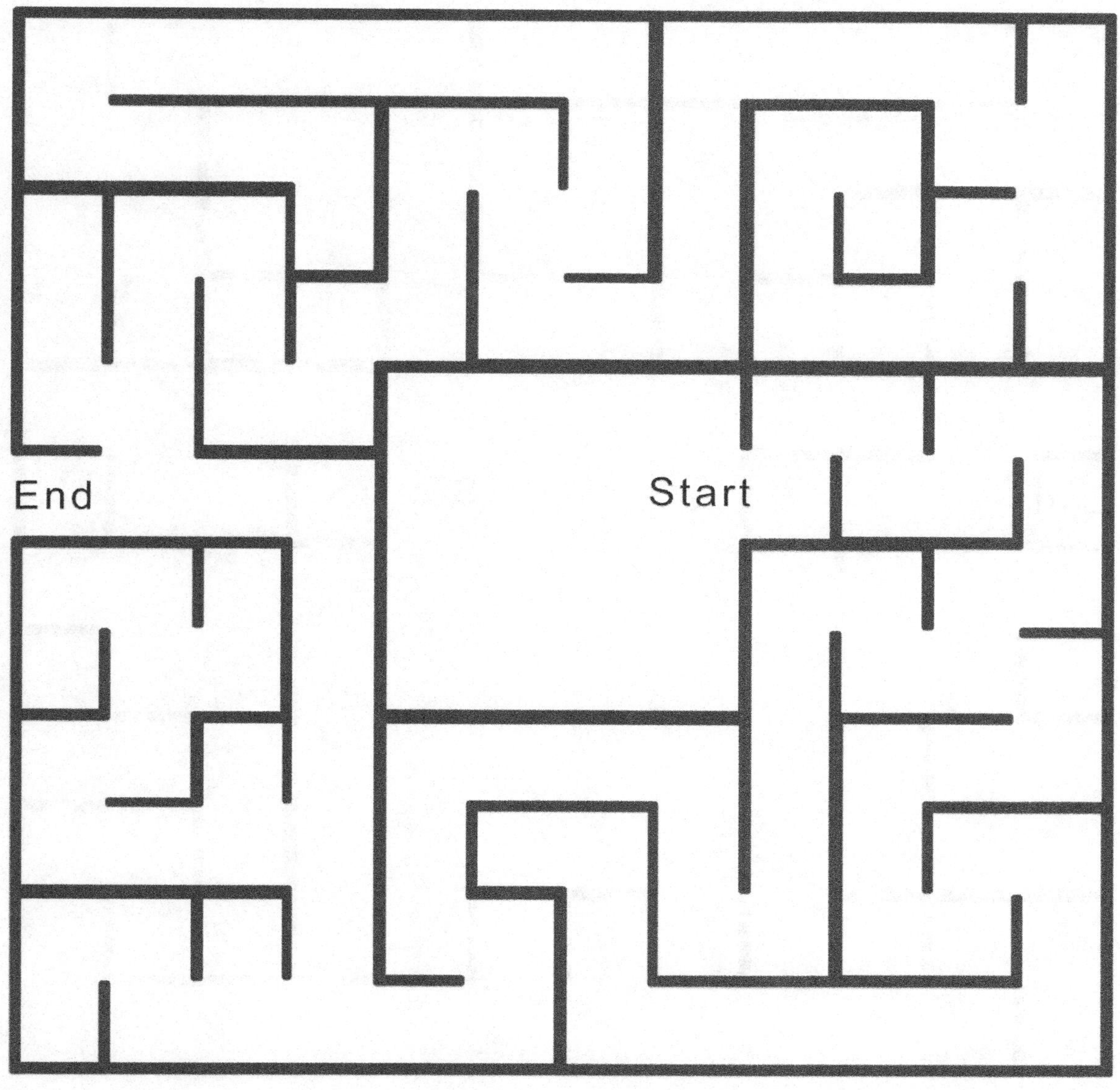

Start time: __________ End time: __________

Total time, maze 1: __________

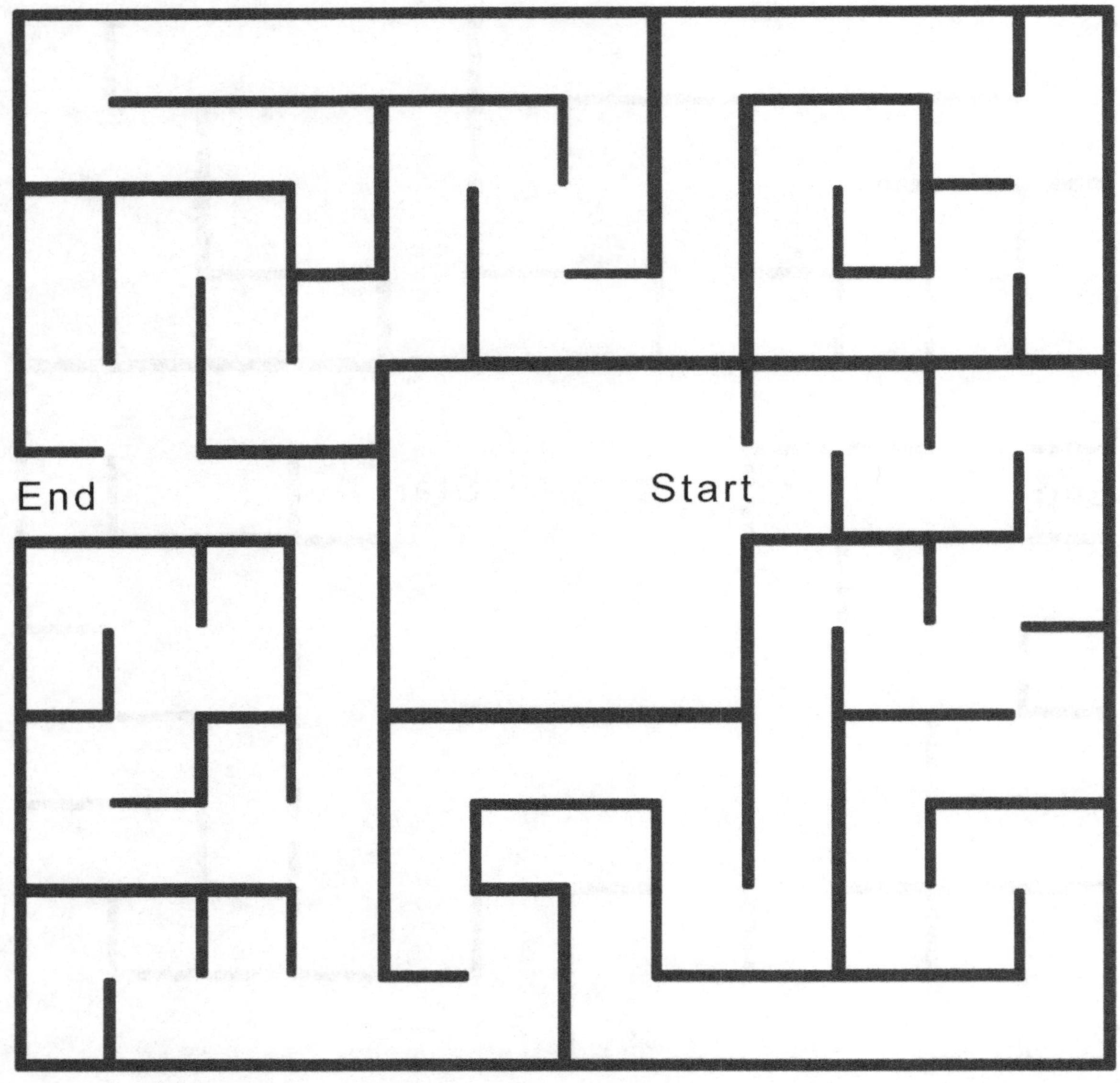

Start time: __________ End time: __________

Total time, maze 2: __________

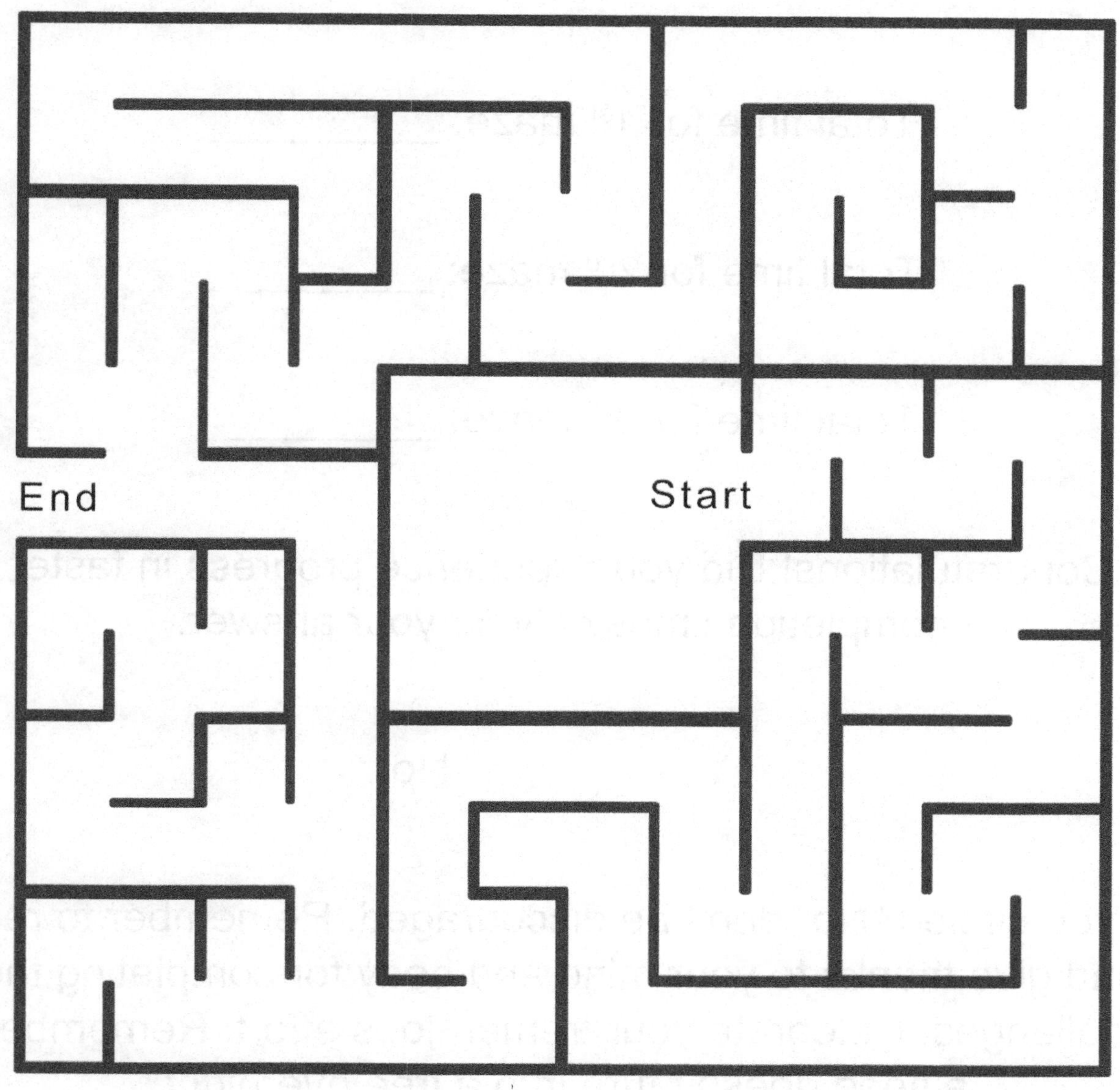

Start time: __________ End time: __________

Total time, maze 3: __________

Total time for 1st maze: __________

Total time for 2nd maze: __________

Total time for 3rd maze: __________

Congratulations! Did you experience progress in faster completion times? Circle your answer.

Yes No

If you circled "No" don't be discouraged. Remember to rest and give thanks to your mind and body for completing the challenges. Celebrate your tremendous effort. Remember, a seed doesn't turn into a tree overnight.

Continuous, unflagging effort, persistence and determination will win. Let not the man be discouraged who has these.

—James Whitcomb Riley

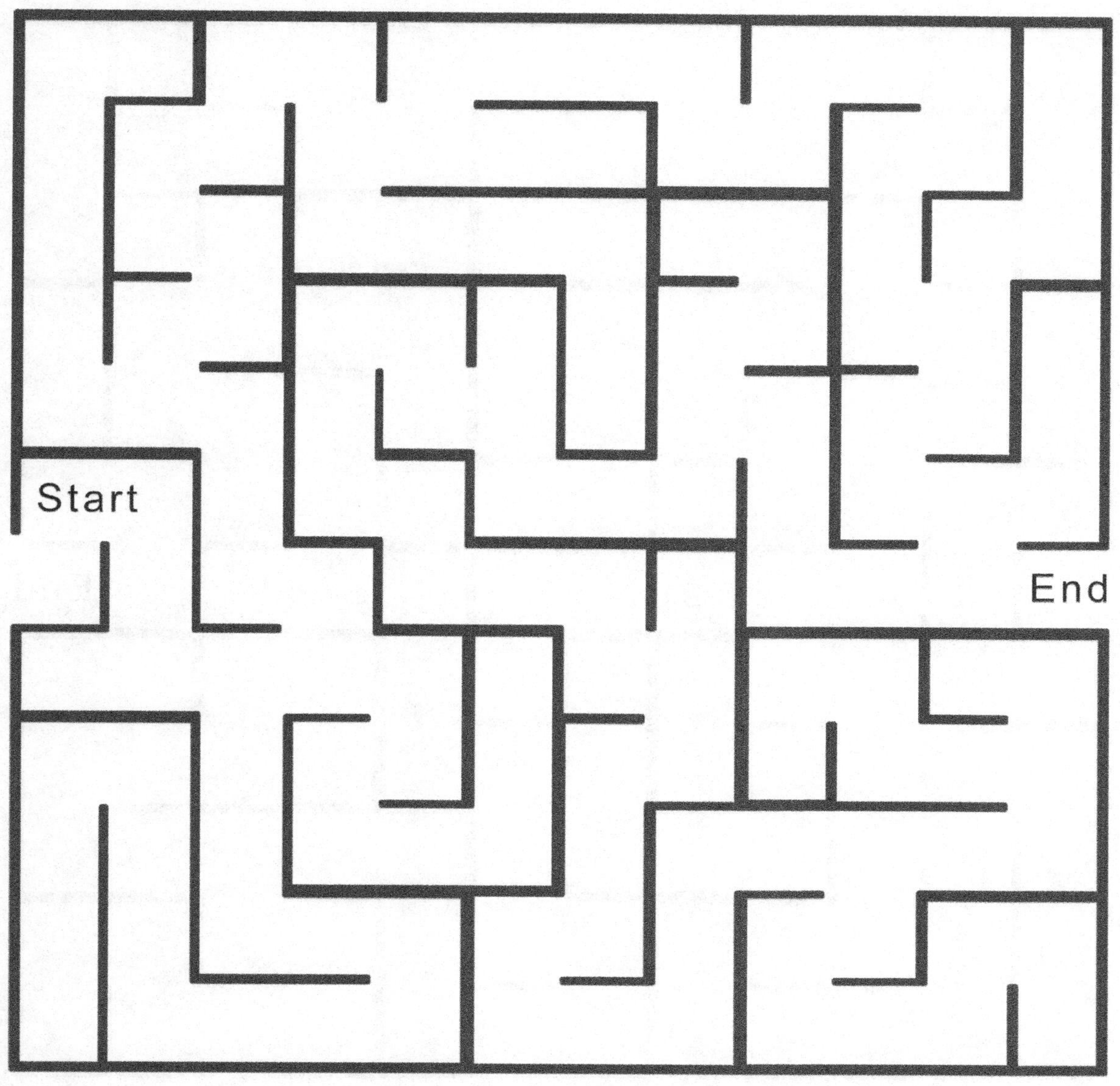

Start time: __________ End time: __________

Total time, maze 1: __________

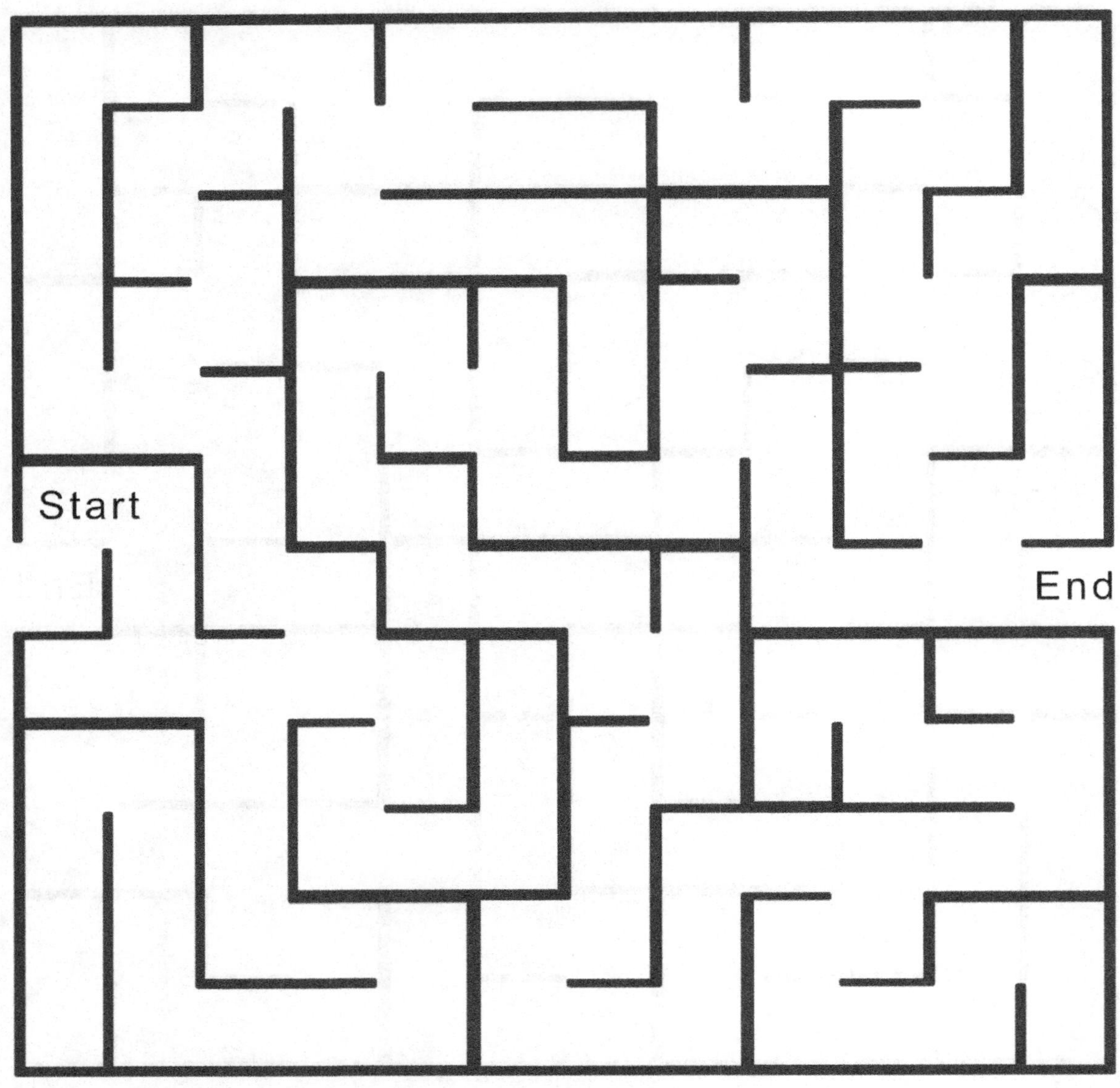

Start time: __________ End time: __________

Total time, maze 2: __________

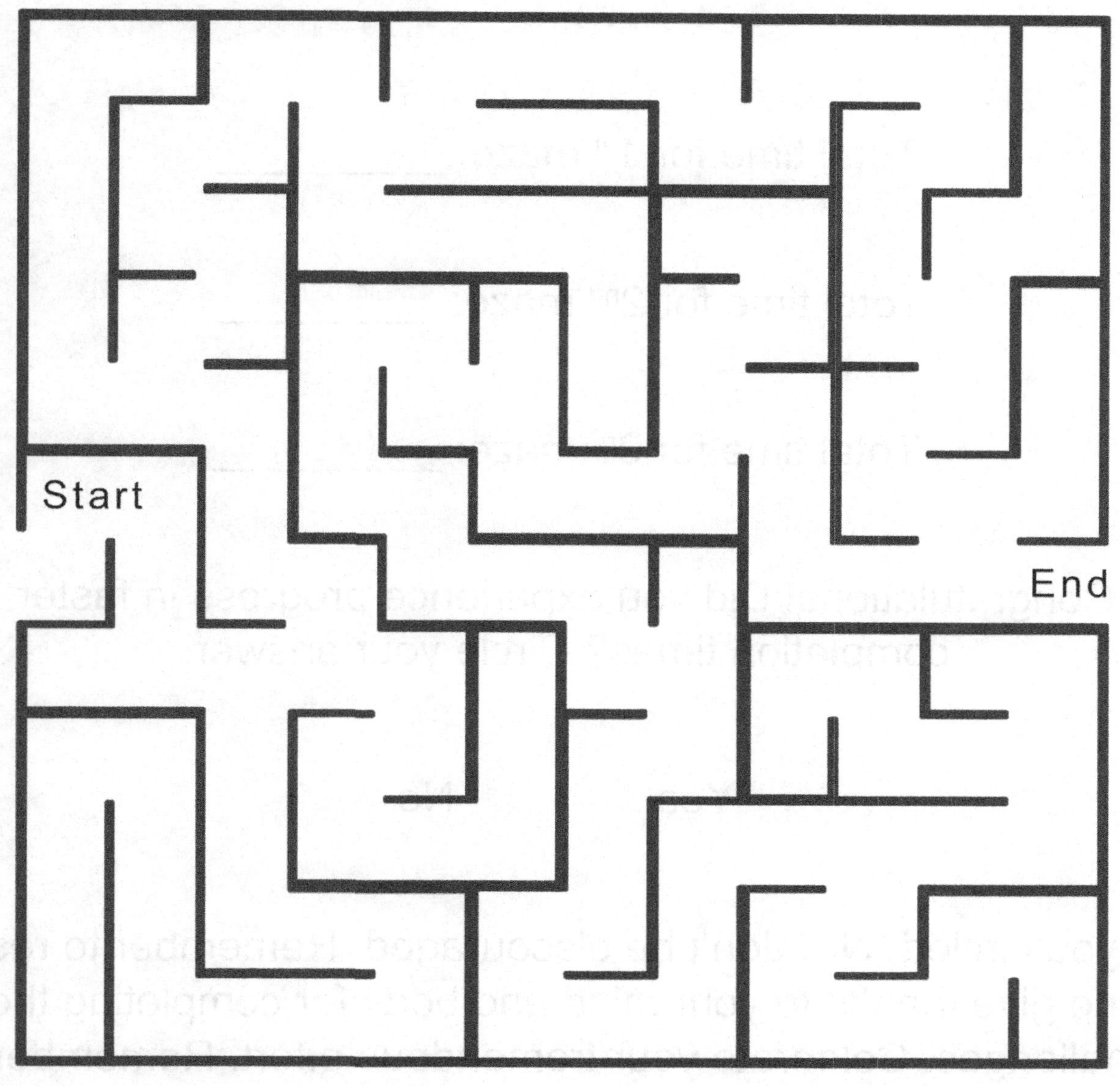

Start time: __________ End time: __________

Total time, maze 3: __________

Total time for 1st maze: __________

Total time for 2nd maze: __________

Total time for 3rd maze: __________

Congratulations! Did you experience progress in faster completion times? Circle your answer.

Yes No

If you circled "No" don't be discouraged. Remember to rest and give thanks to your mind and body for completing the challenges. Celebrate your tremendous effort. Remember, a seed doesn't turn into a tree overnight.

What is important is to believe in something so strongly that you're never discouraged.

—*Salma Hayek*

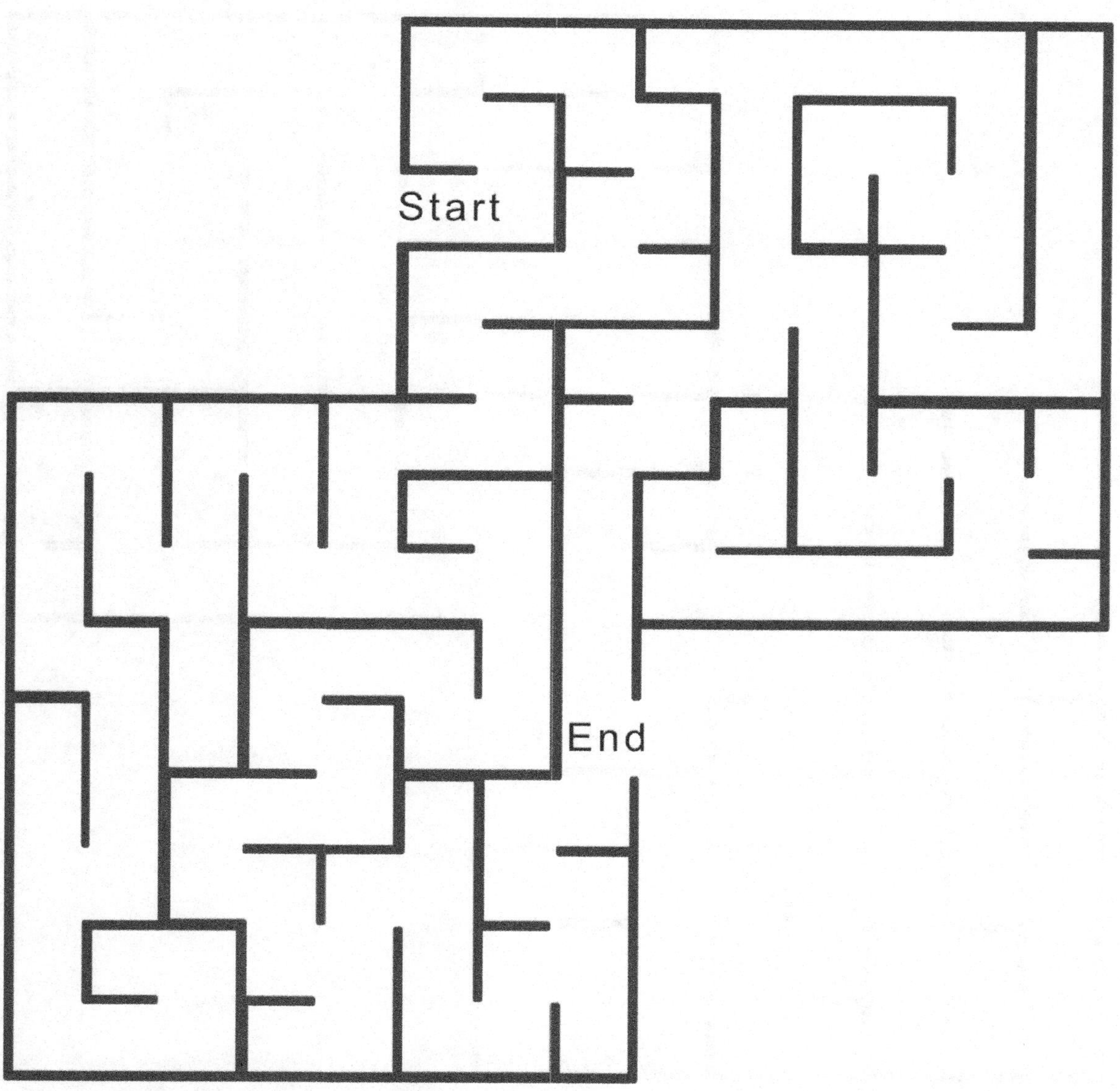

Start time: __________ End time: __________

Total time, maze 1: __________

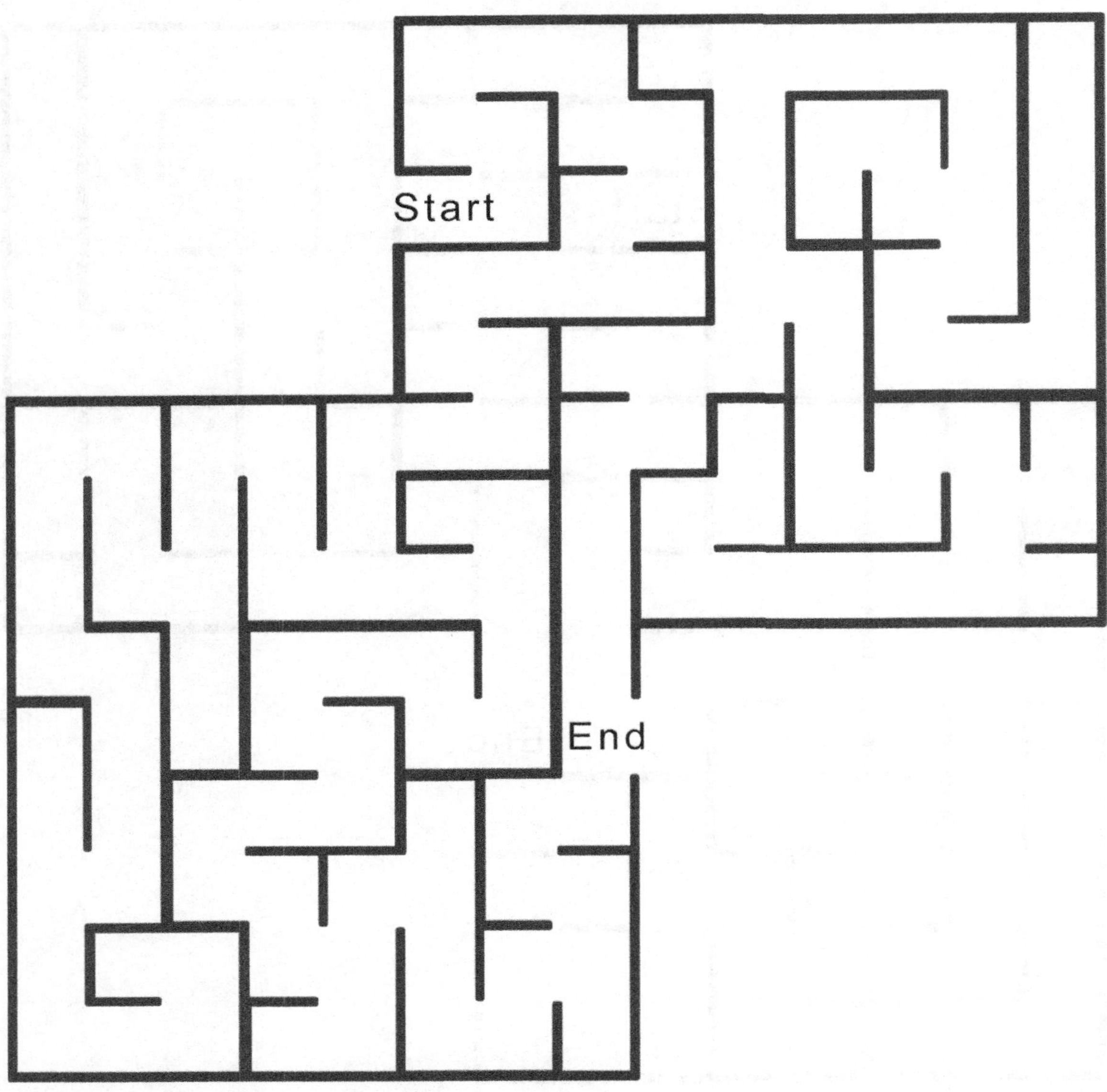

Start time: __________ End time: __________

Total time, maze 2: __________

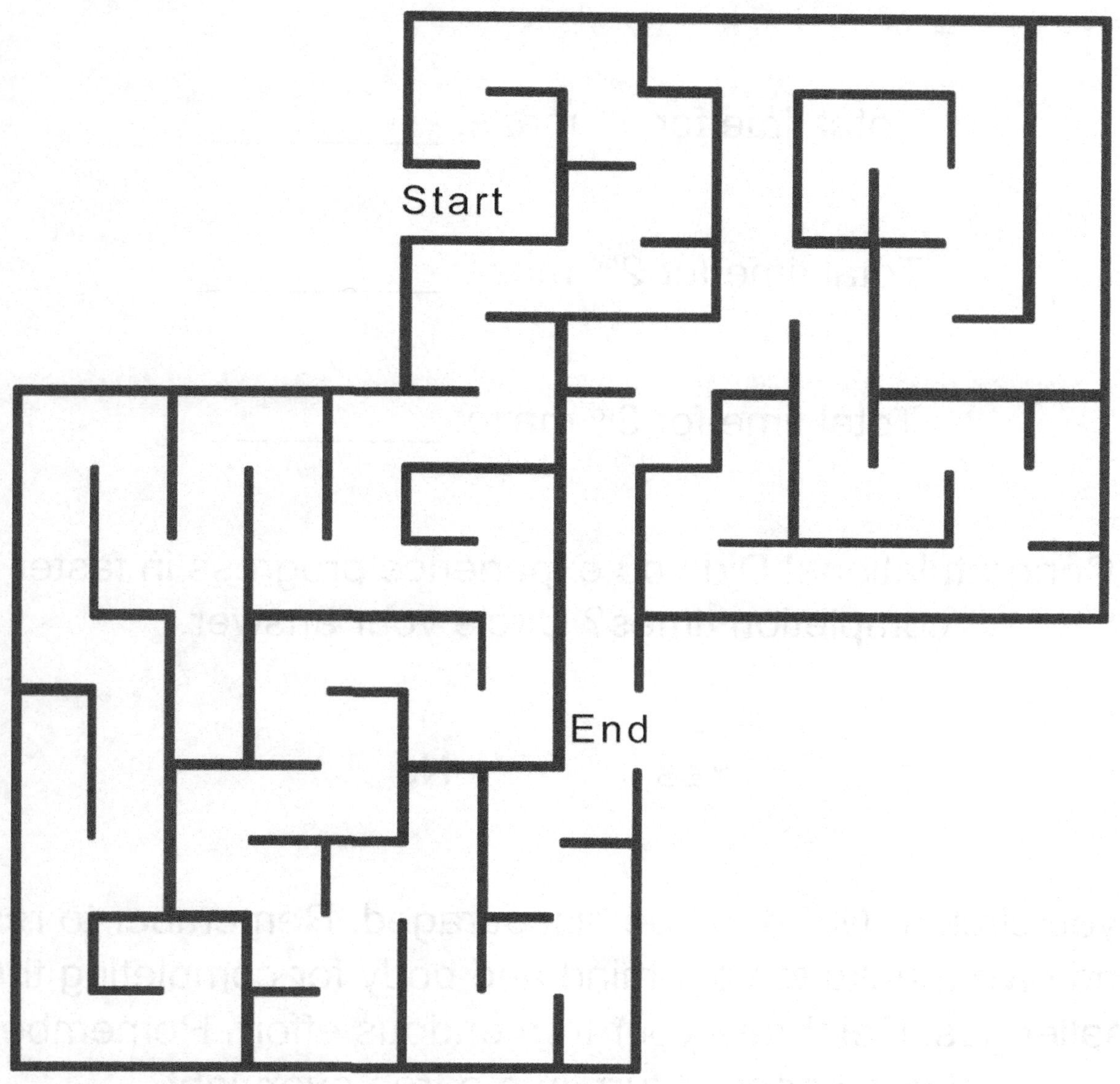

Start time: __________ End time: __________

Total time, maze 3: __________

Total time for 1st maze: __________

Total time for 2nd maze: __________

Total time for 3rd maze: __________

Congratulations! Did you experience progress in faster completion times? Circle your answer.

Yes No

If you circled "No" don't be discouraged. Remember to rest and give thanks to your mind and body for completing the challenges. Celebrate your tremendous effort. Remember, a seed doesn't turn into a tree overnight.

Stop beating yourself up. You are a work in progress - which means you get there a little at a time, not all at once.

—*Unknown*

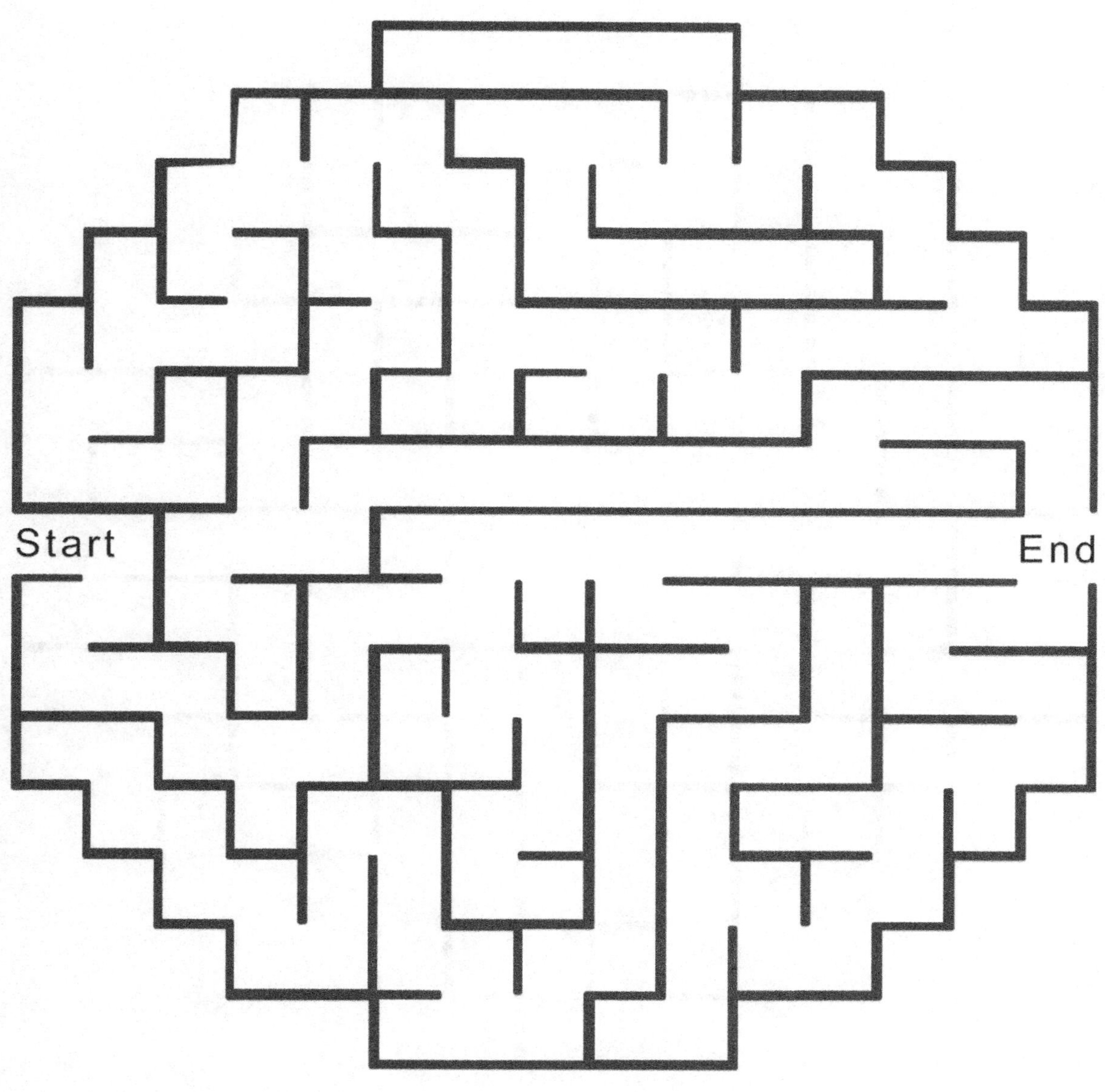

Start time: __________ End time: __________

Total time, maze 1: __________

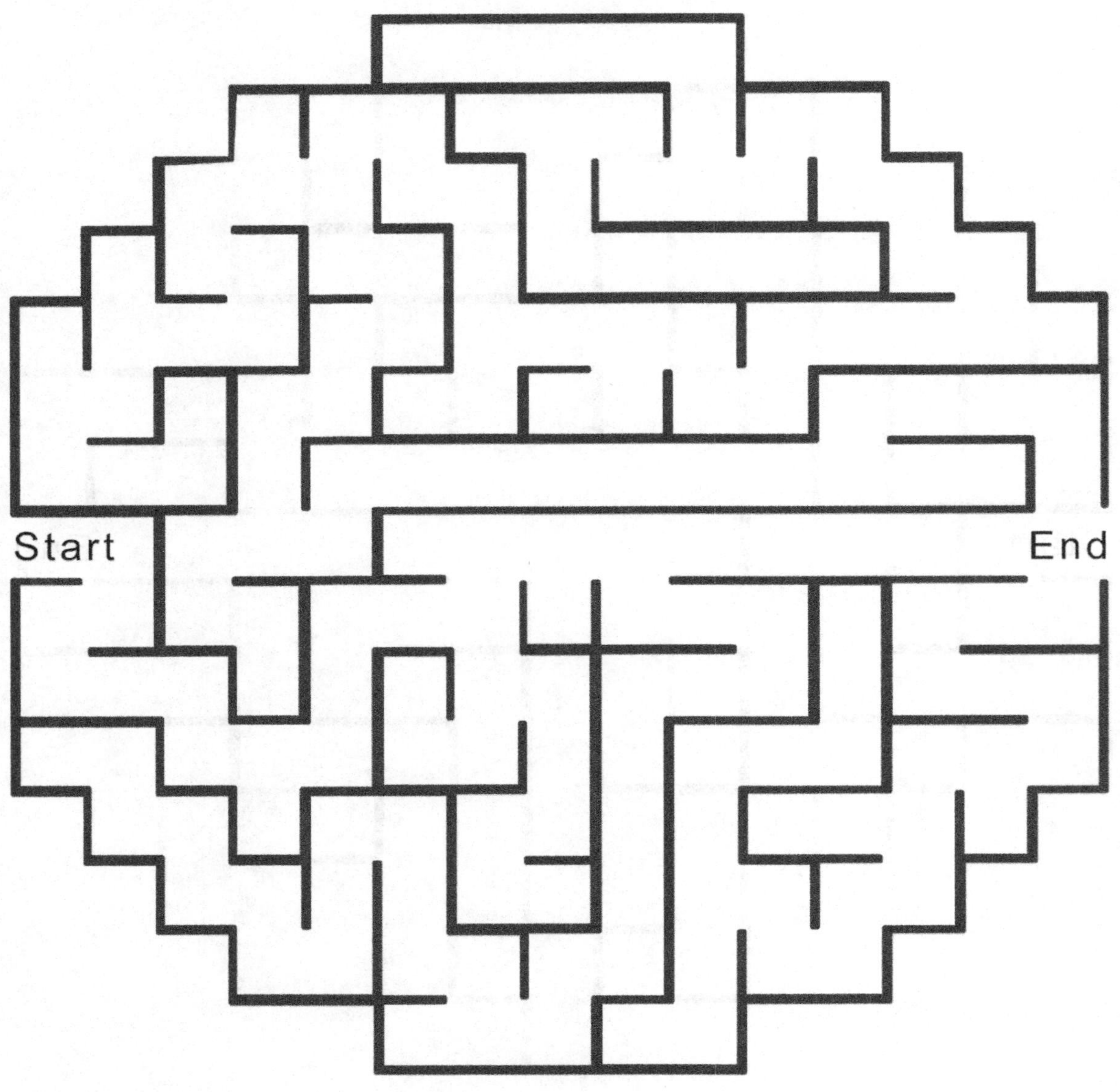

Start time: __________ End time: __________

Total time, maze 2: __________

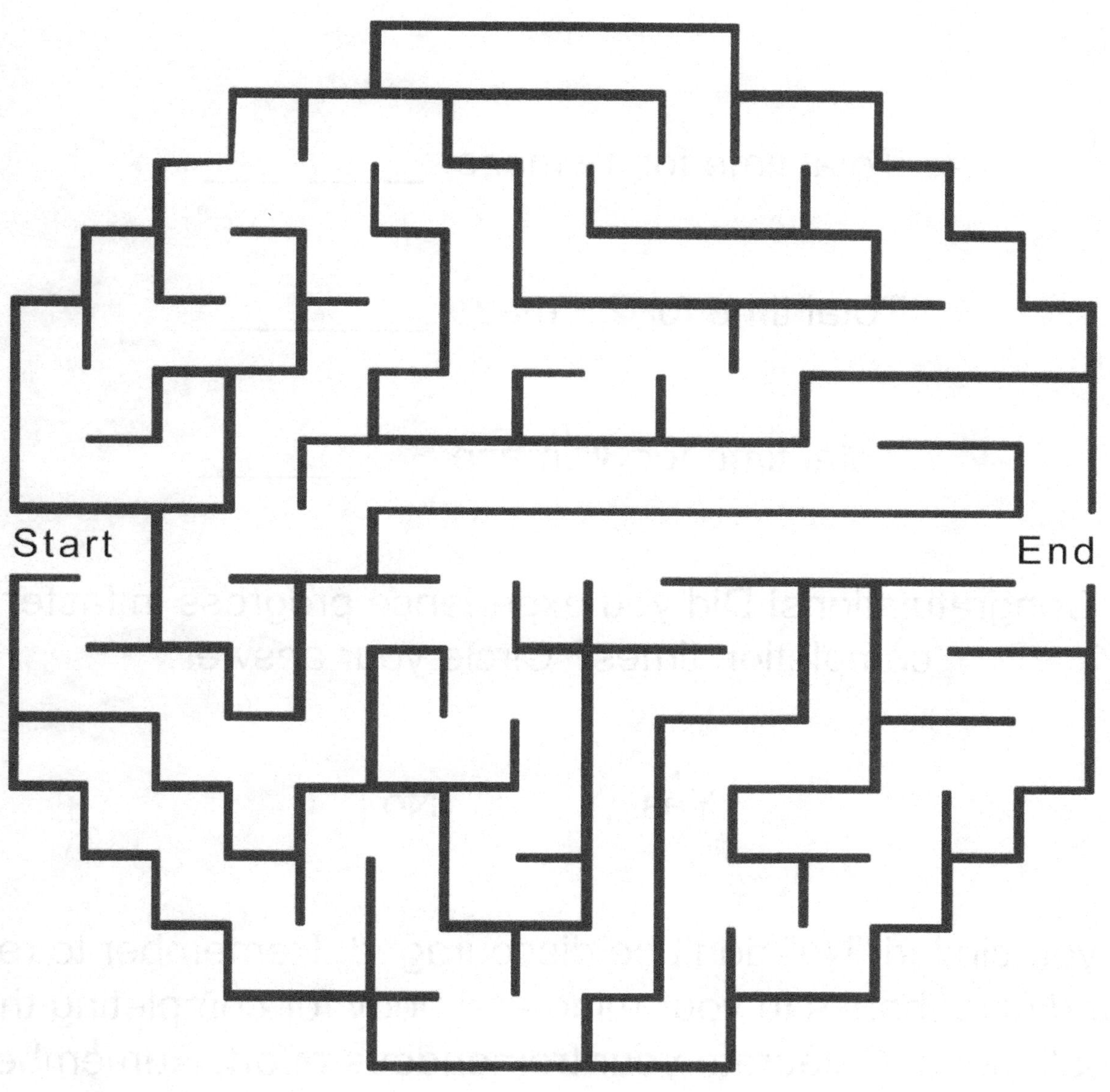

Start time: __________ End time: __________

Total time, maze 3: __________

Total time for 1st maze: __________

Total time for 2nd maze: __________

Total time for 3rd maze: __________

Congratulations! Did you experience progress in faster completion times? Circle your answer.

Yes No

If you circled “No” don’t be discouraged. Remember to rest and give thanks to your mind and body for completing the challenges. Celebrate your tremendous effort. Remember, a seed doesn’t turn into a tree overnight.

Yesterday I was clever so I wanted to change the world. Today I am wise, so I am changing myself.

—*Rumi*

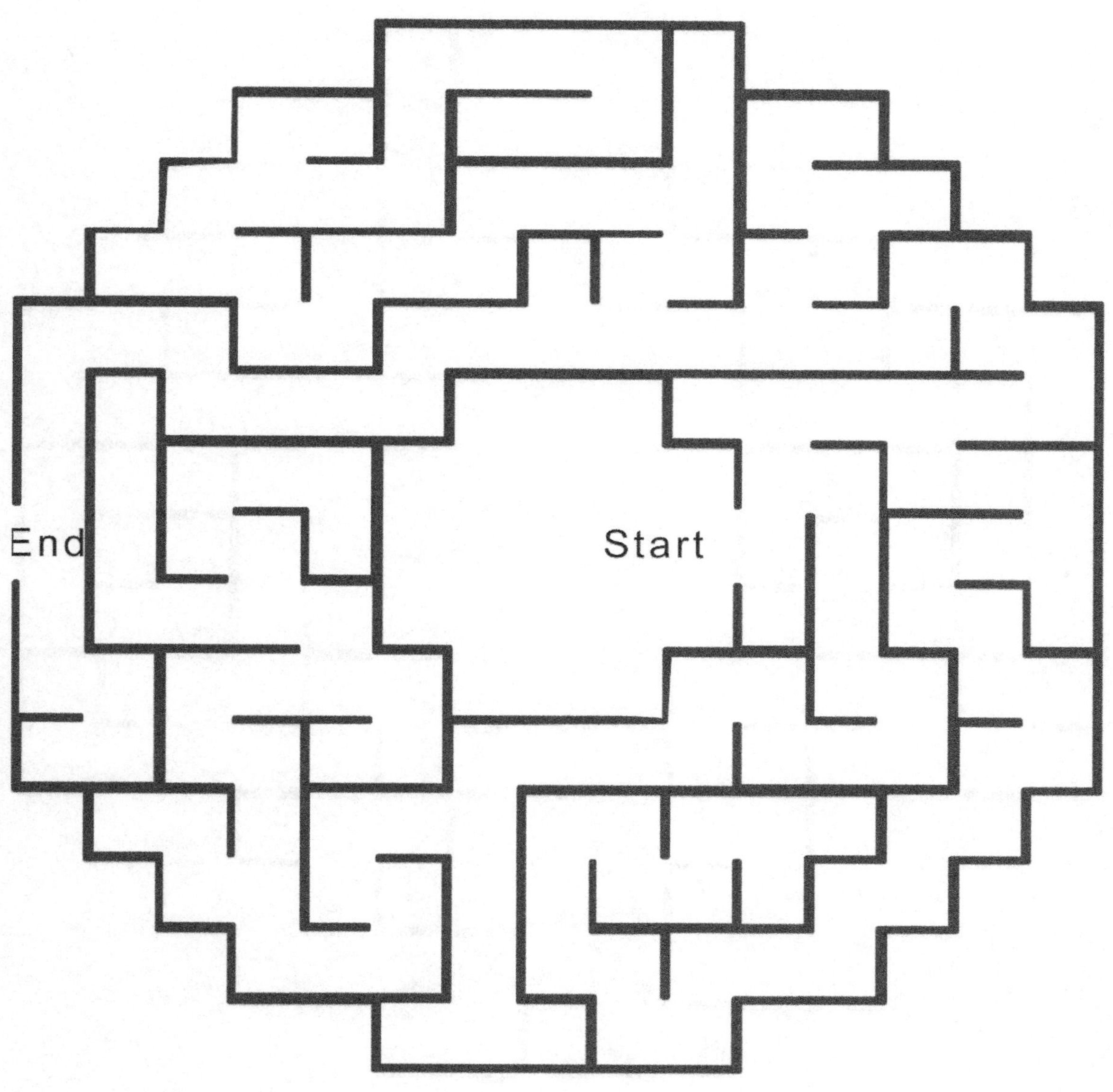

Start time: __________ End time: __________

Total time, maze 1: __________

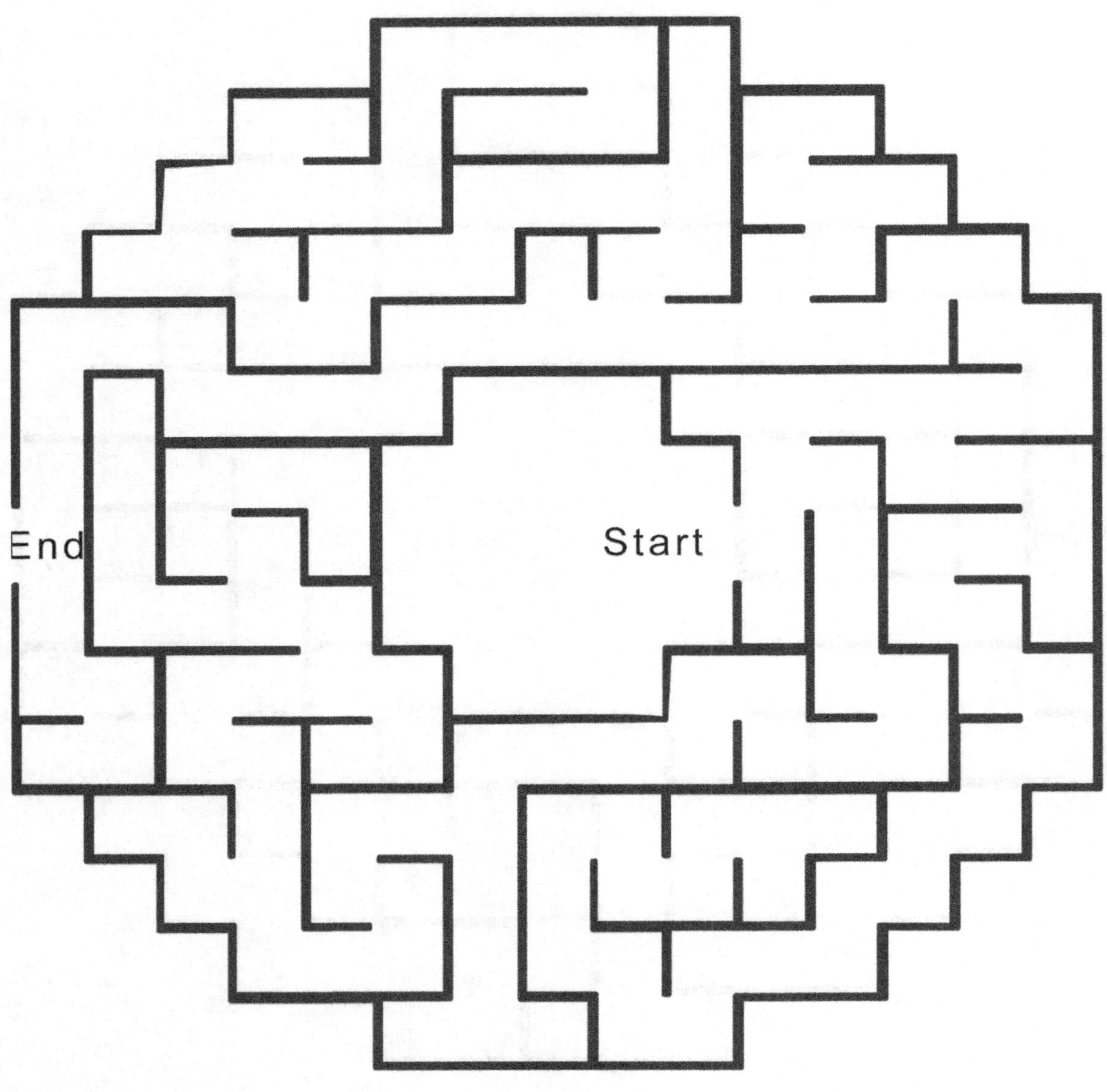

Start time: __________ End time: __________

Total time, maze 2: __________

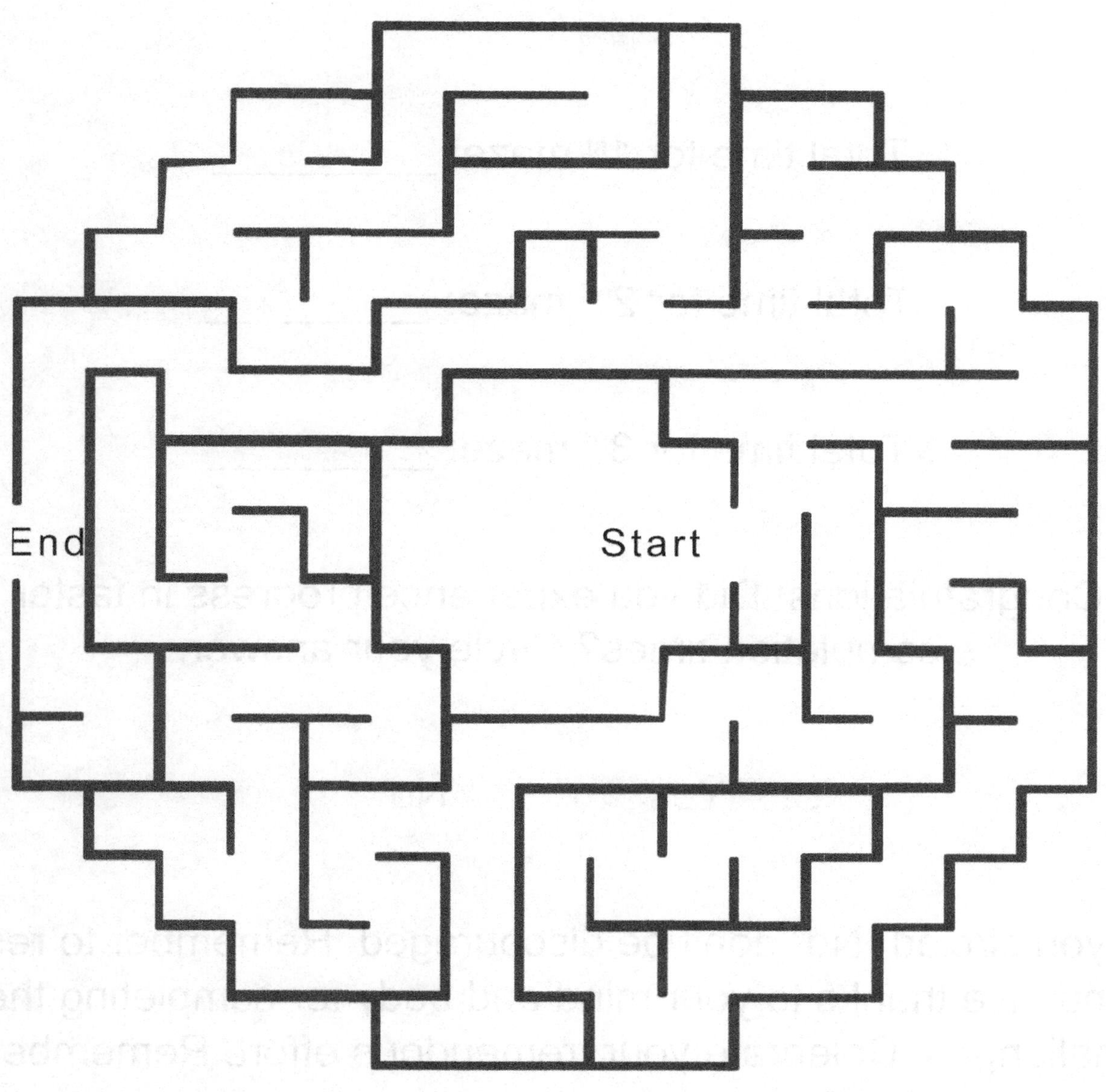

Start time: __________ End time: __________

Total time, maze 3: __________

Total time for 1st maze: __________

Total time for 2nd maze: __________

Total time for 3rd maze: __________

Congratulations! Did you experience progress in faster completion times? Circle your answer.

Yes No

If you circled "No" don't be discouraged. Remember to rest and give thanks to your mind and body for completing the challenges. Celebrate your tremendous effort. Remember, a seed doesn't turn into a tree overnight.

If you really want to do something, you'll find a way. If you don't, you'll find an excuse.

—Jim Rohn

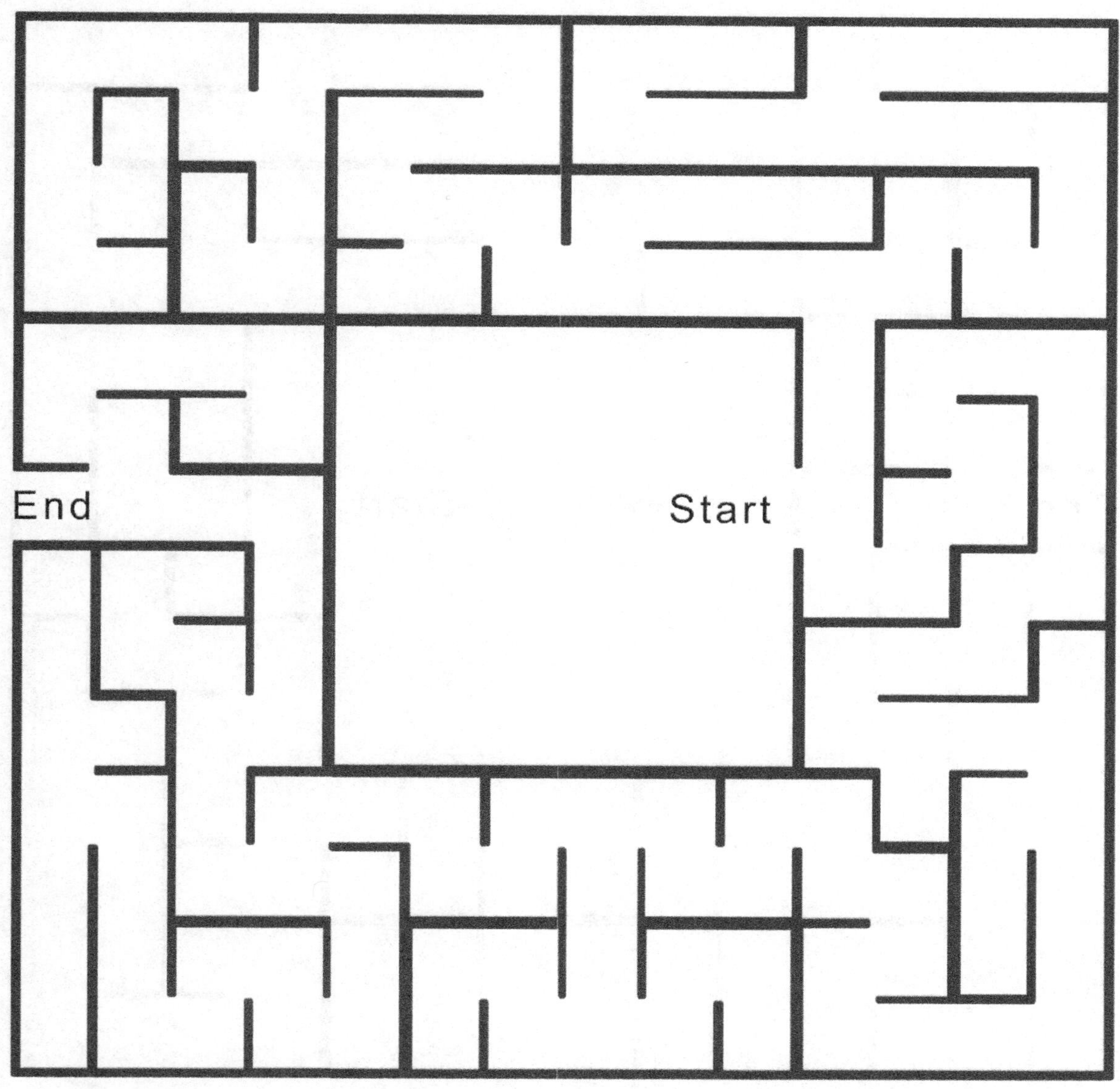

Start time: __________ End time: __________

Total time, maze 1: __________

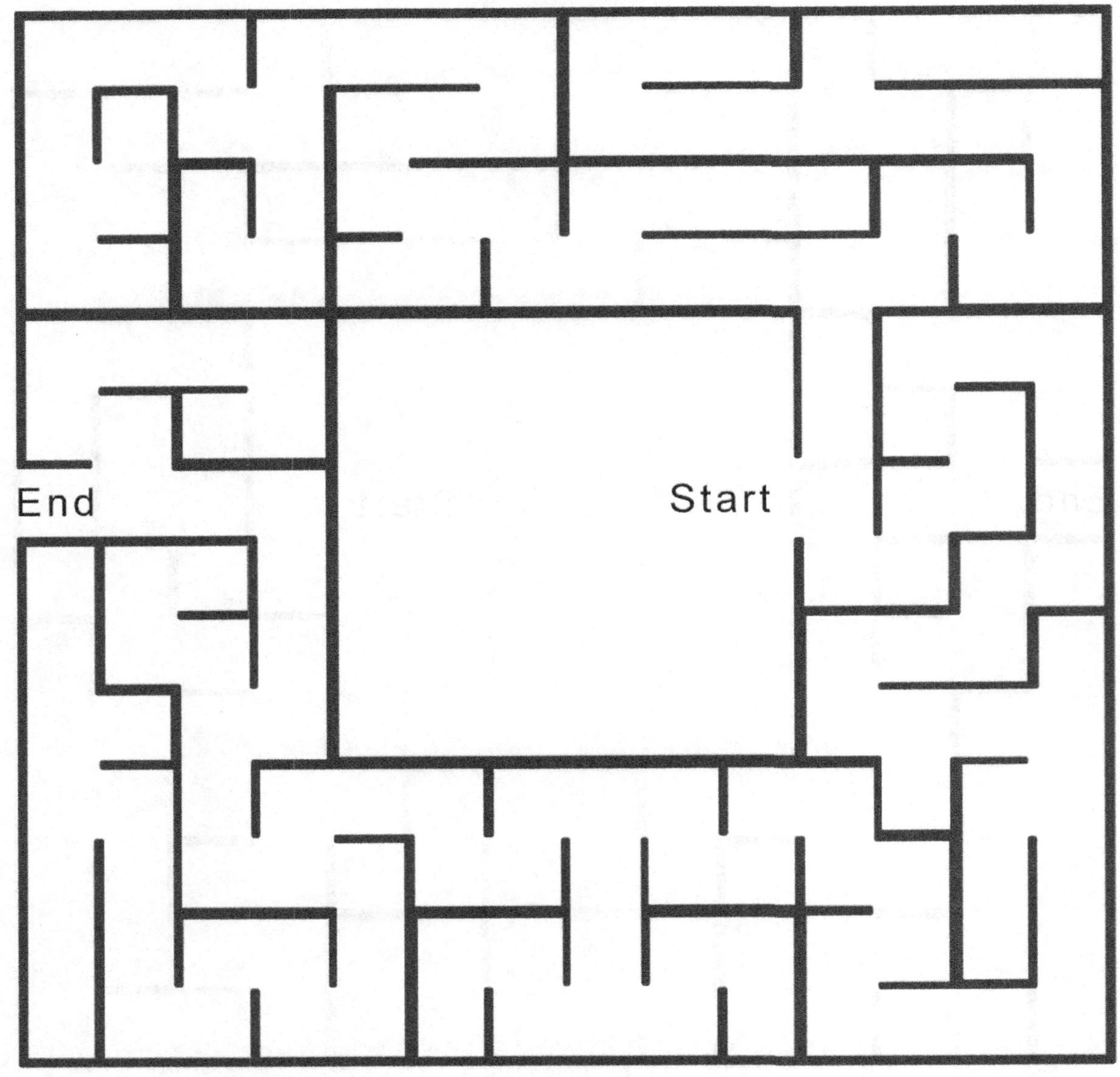

Start time: __________ End time: __________

Total time, maze 2: __________

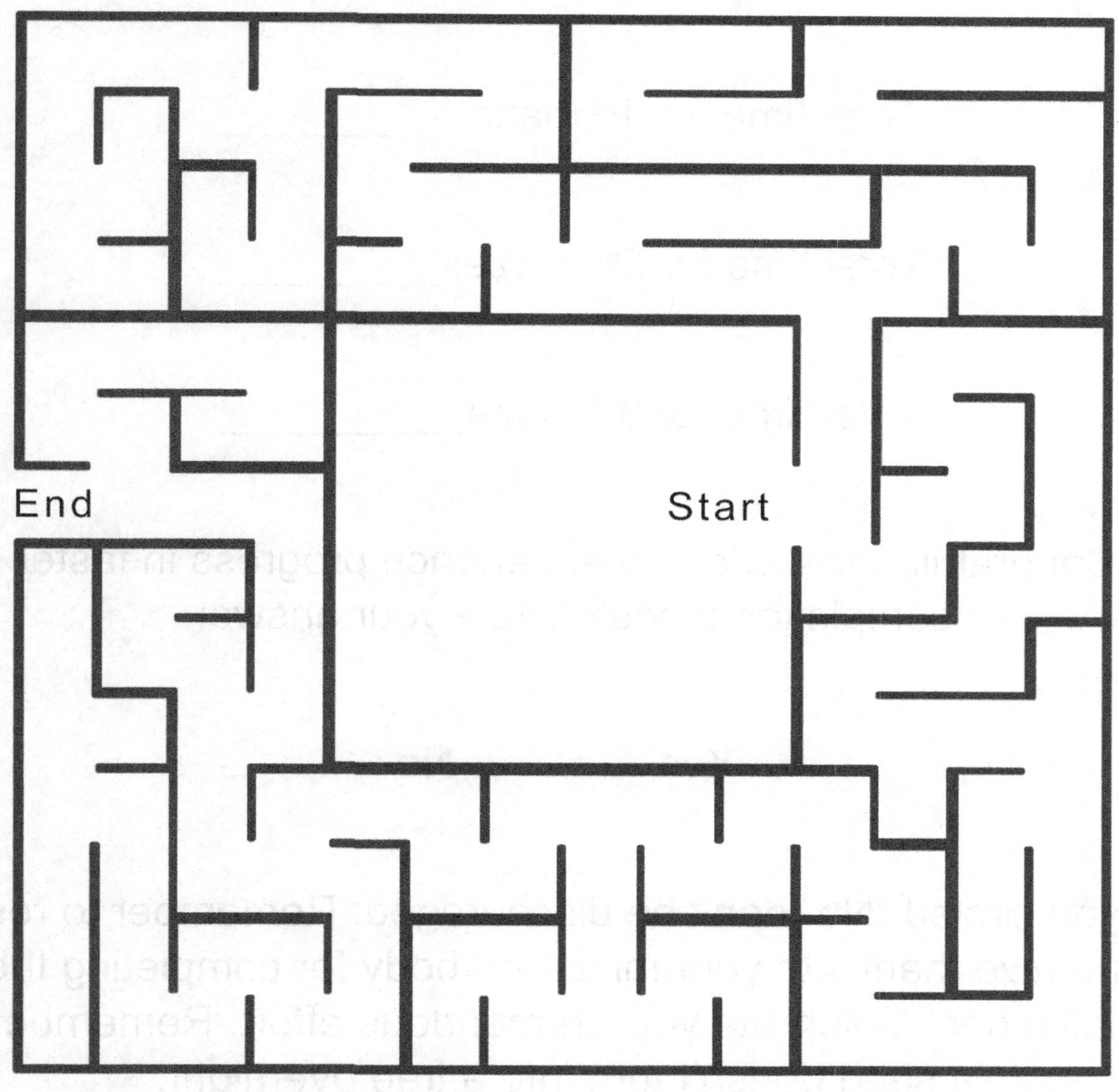

Start time: __________ End time: __________

Total time, maze 3: __________

Total time for 1st maze: __________

Total time for 2nd maze: __________

Total time for 3rd maze: __________

Congratulations! Did you experience progress in faster completion times? Circle your answer.

Yes No

If you circled "No" don't be discouraged. Remember to rest and give thanks to your mind and body for completing the challenges. Celebrate your tremendous effort. Remember, a seed doesn't turn into a tree overnight.

F.E.A.R: has two meanings: 1). Forget Everything And Run or 2). Face Everything And Rise; the choice is yours!

—Zig Ziglar

The soul always knows what to do to heal itself,
the challenge is to silence the mind.

—Caroline Myss

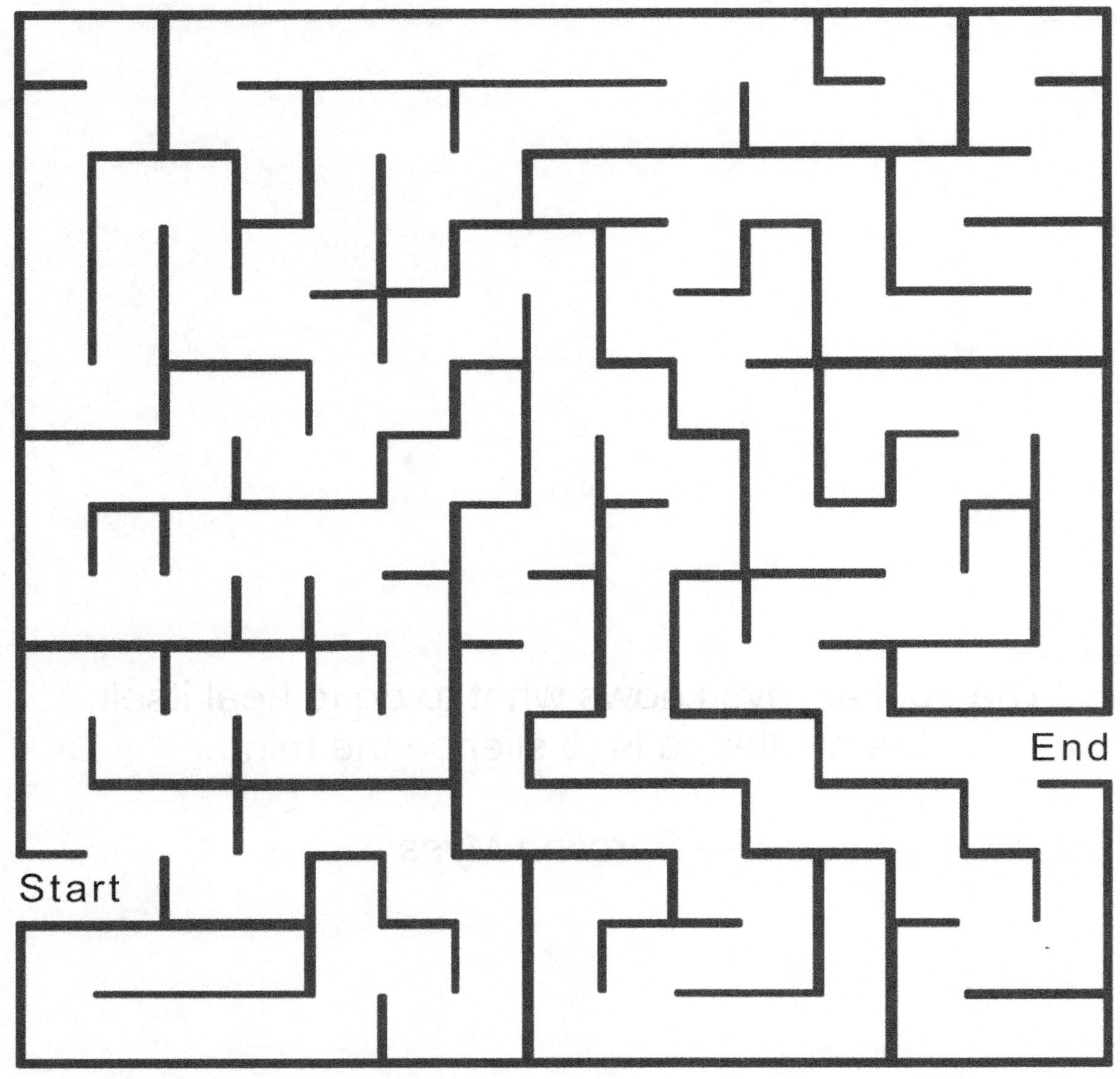

Start time: __________ End time: __________

Total time, maze 1: __________

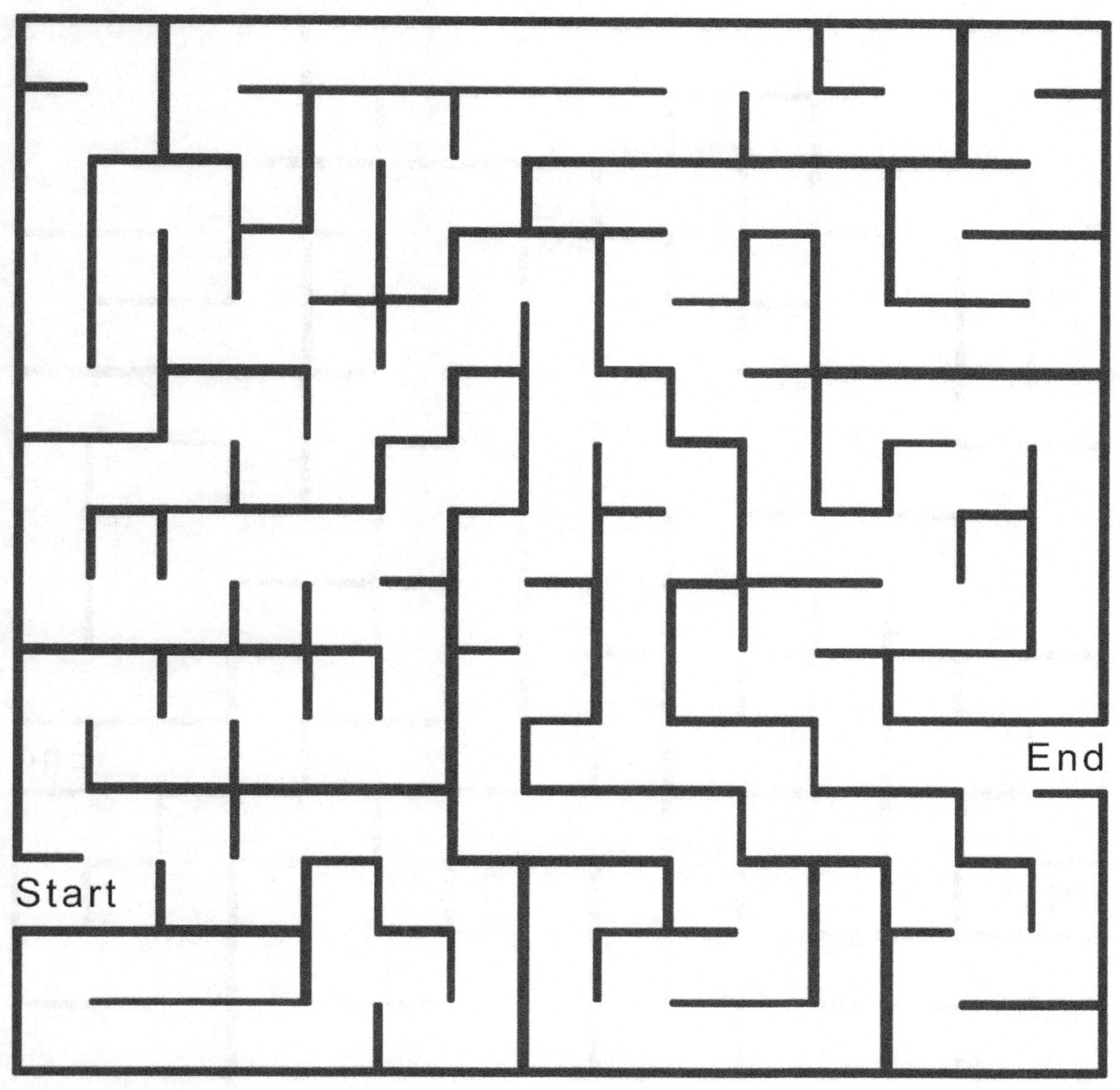

Start time: __________ End time: __________

Total time, maze 2: __________

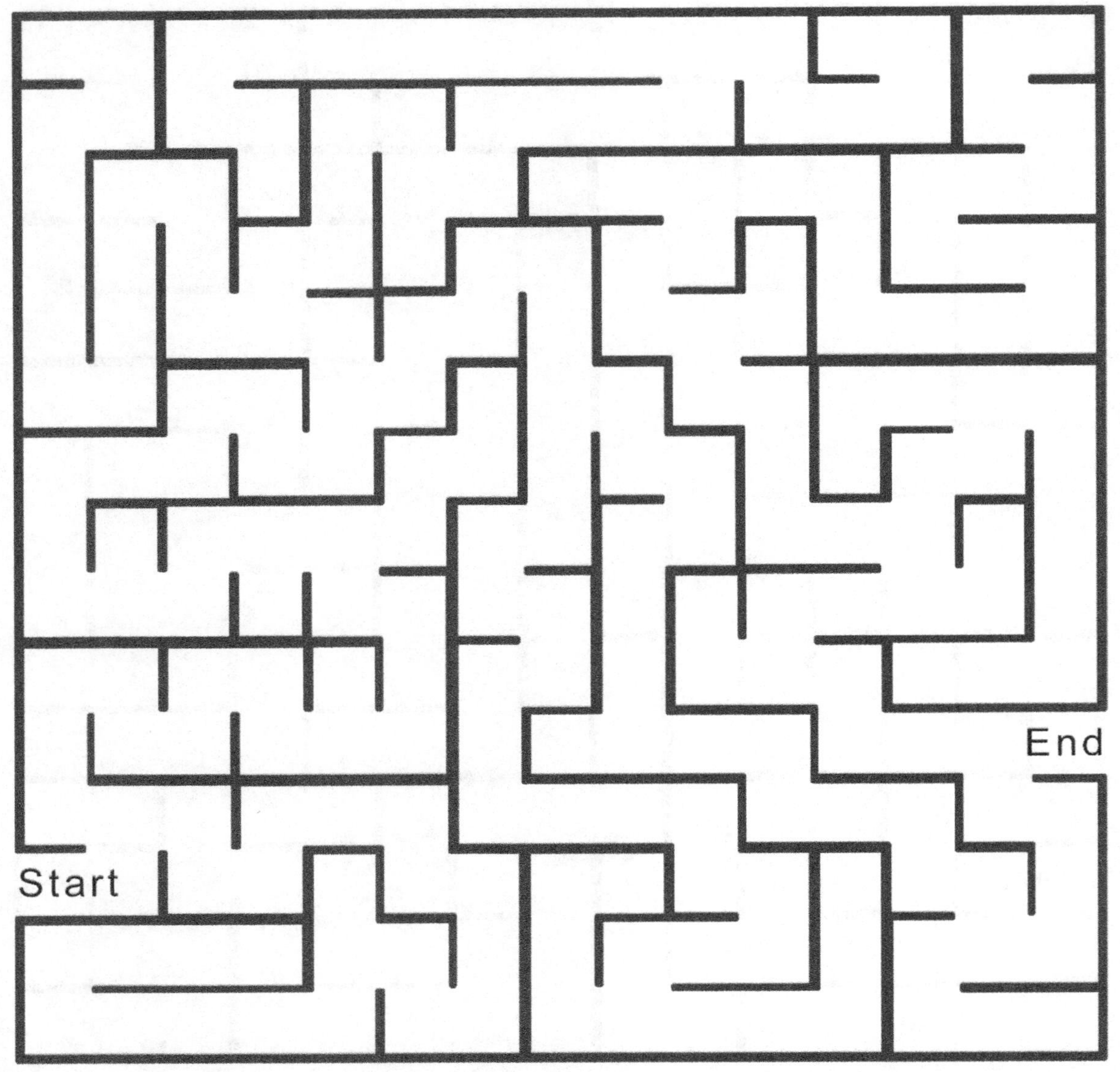

Start time: __________ End time: __________

Total time, maze 3: __________

Total time for 1st maze: __________

Total time for 2nd maze: __________

Total time for 3rd maze: __________

Congratulations! Did you experience progress in faster completion times? Circle your answer.

Yes No

If you circled "No" don't be discouraged. Remember to rest and give thanks to your mind and body for completing the challenges. Celebrate your tremendous effort. Remember, a seed doesn't turn into a tree overnight.

Life is like a camera… focus on what's important, capture the good times, develop from the negatives, and if things don't work out, take another shot.

—*Unknown*

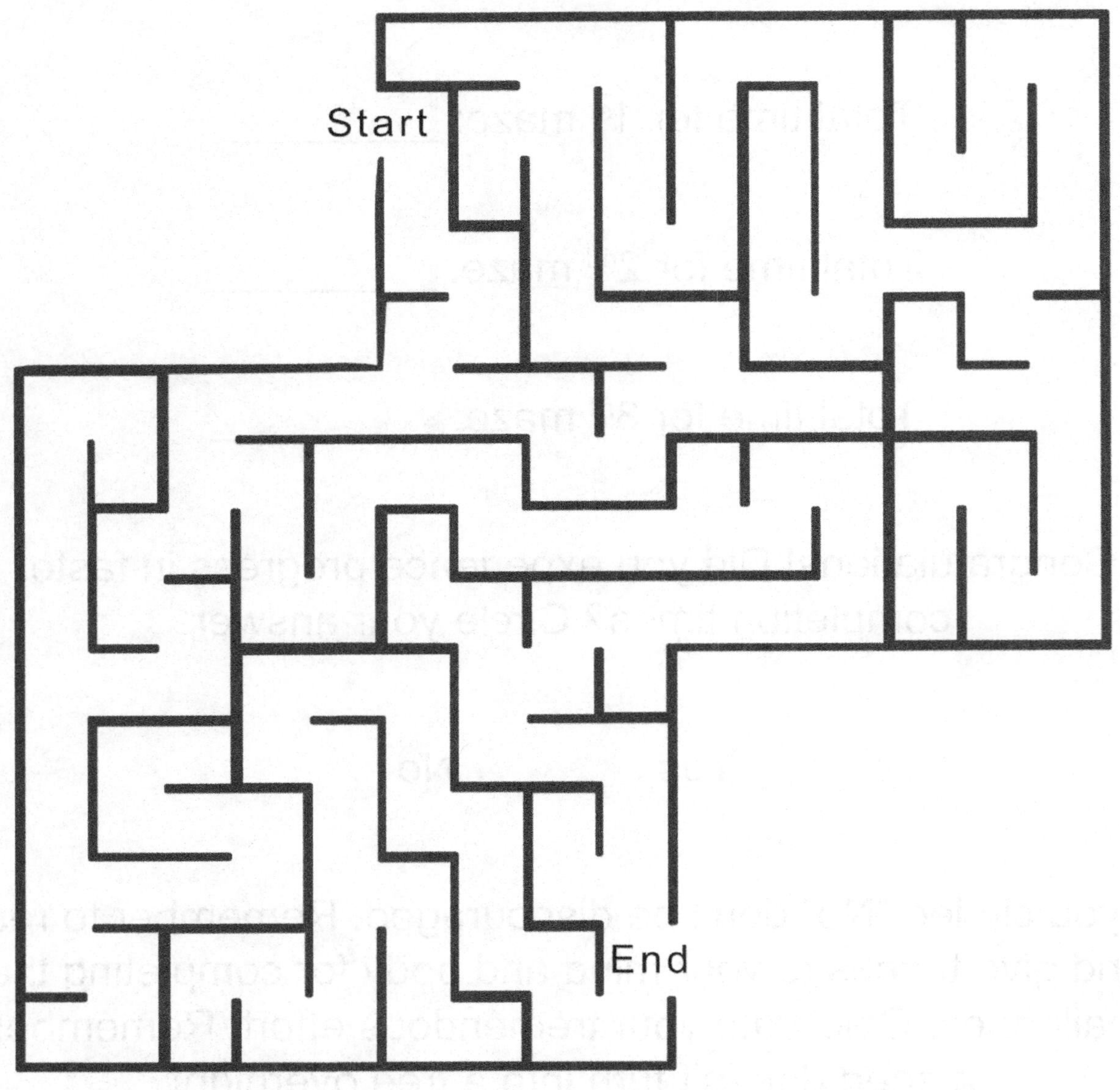

Start time: __________ End time: __________

Total time, maze 1: __________

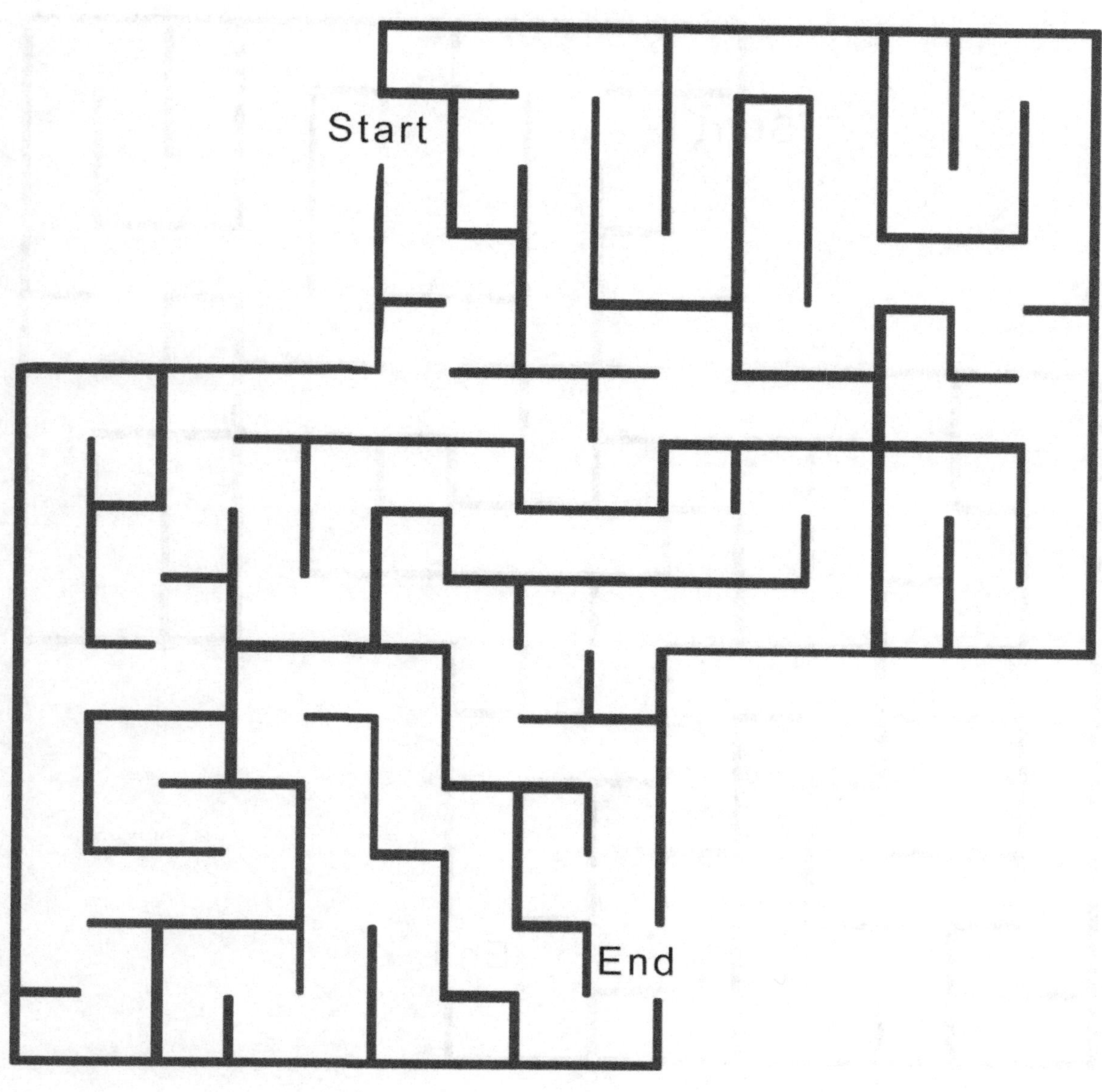

Start time: __________ End time: __________

Total time, maze 2: __________

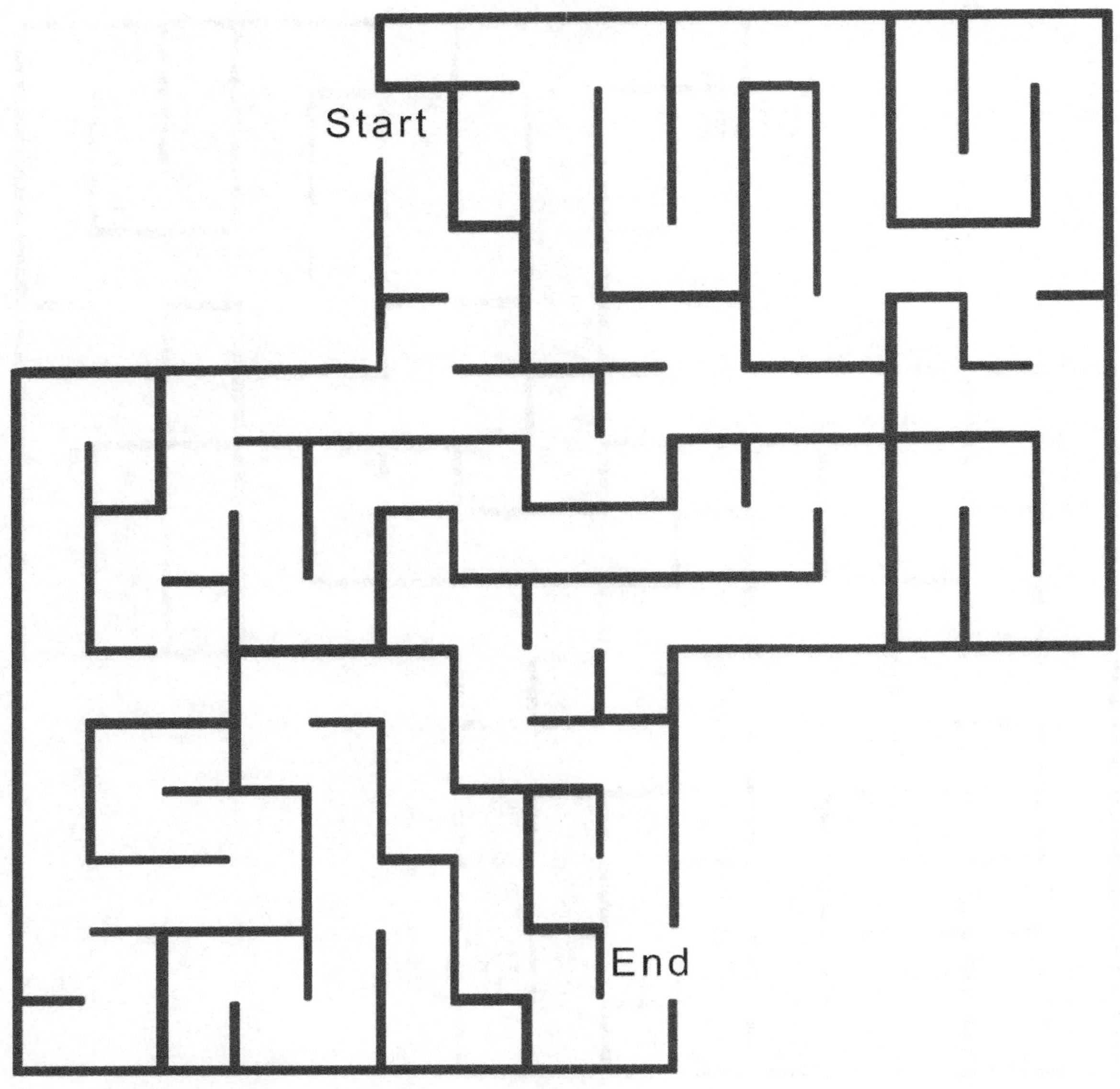

Start time: __________ End time: __________

Total time, maze 3: __________

Total time for 1st maze: __________

Total time for 2nd maze: __________

Total time for 3rd maze: __________

Congratulations! Did you experience progress in faster completion times? Circle your answer.

Yes No

If you circled "No" don't be discouraged. Remember to rest and give thanks to your mind and body for completing the challenges. Celebrate your tremendous effort. Remember, a seed doesn't turn into a tree overnight.

Keep watering, keep planting, keep cultivating, and one day your garden will bloom.

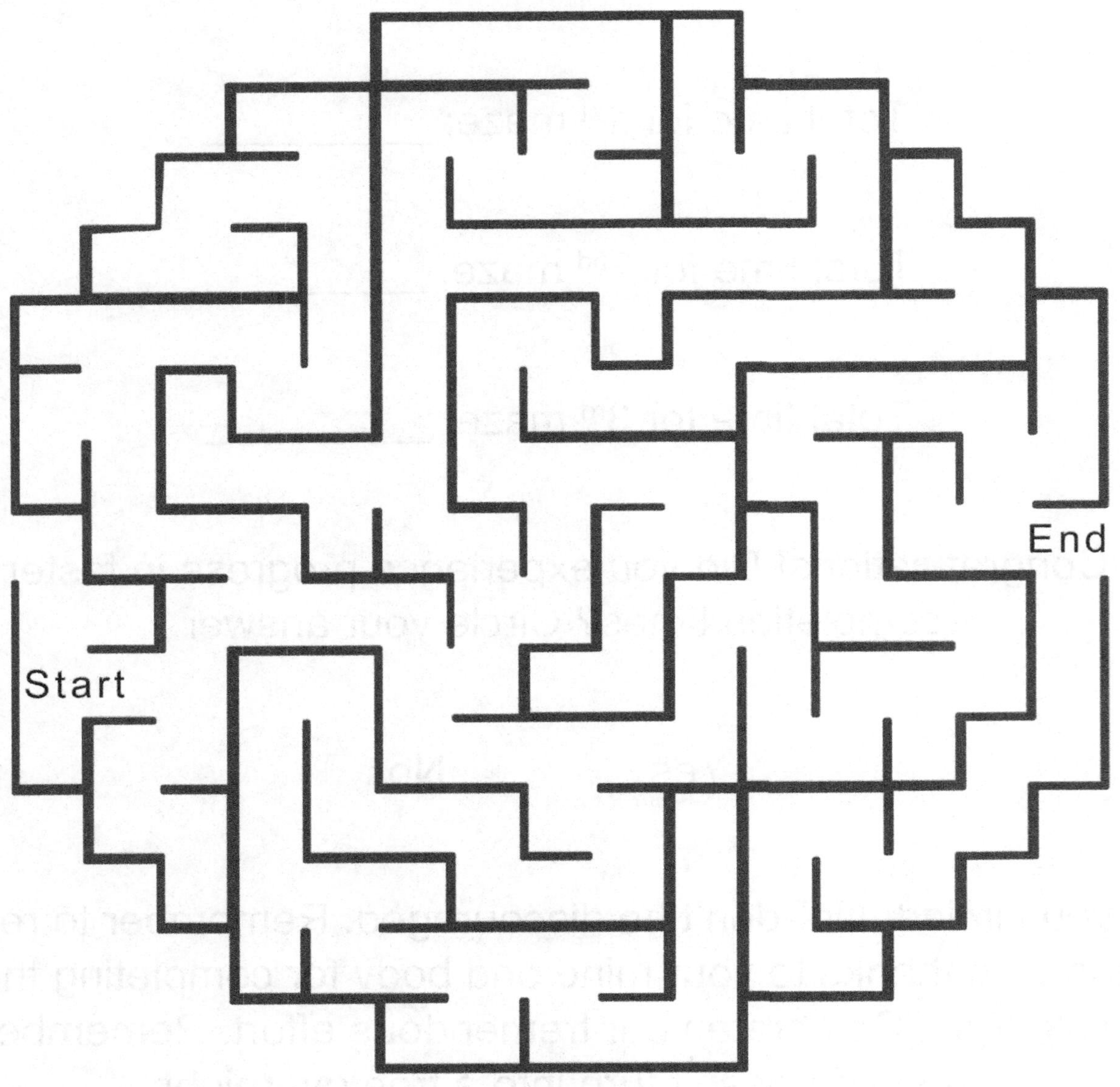

Start time: __________ End time: __________

Total time, maze 1: __________

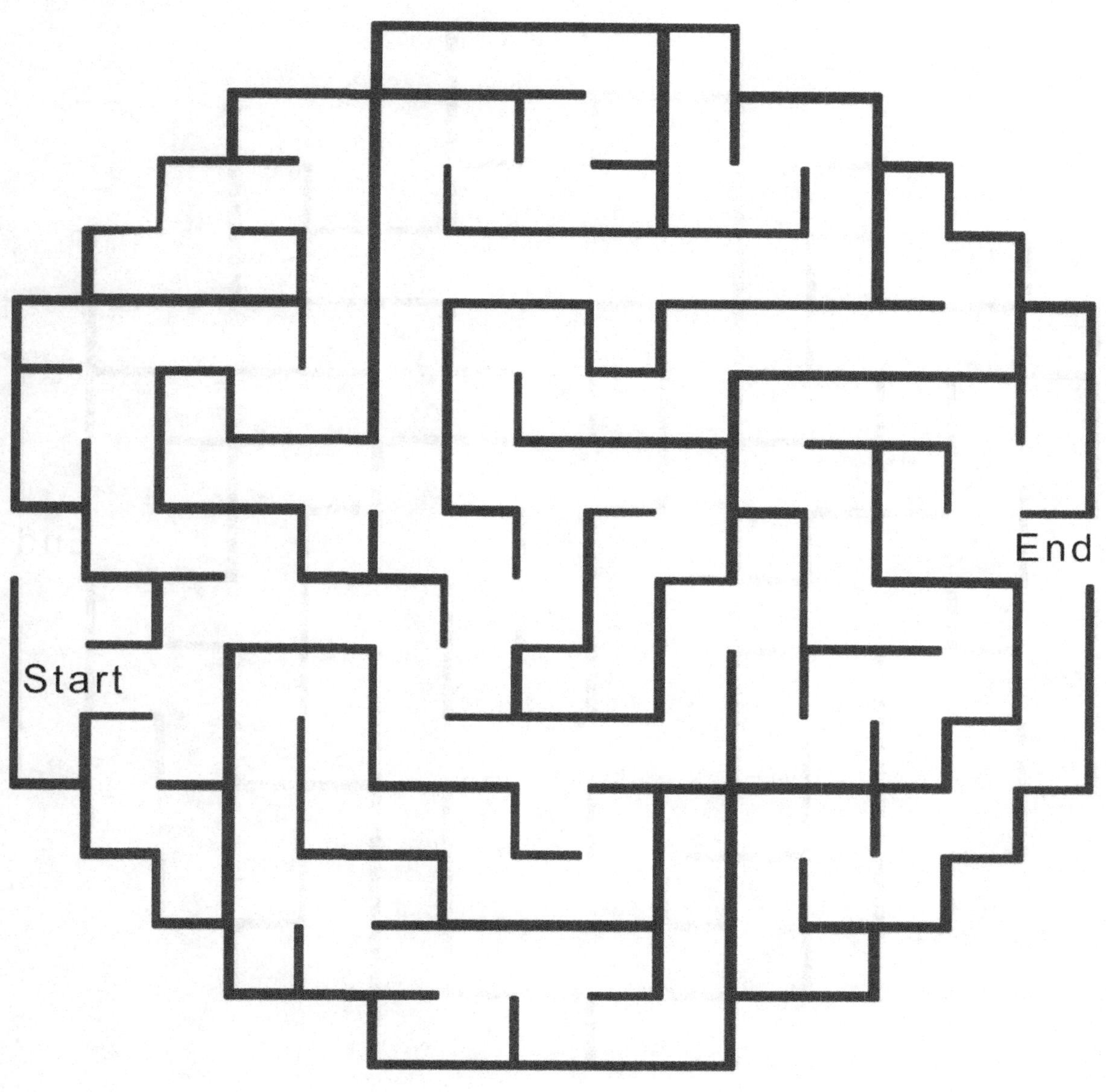

Start time: __________ End time: __________

Total time, maze 2: __________

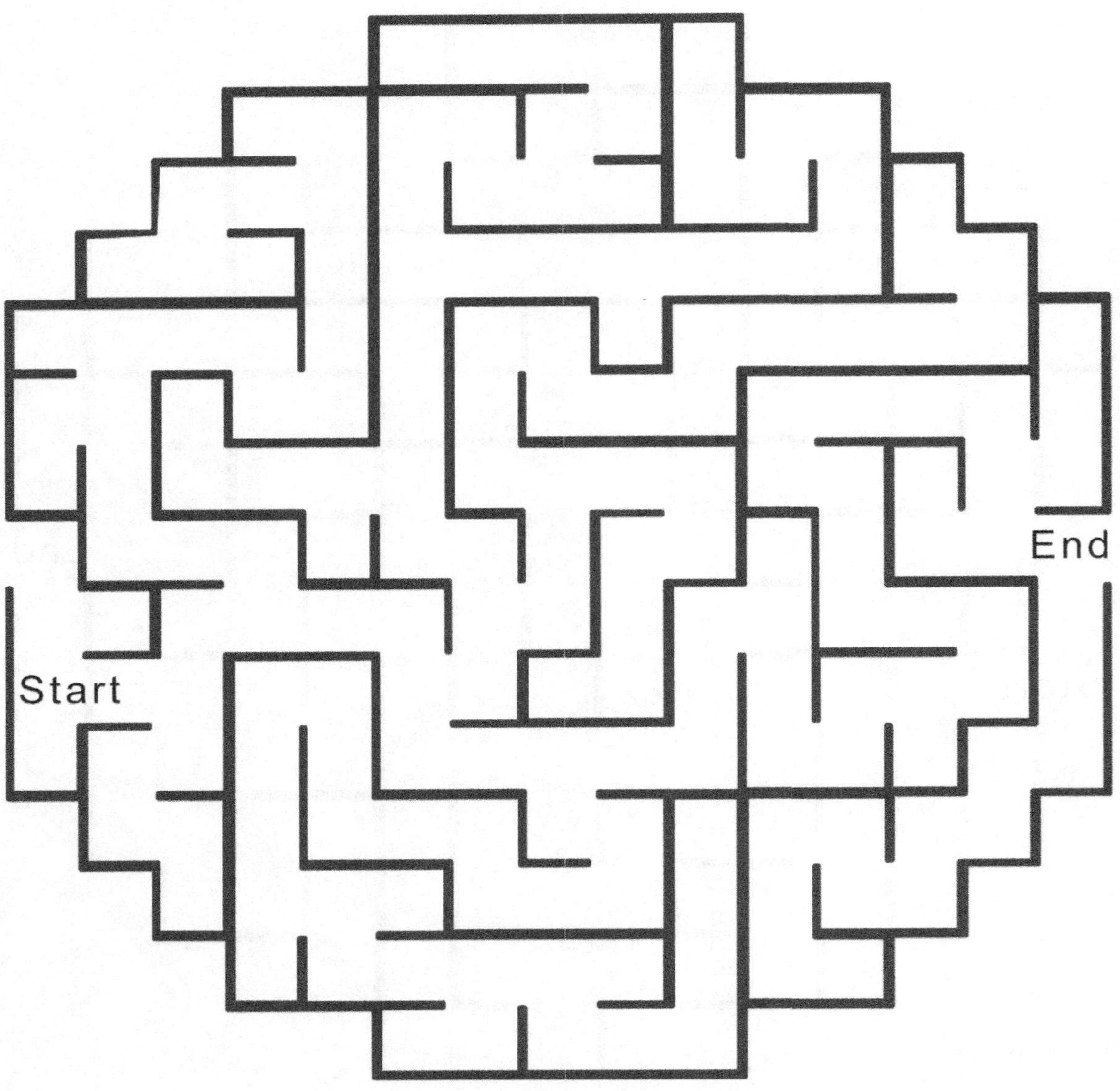

Start time: __________ End time: __________

Total time, maze 3: __________

Total time for 1st maze: __________

Total time for 2nd maze: __________

Total time for 3rd maze: __________

Congratulations! Did you experience progress in faster completion times? Circle your answer.

Yes No

If you circled "No" don't be discouraged. Remember to rest and give thanks to your mind and body for completing the challenges. Celebrate your tremendous effort. Remember, a seed doesn't turn into a tree overnight.

One of the things I learned the hard way was that it doesn't pay to get discouraged. Keeping busy and making optimism a way of life can restore your faith in yourself.

—Lucille Ball

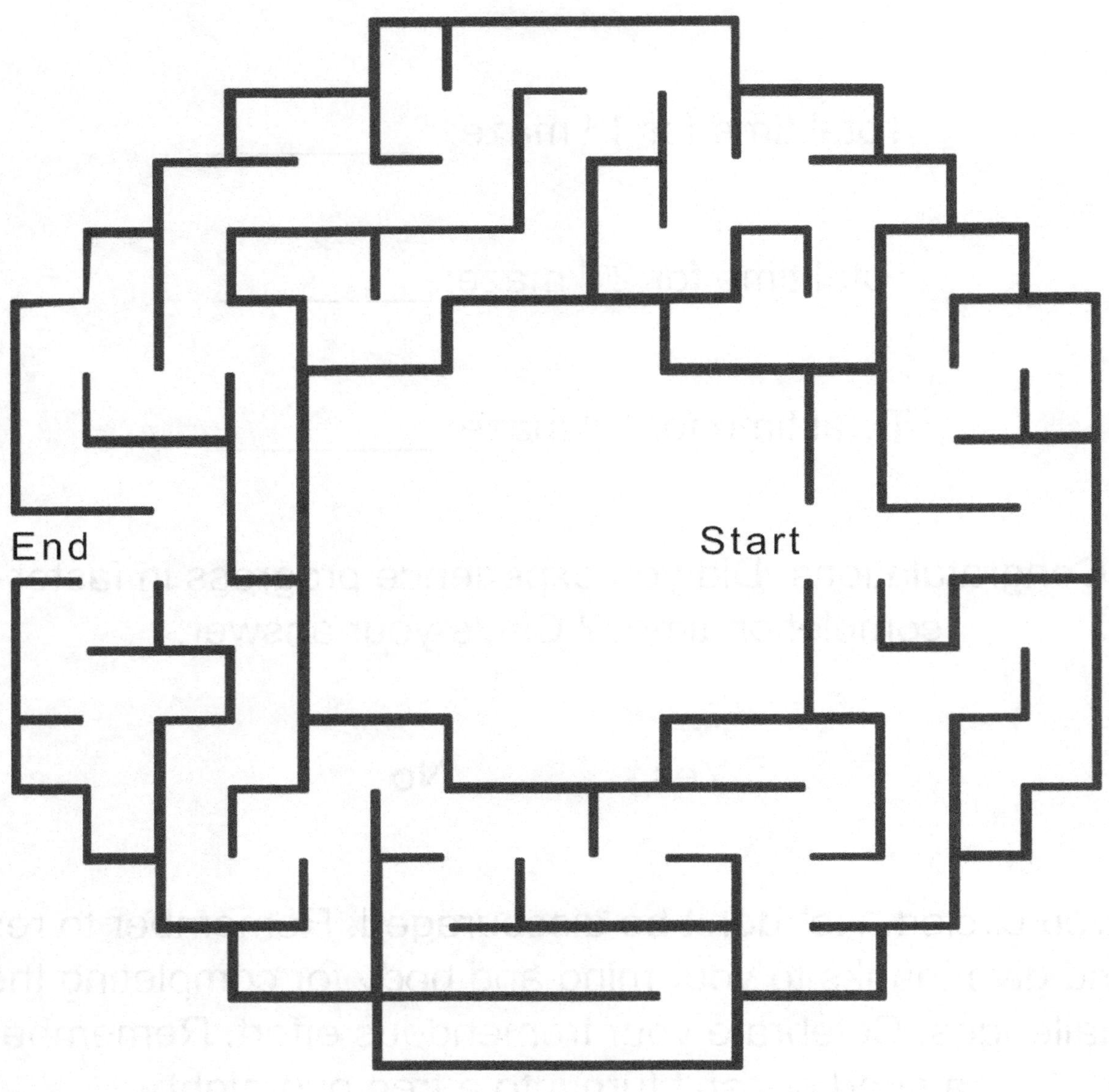

Start time: __________ End time: __________

Total time, maze 1: __________

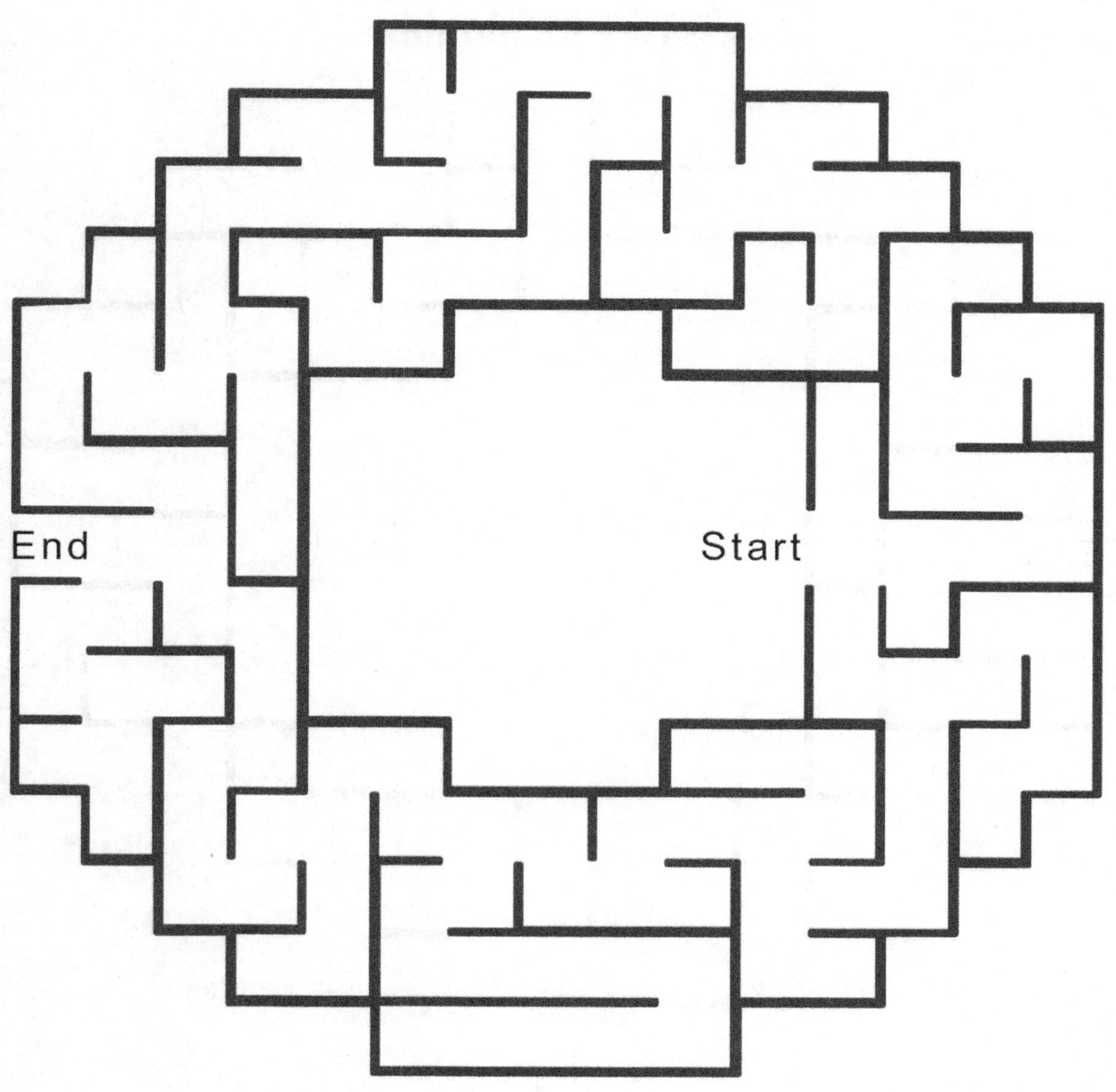

Start time: __________ End time: __________

Total time, maze 2: __________

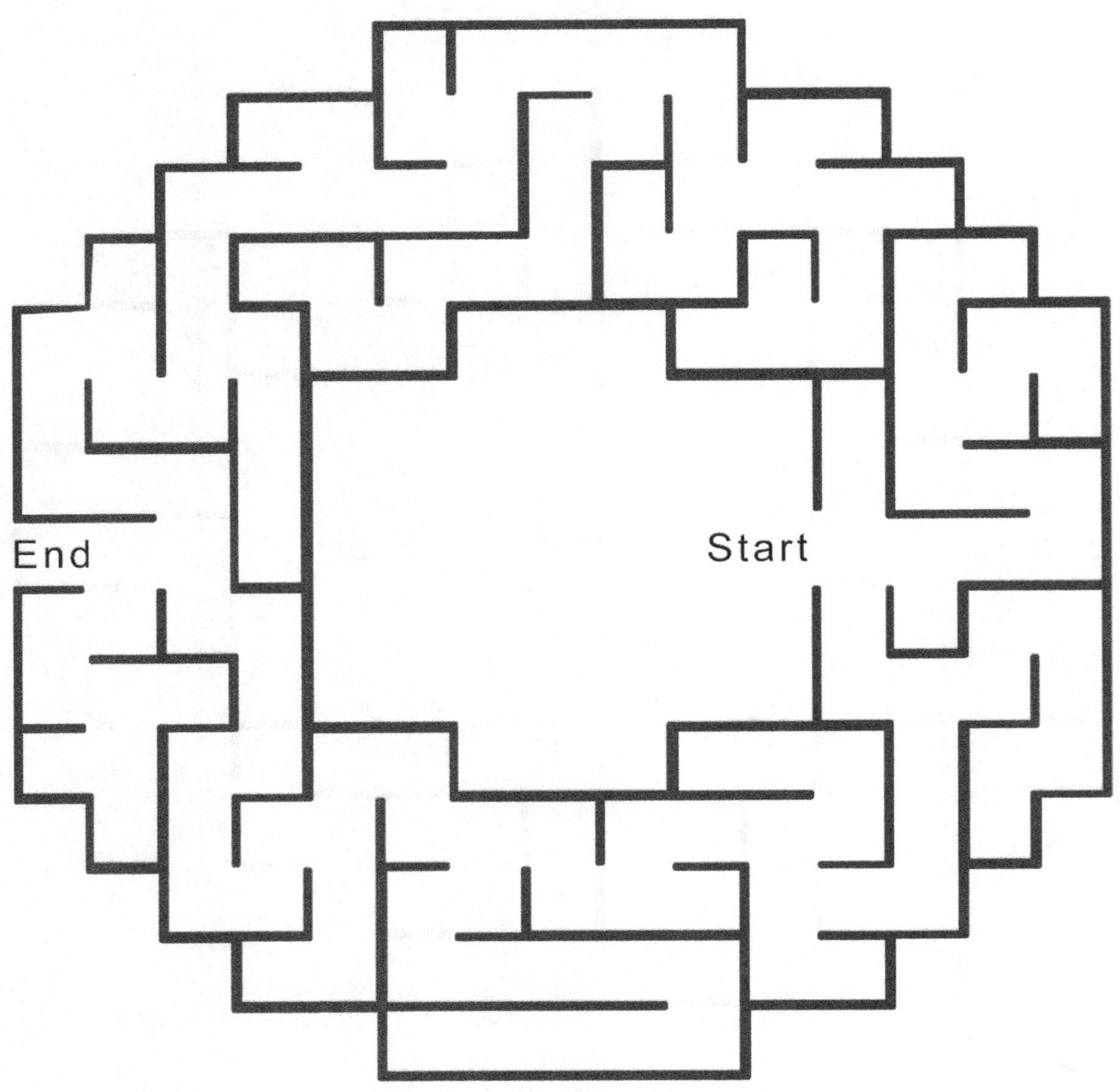

Start time: __________ End time: __________

Total time, maze 3: __________

Total time for 1st maze: __________

Total time for 2nd maze: __________

Total time for 3rd maze: __________

Congratulations! Did you experience progress in faster completion times? Circle your answer.

Yes No

If you circled "No" don't be discouraged. Remember to rest and give thanks to your mind and body for completing the challenges. Celebrate your tremendous effort. Remember, a seed doesn't turn into a tree overnight.

Edison failed 10,000 times before he made the electric light. Do not be discouraged if you fail a few times.

—Napoleon Hill

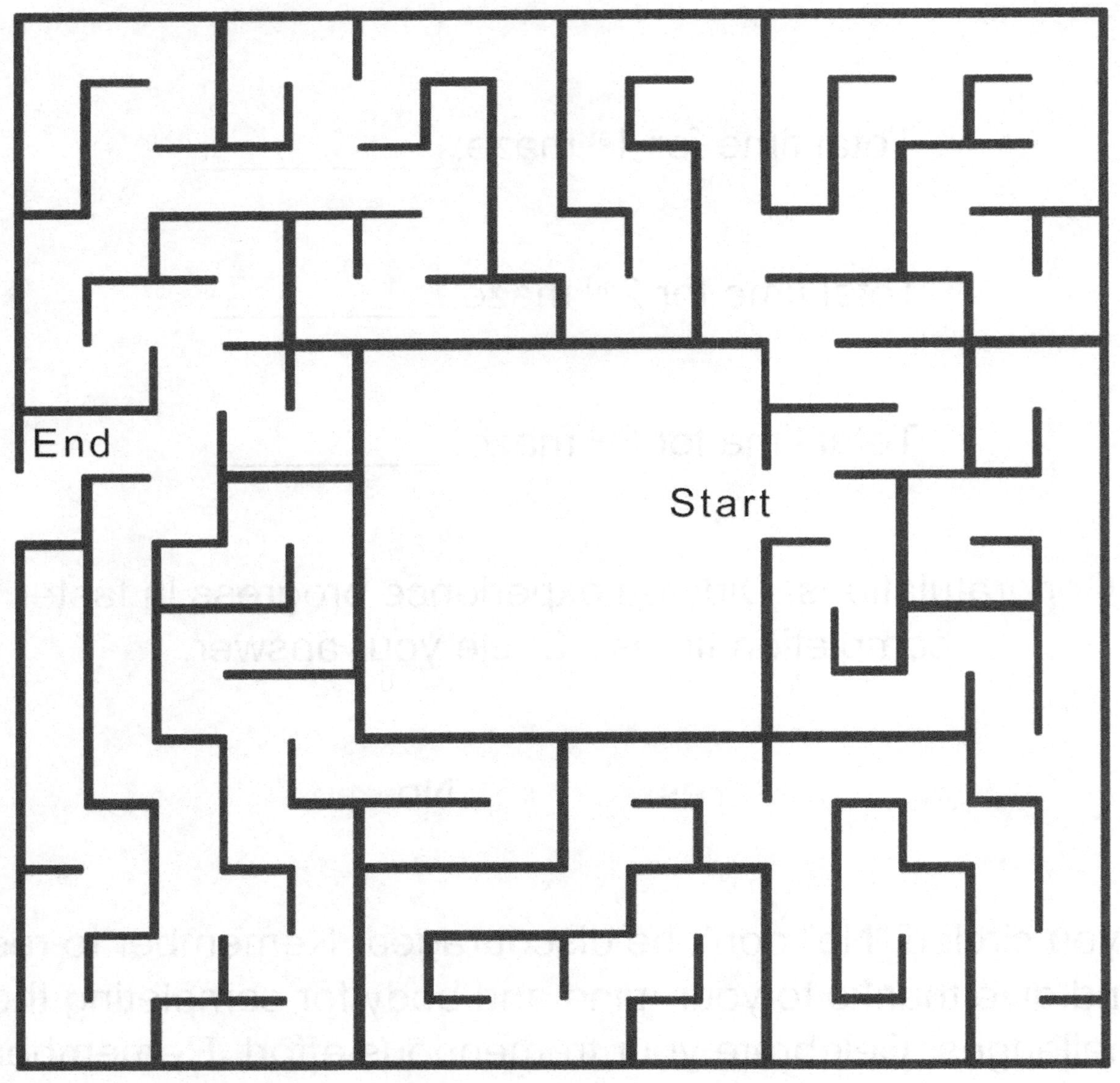

Start time: __________ End time: __________

Total time, maze 1: __________

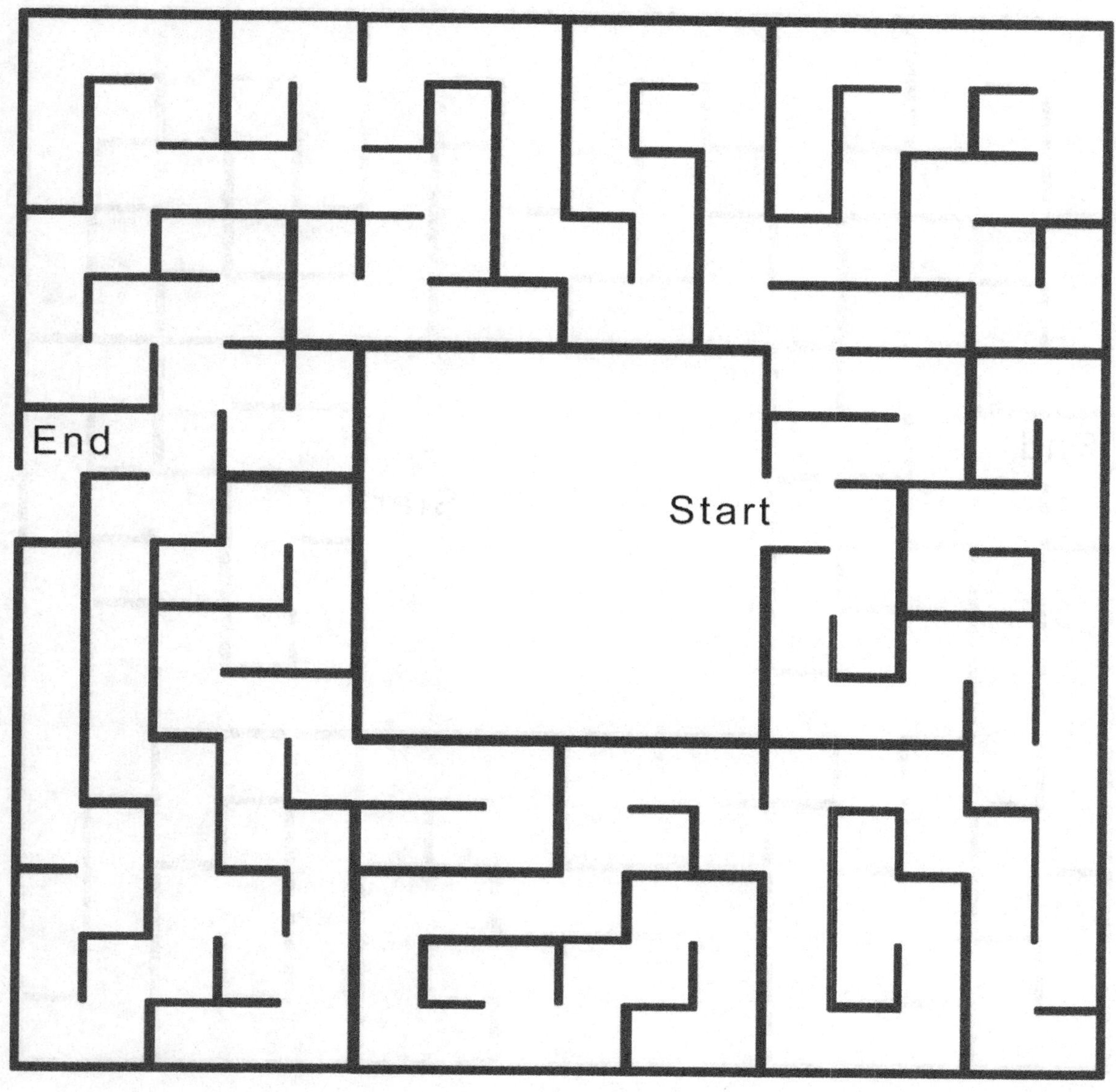

Start time: __________ End time: __________

Total time, maze 2: __________

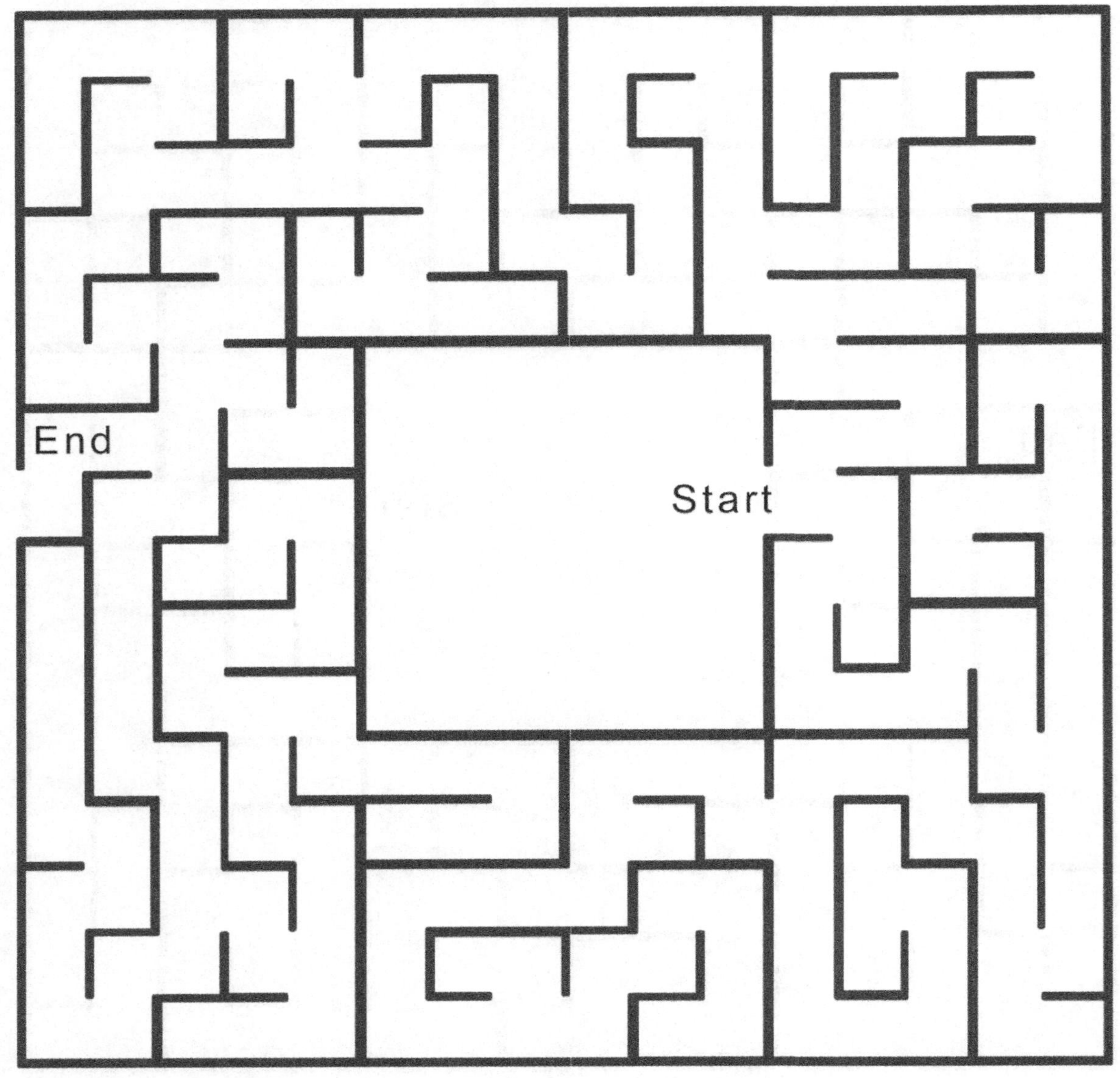

Start time: __________ End time: __________

Total time, maze 3: __________

Total time for 1st maze: __________

Total time for 2nd maze: __________

Total time for 3rd maze: __________

Congratulations! Did you experience progress in faster completion times? Circle your answer.

Yes No

If you circled "No" don't be discouraged. Remember to rest and give thanks to your mind and body for completing the challenges. Celebrate your tremendous effort. Remember, a seed doesn't turn into a tree overnight.

A man can get discouraged many times but he is not a failure until he begins to blame somebody else and stops trying.

—*John Burroughs*

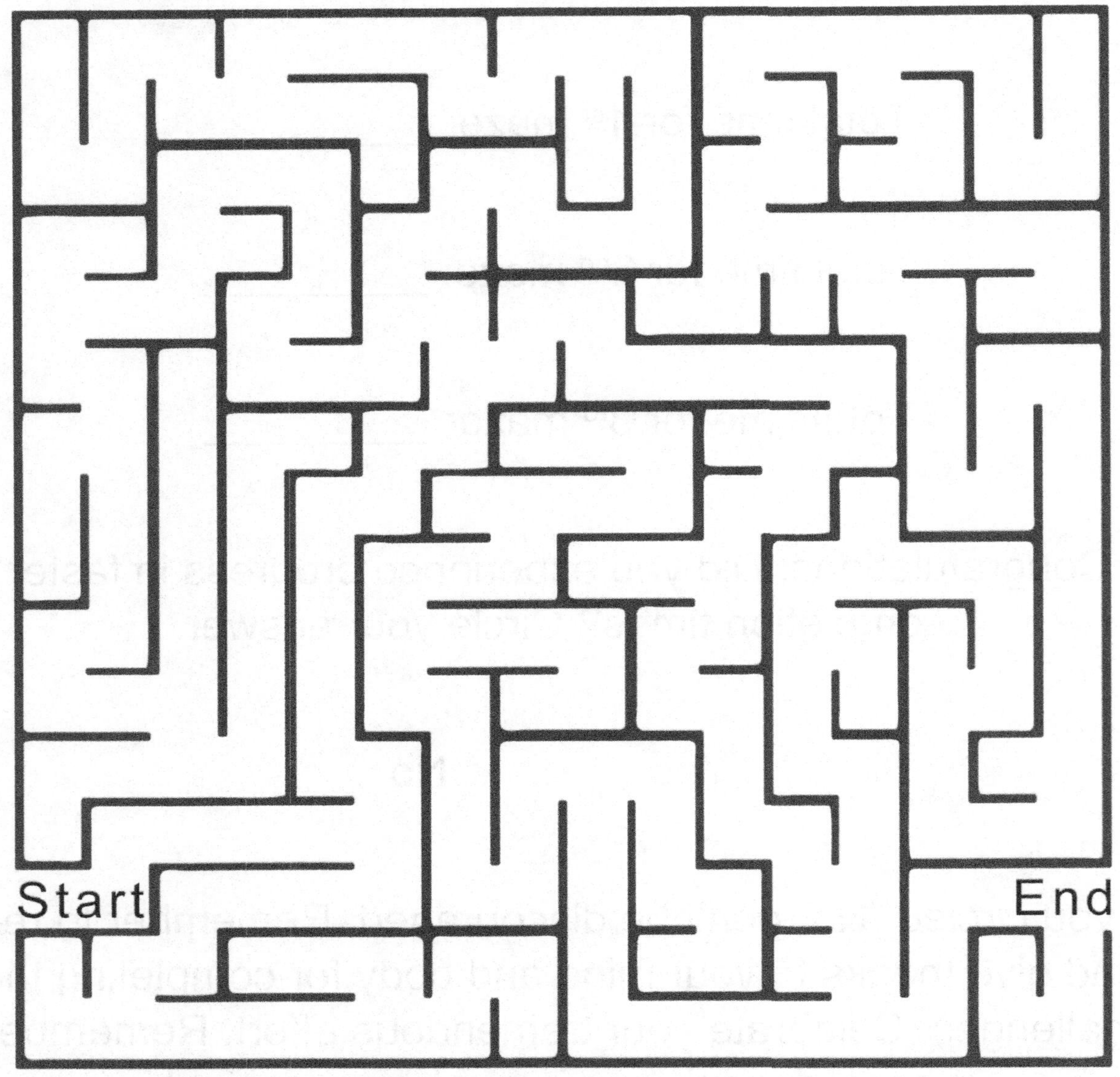

Start time: __________ End time: __________

Total time, maze 1: __________

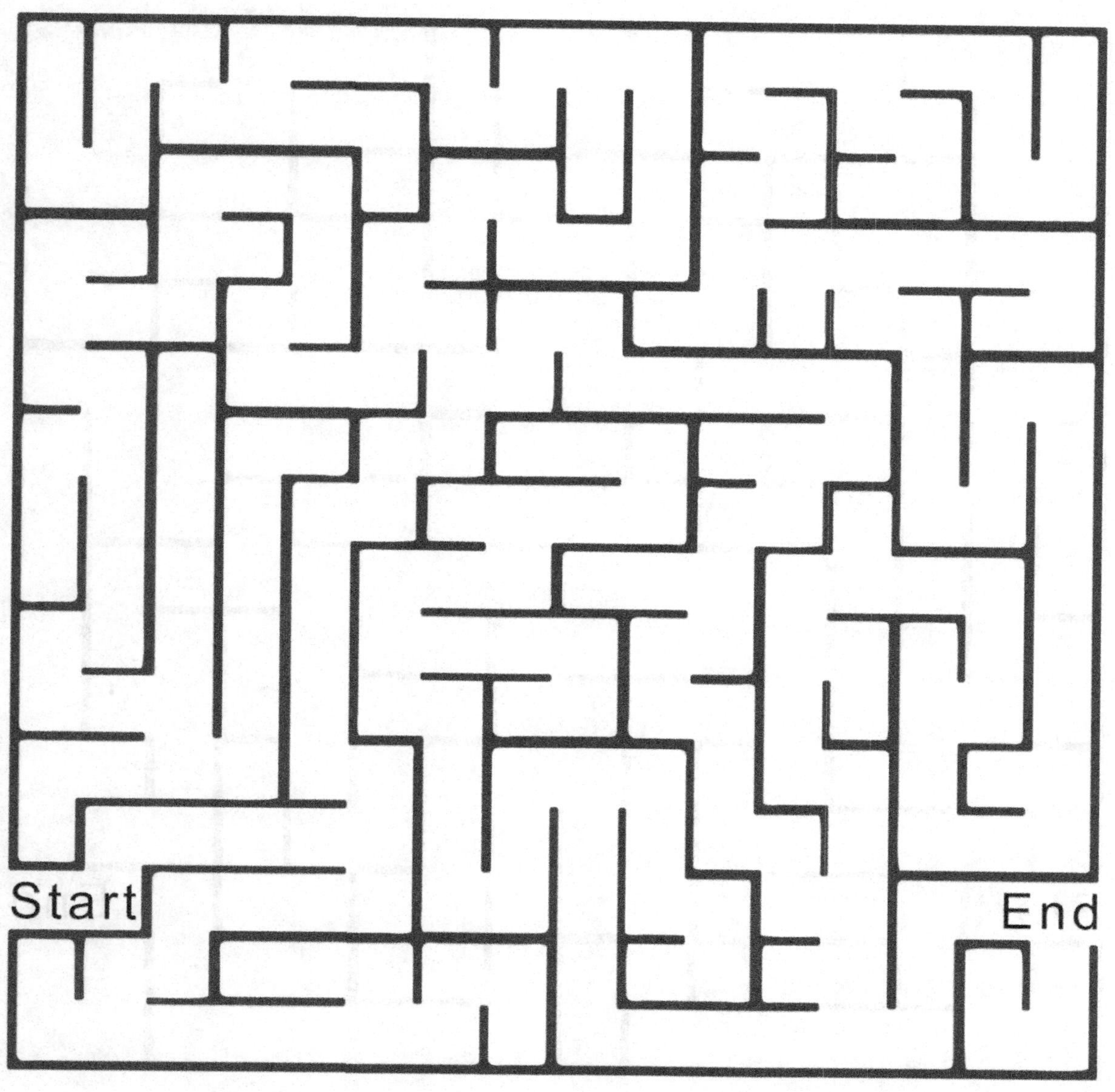

Start time: __________ End time: __________

Total time, maze 2: __________

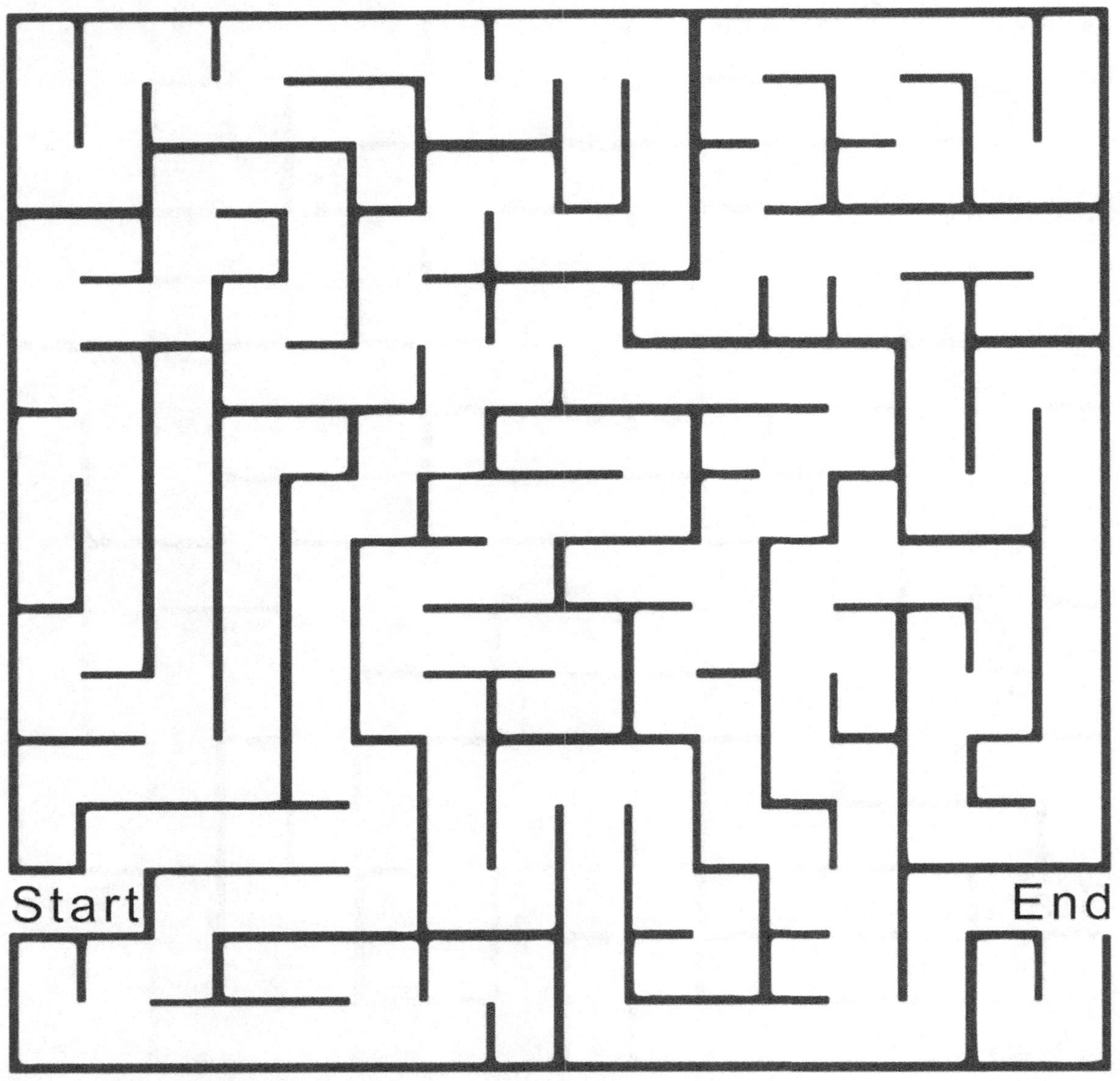

Start time: __________ End time: __________

Total time, maze 3: __________

Total time for 1st maze: __________

Total time for 2nd maze: __________

Total time for 3rd maze: __________

Congratulations! Did you experience progress in faster completion times? Circle your answer.

Yes No

If you circled “No” don’t be discouraged. Remember to rest and give thanks to your mind and body for completing the challenges. Celebrate your tremendous effort. Remember, a seed doesn’t turn into a tree overnight.

Continuous, unflagging effort, persistence and determination will win. Let not the man be discouraged who has these.

—James Whitcomb Riley

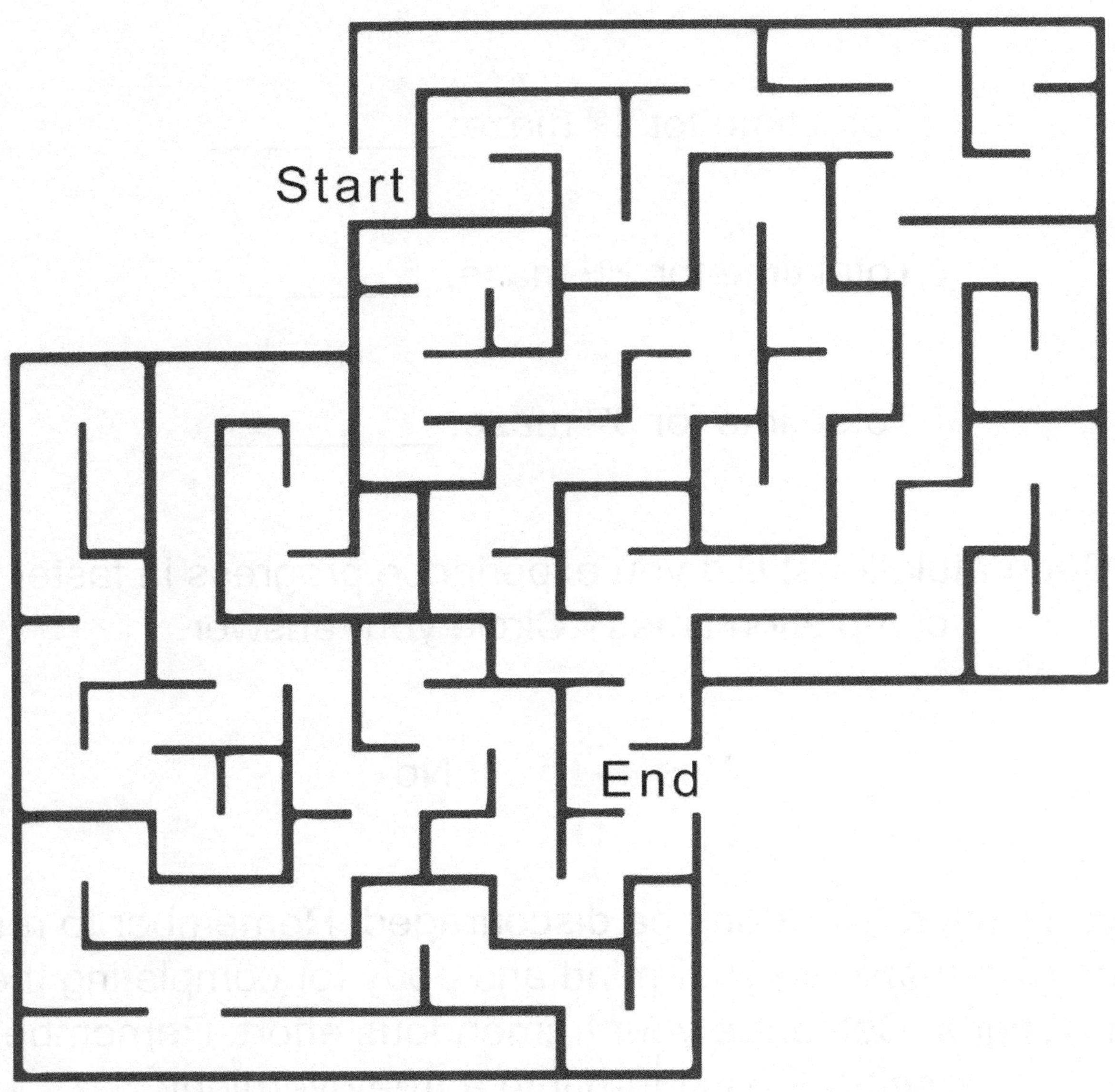

Start time: __________ End time: __________

Total time, maze 1: __________

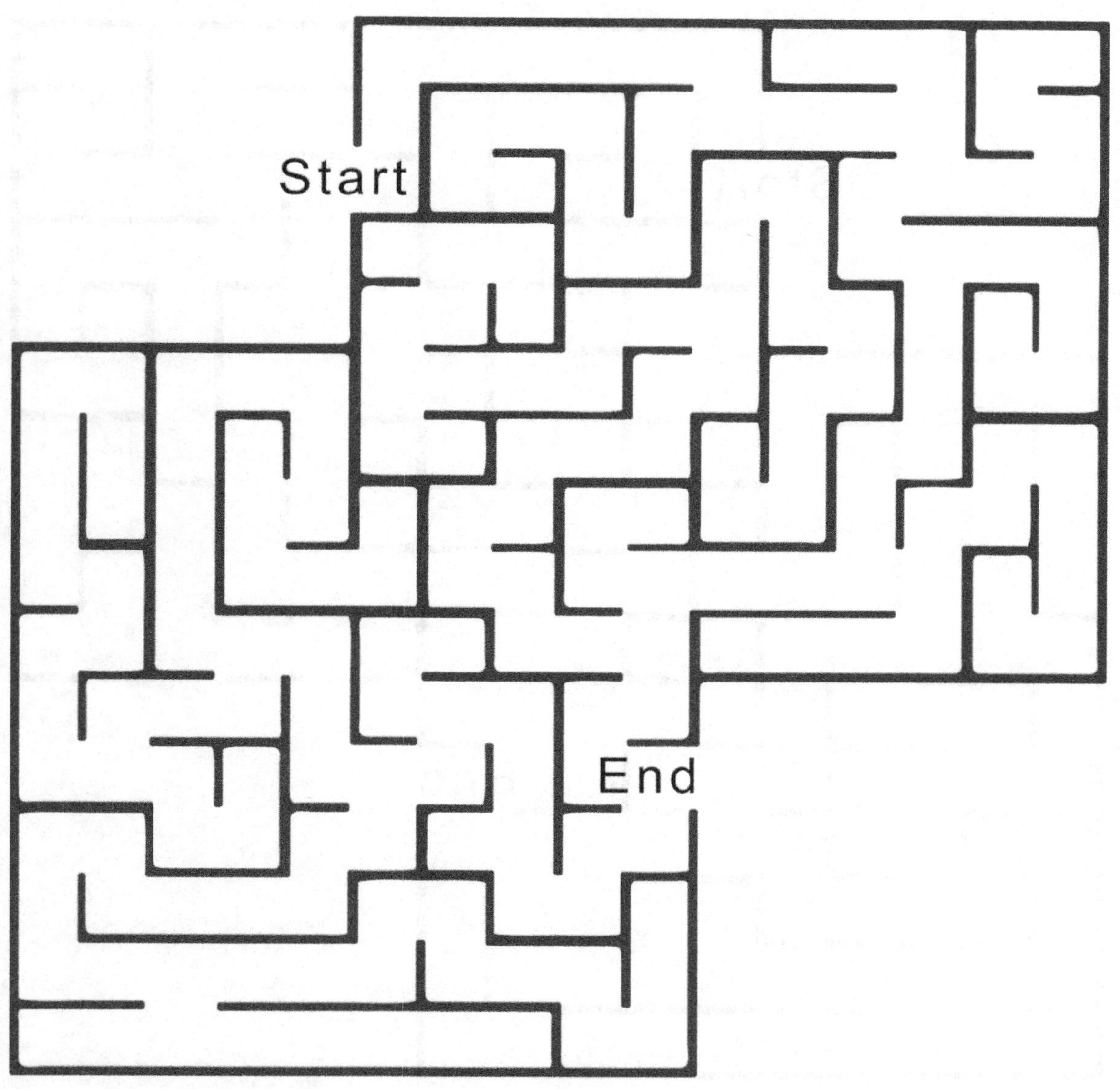

Start time: __________ End time: __________

Total time, maze 2: __________

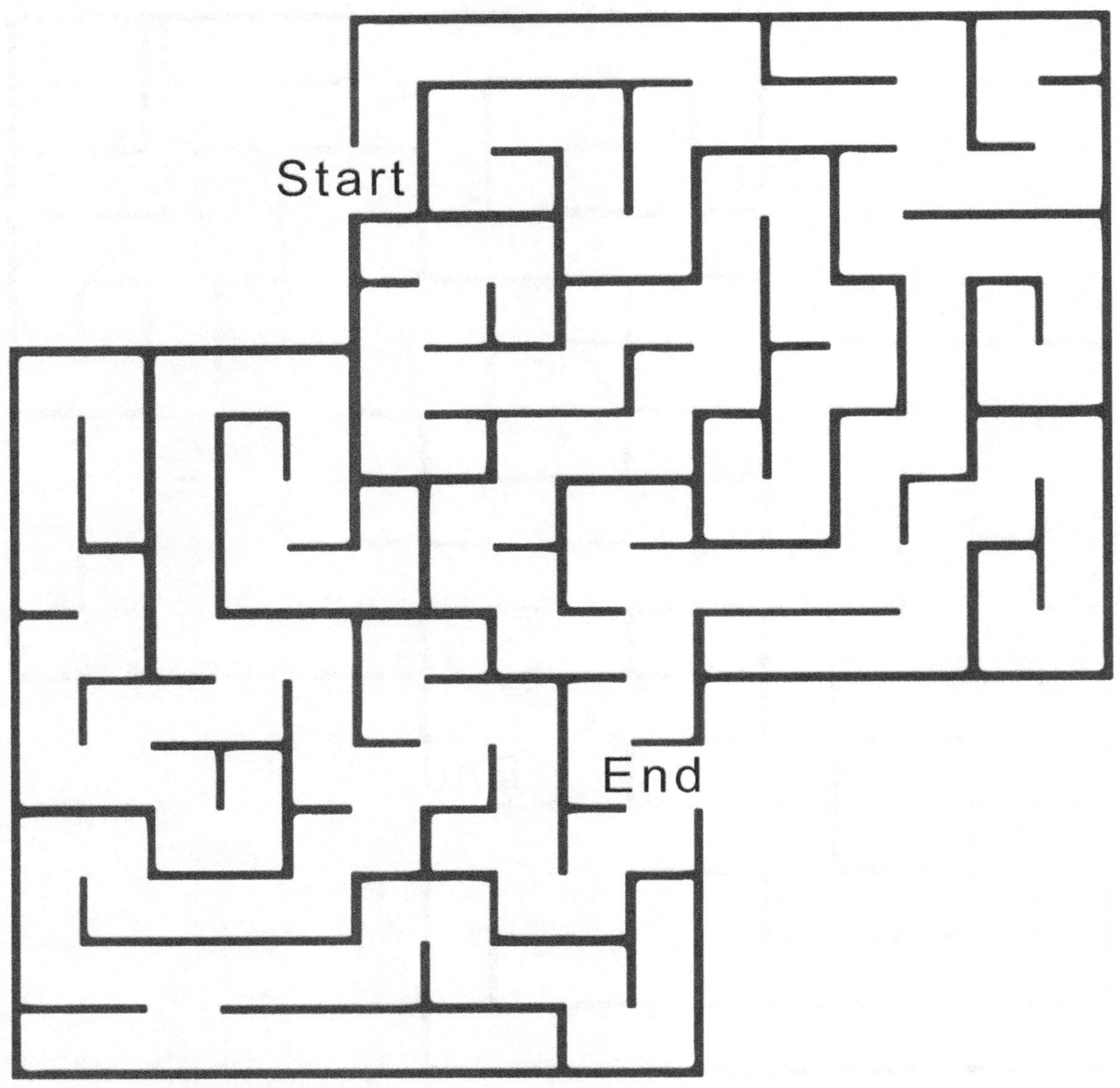

Start time: __________ End time: __________

Total time, maze 3: __________

Total time for 1st maze: __________

Total time for 2nd maze: __________

Total time for 3rd maze: __________

Congratulations! Did you experience progress in faster completion times? Circle your answer.

Yes No

If you circled "No" don't be discouraged. Remember to rest and give thanks to your mind and body for completing the challenges. Celebrate your tremendous effort. Remember, a seed doesn't turn into a tree overnight.

What is important is to believe in something so strongly that you're never discouraged.

—*Salma Hayek*

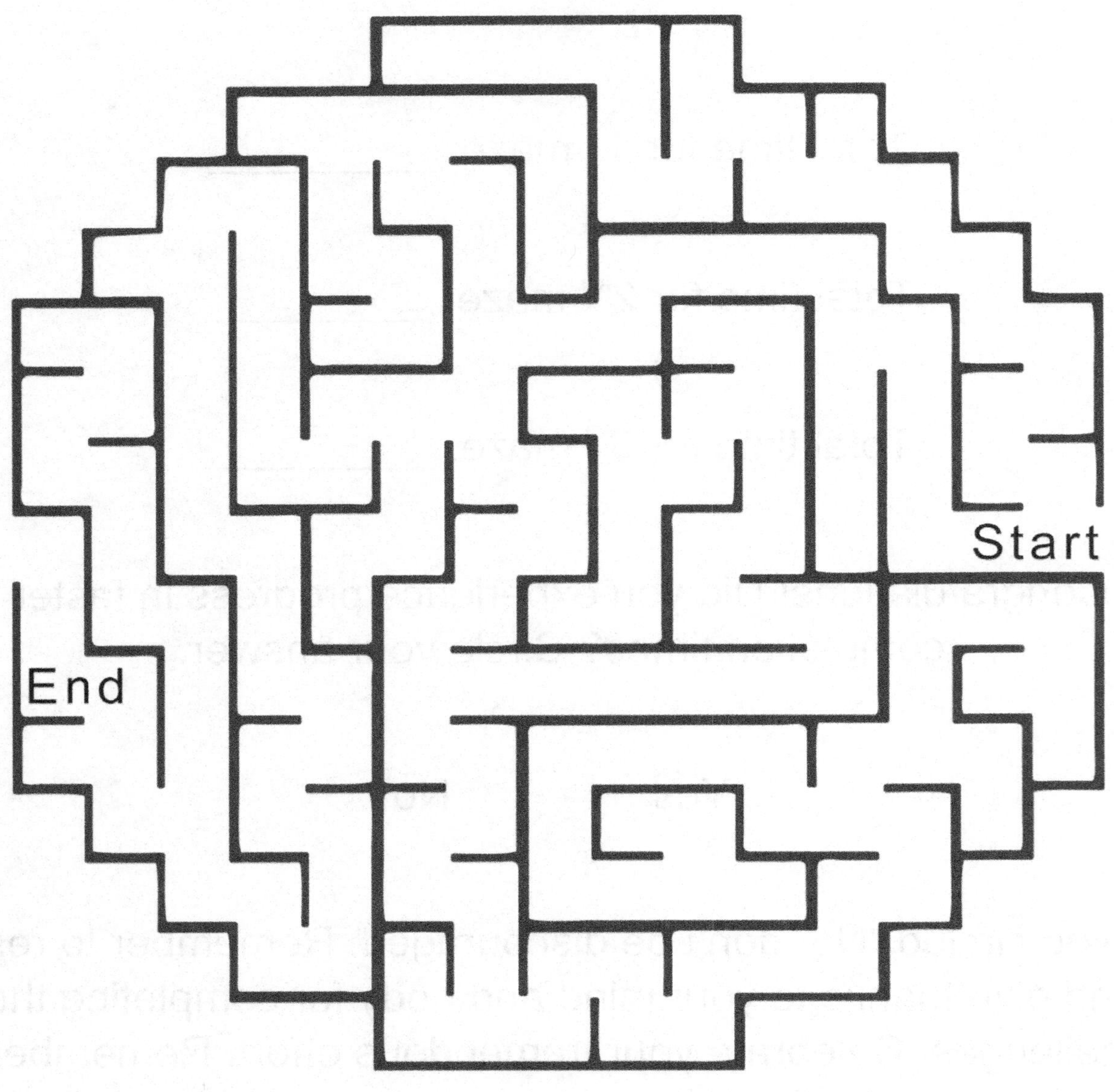

Start time: __________ End time: __________

Total time, maze 1: __________

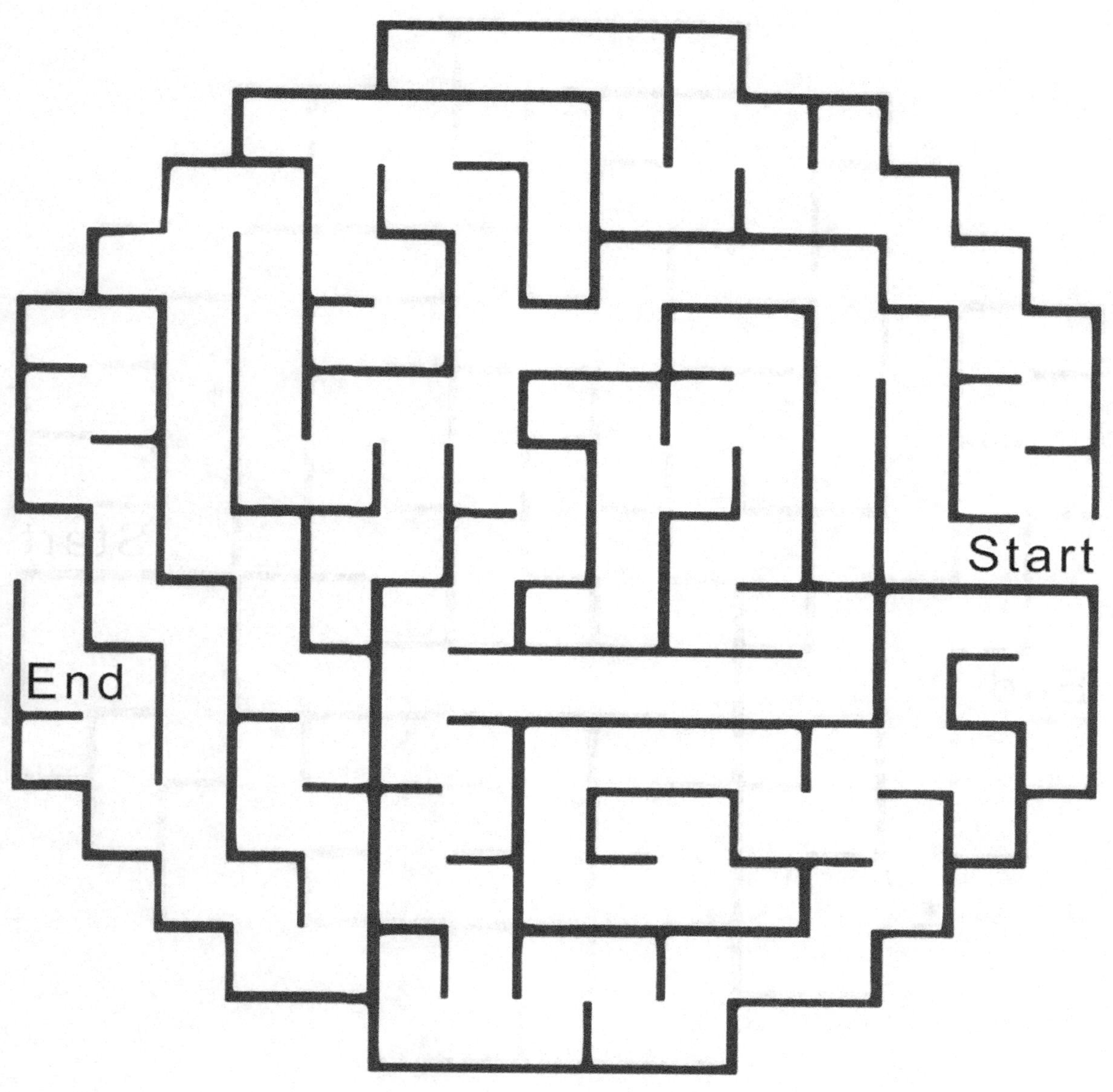

Start time: __________ End time: __________

Total time, maze 2: __________

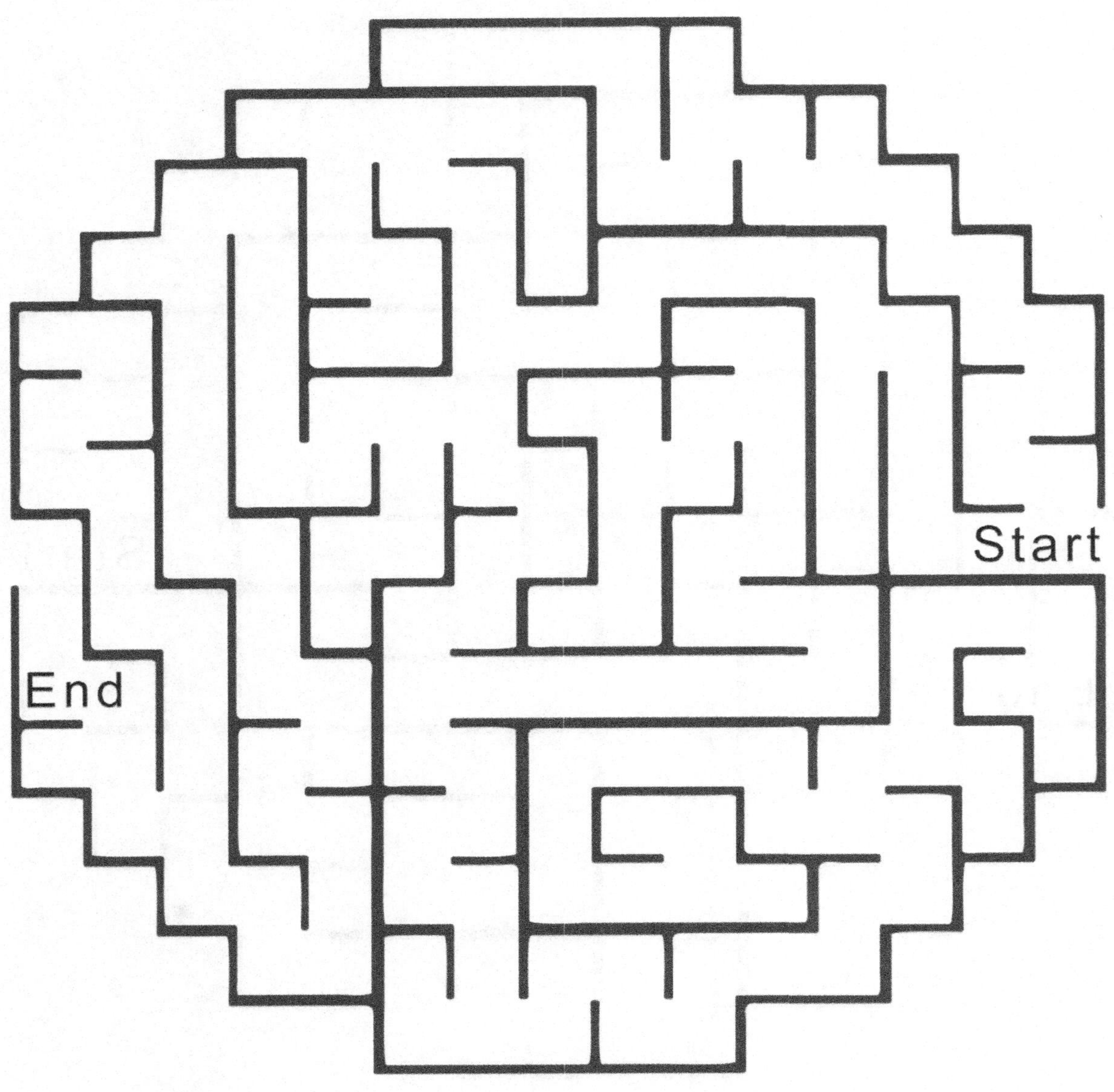

Start time: __________ End time: __________

Total time, maze 3: __________

Total time for 1st maze: __________

Total time for 2nd maze: __________

Total time for 3rd maze: __________

Congratulations! Did you experience progress in faster completion times? Circle your answer.

Yes No

If you circled "No" don't be discouraged. Remember to rest and give thanks to your mind and body for completing the challenges. Celebrate your tremendous effort. Remember, a seed doesn't turn into a tree overnight.

Stop beating yourself up. You are a work in progress - which means you get there a little at a time, not all at once.

—*Unknown*

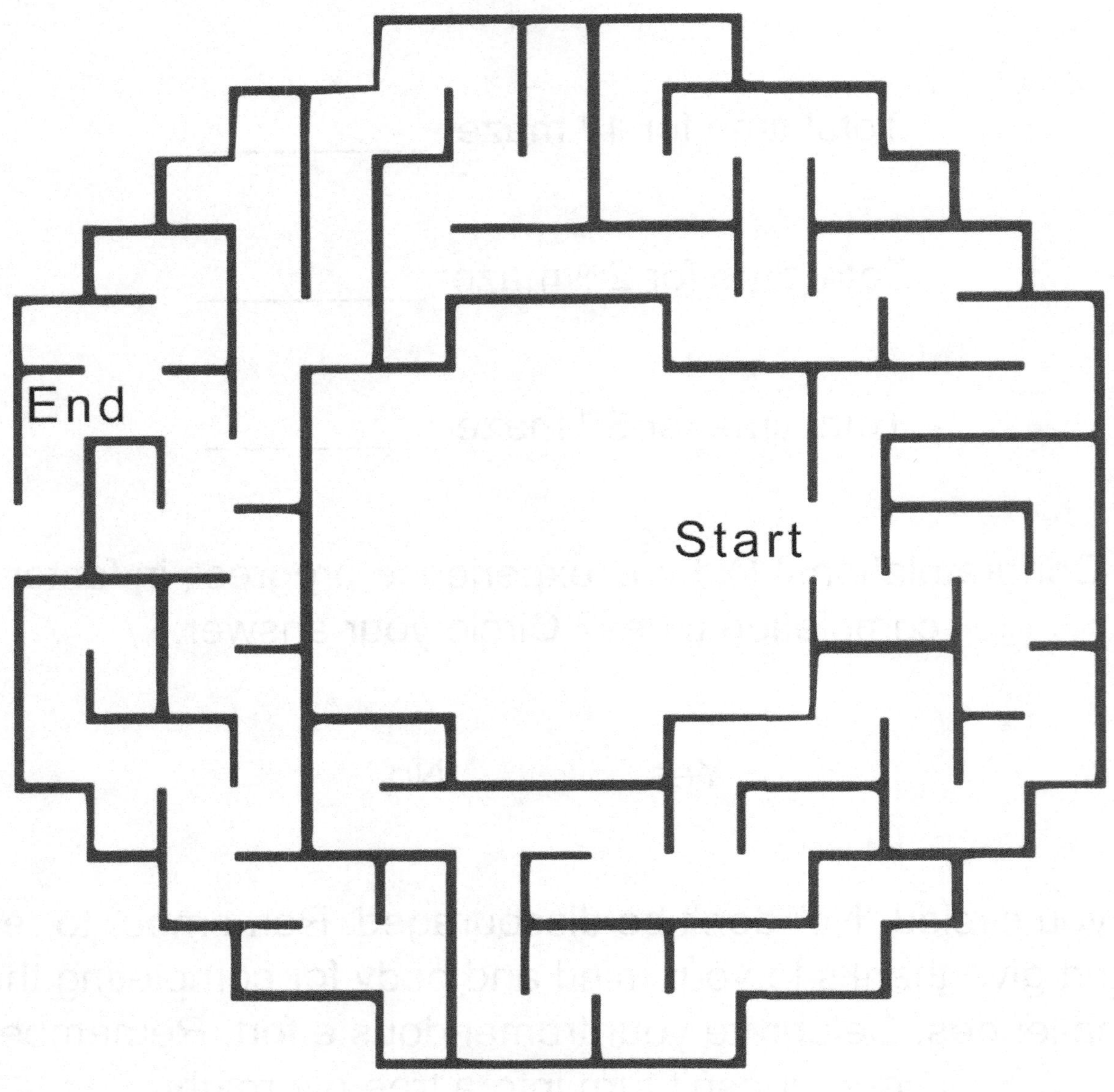

Start time: __________ End time: __________

Total time, maze 1: __________

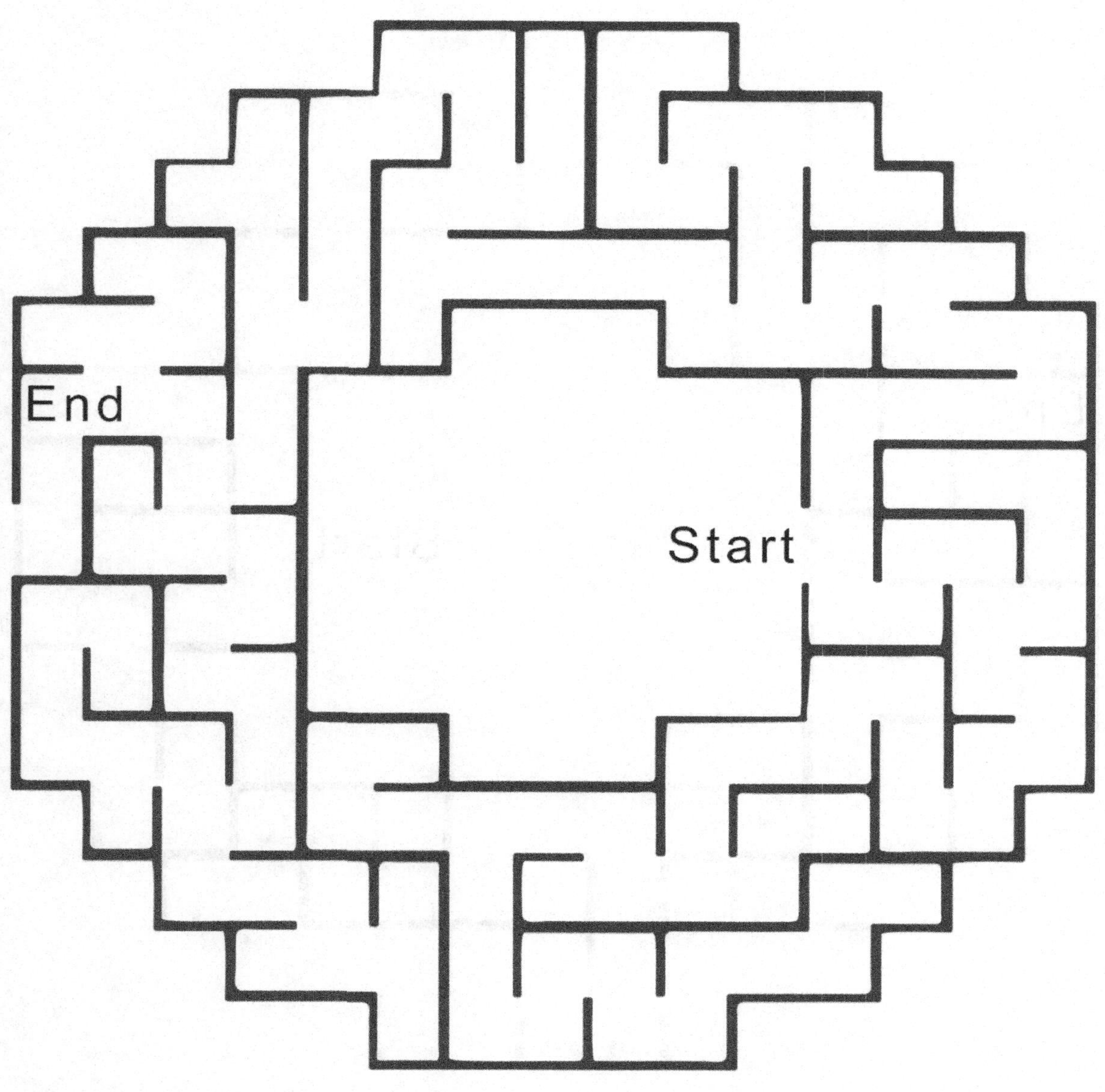

Start time: __________ End time: __________

Total time, maze 2: __________

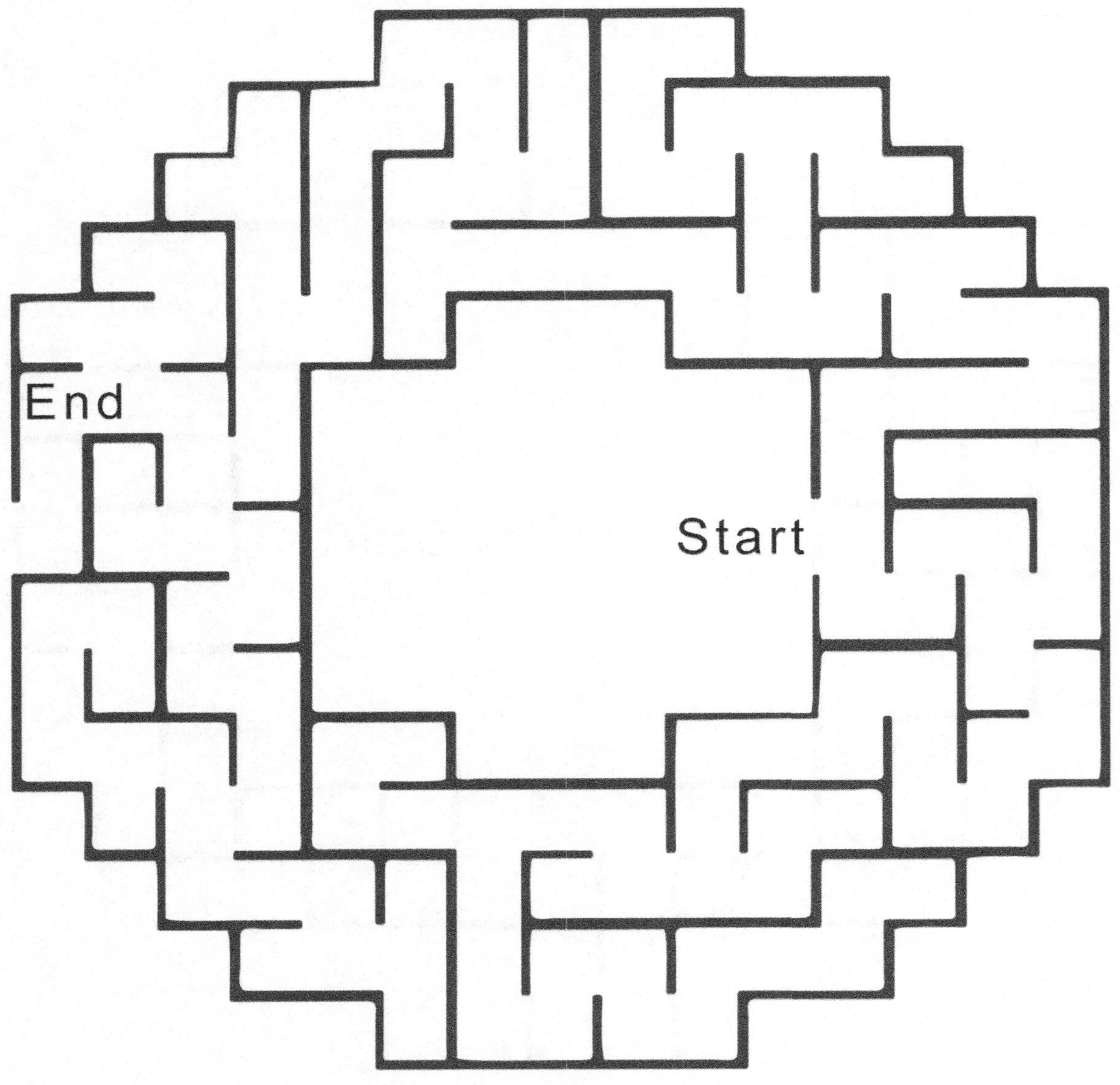

Start time: __________ End time: __________

Total time, maze 3: __________

Total time for 1st maze: __________

Total time for 2nd maze: __________

Total time for 3rd maze: __________

Congratulations! Did you experience progress in faster completion times? Circle your answer.

Yes No

If you circled "No" don't be discouraged. Remember to rest and give thanks to your mind and body for completing the challenges. Celebrate your tremendous effort. Remember, a seed doesn't turn into a tree overnight.

Yesterday I was clever so I wanted to change the world. Today I am wise, so I am changing myself.

—*Rumi*

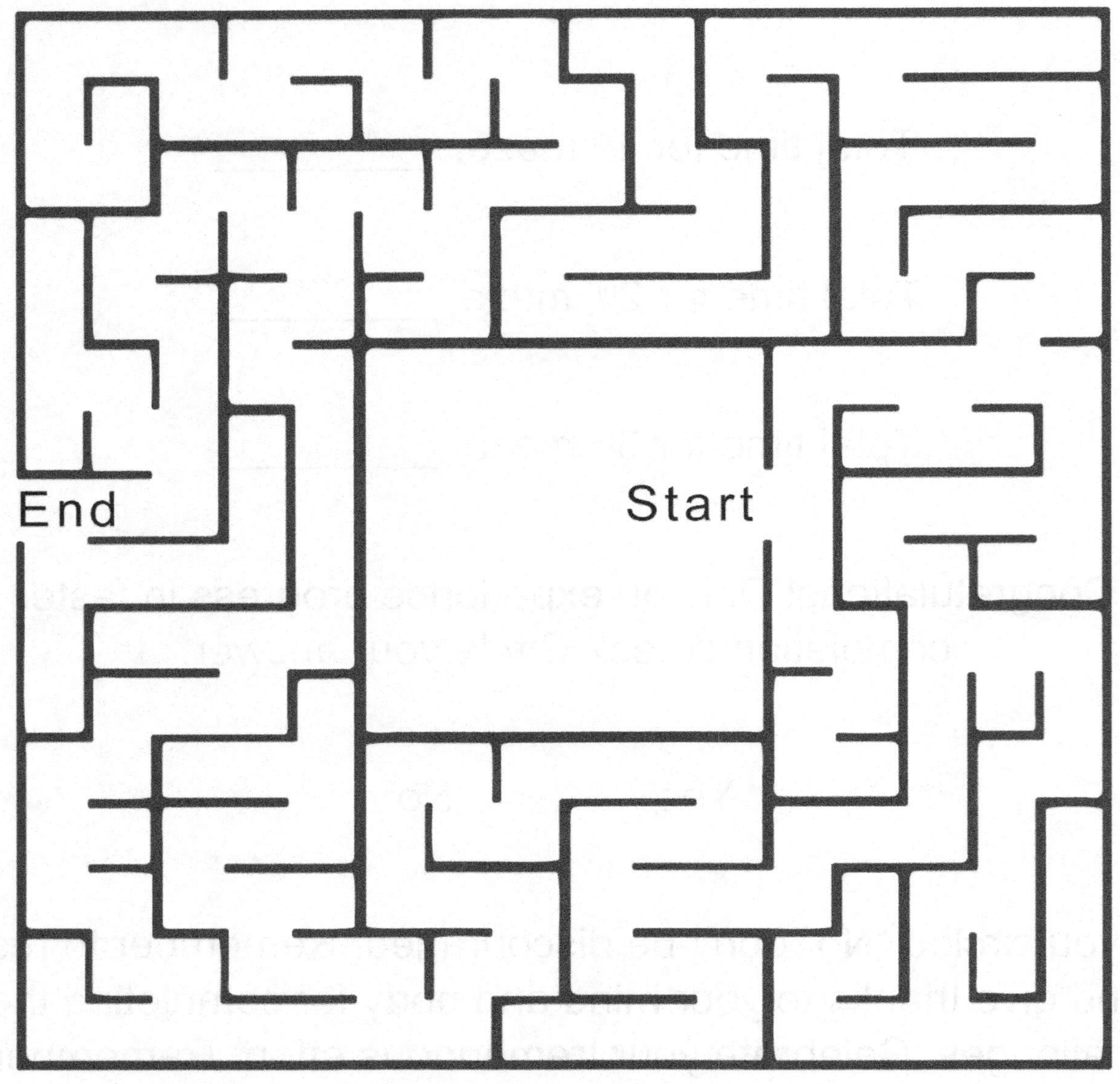

Start time: __________ End time: __________

Total time, maze 1: __________

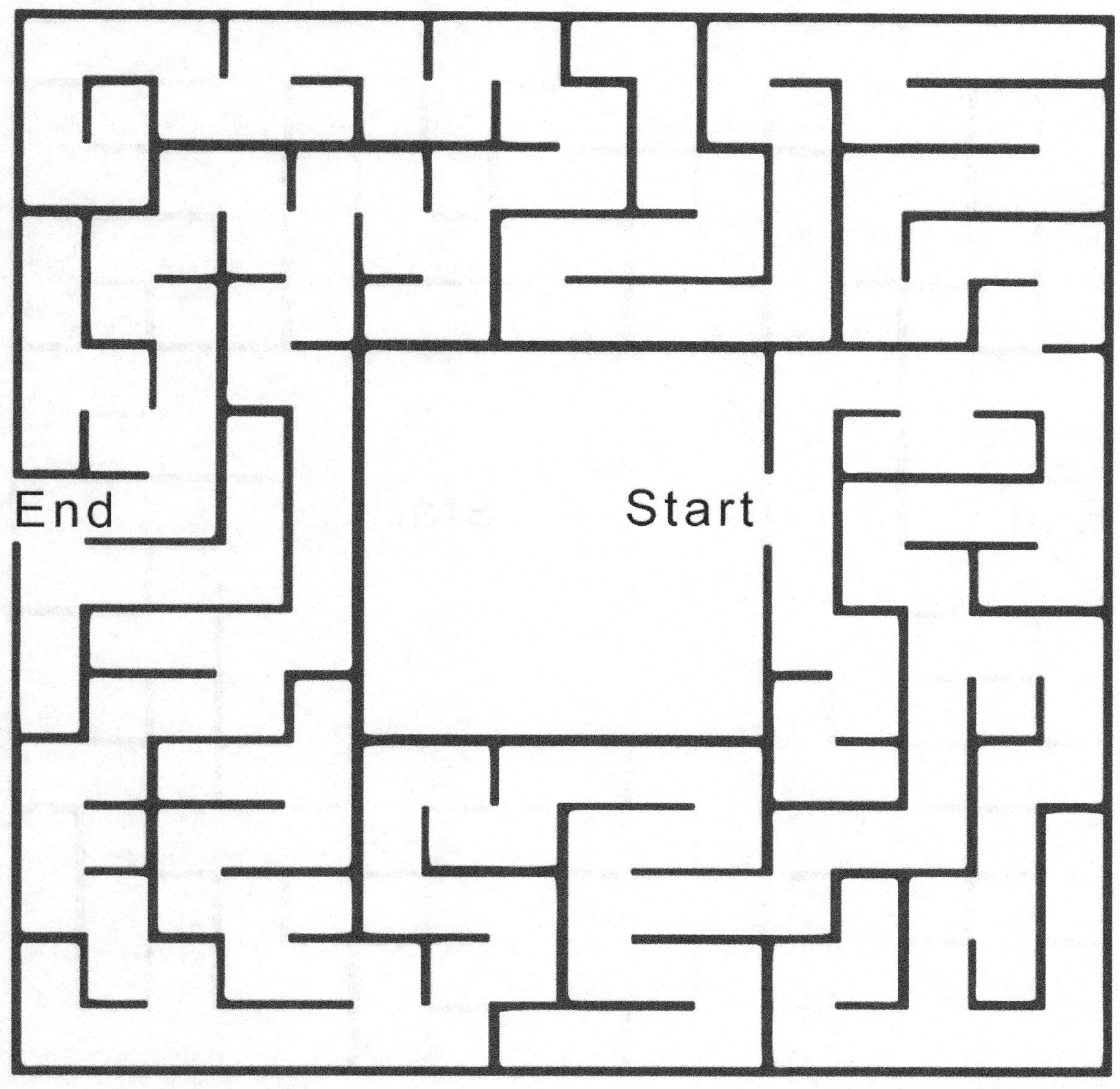

Start time: __________ End time: __________

Total time, maze 2: __________

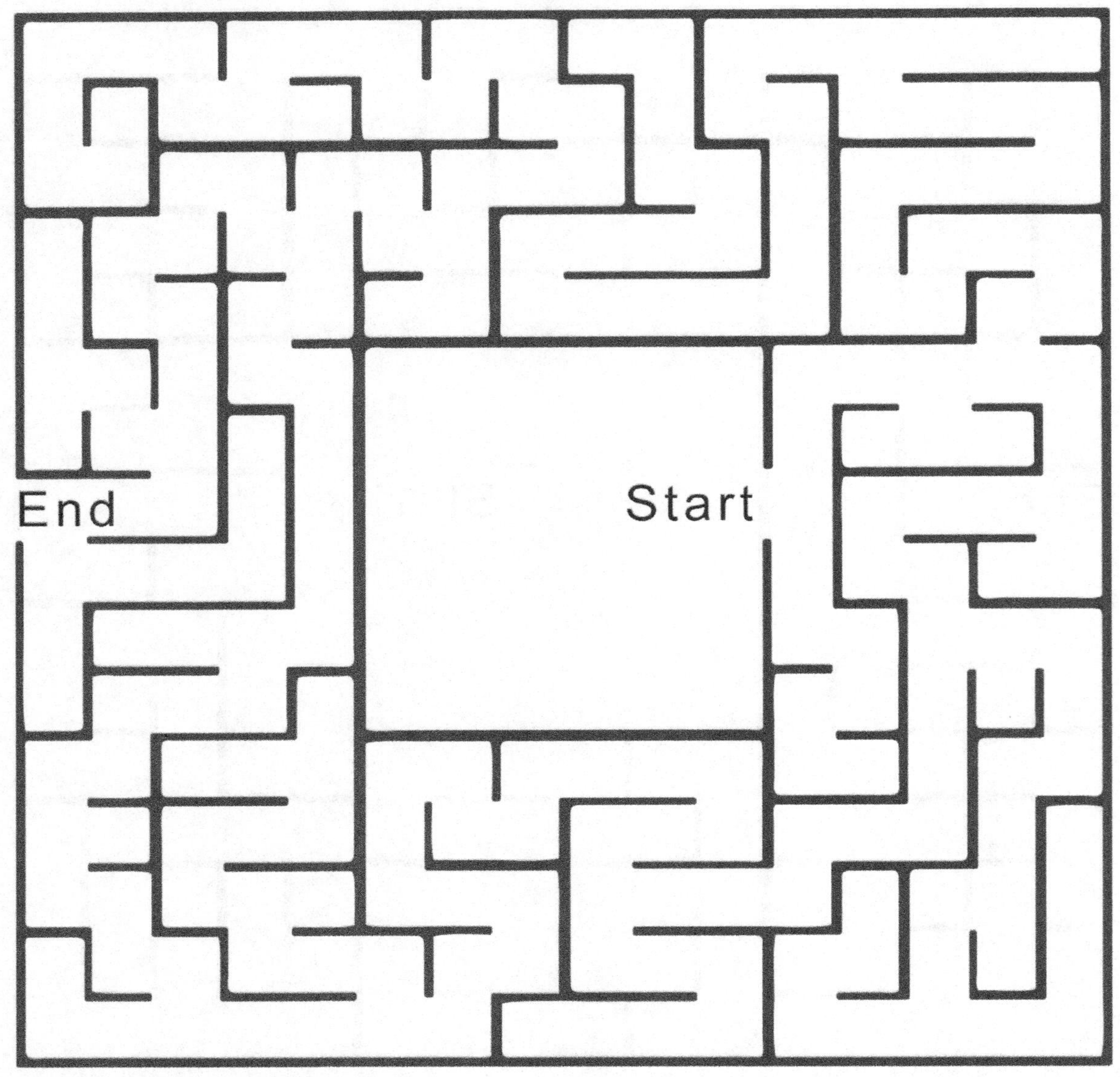

Start time: __________ End time: __________

Total time, maze 3: __________

Total time for 1st maze: __________

Total time for 2nd maze: __________

Total time for 3rd maze: __________

Congratulations! Did you experience progress in faster completion times? Circle your answer.

Yes No

If you circled "No" don't be discouraged. Remember to rest and give thanks to your mind and body for completing the challenges. Celebrate your tremendous effort. Remember, a seed doesn't turn into a tree overnight.

If you really want to do something, you'll find a way. If you don't, you'll find an excuse.

—Jim Rohn

She stood in the storm, and when the wind did not blow her away, she adjusted her sails.

—Elizabeth Edwards

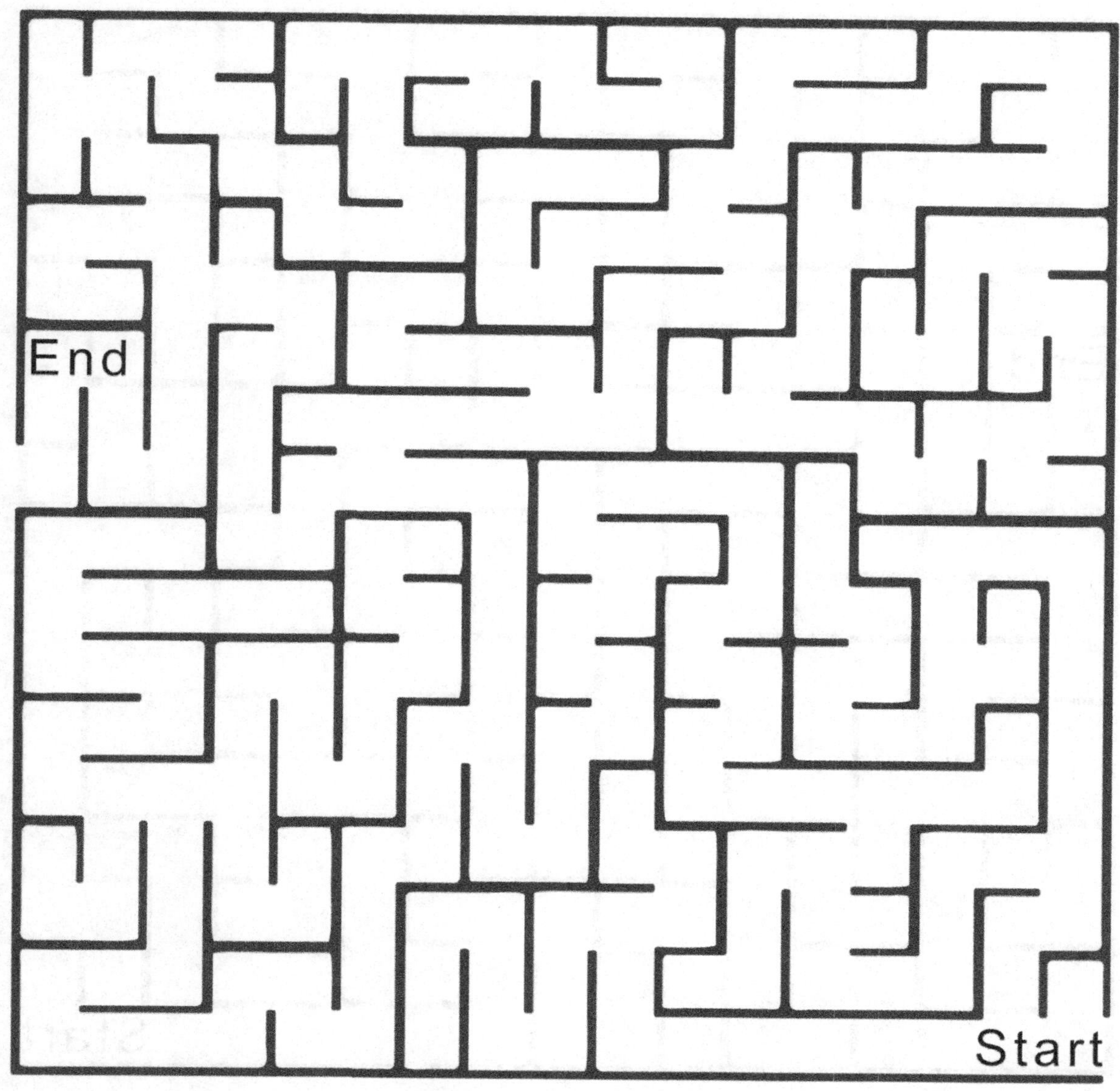

Start time: __________ End time: __________

Total time, maze 1: __________

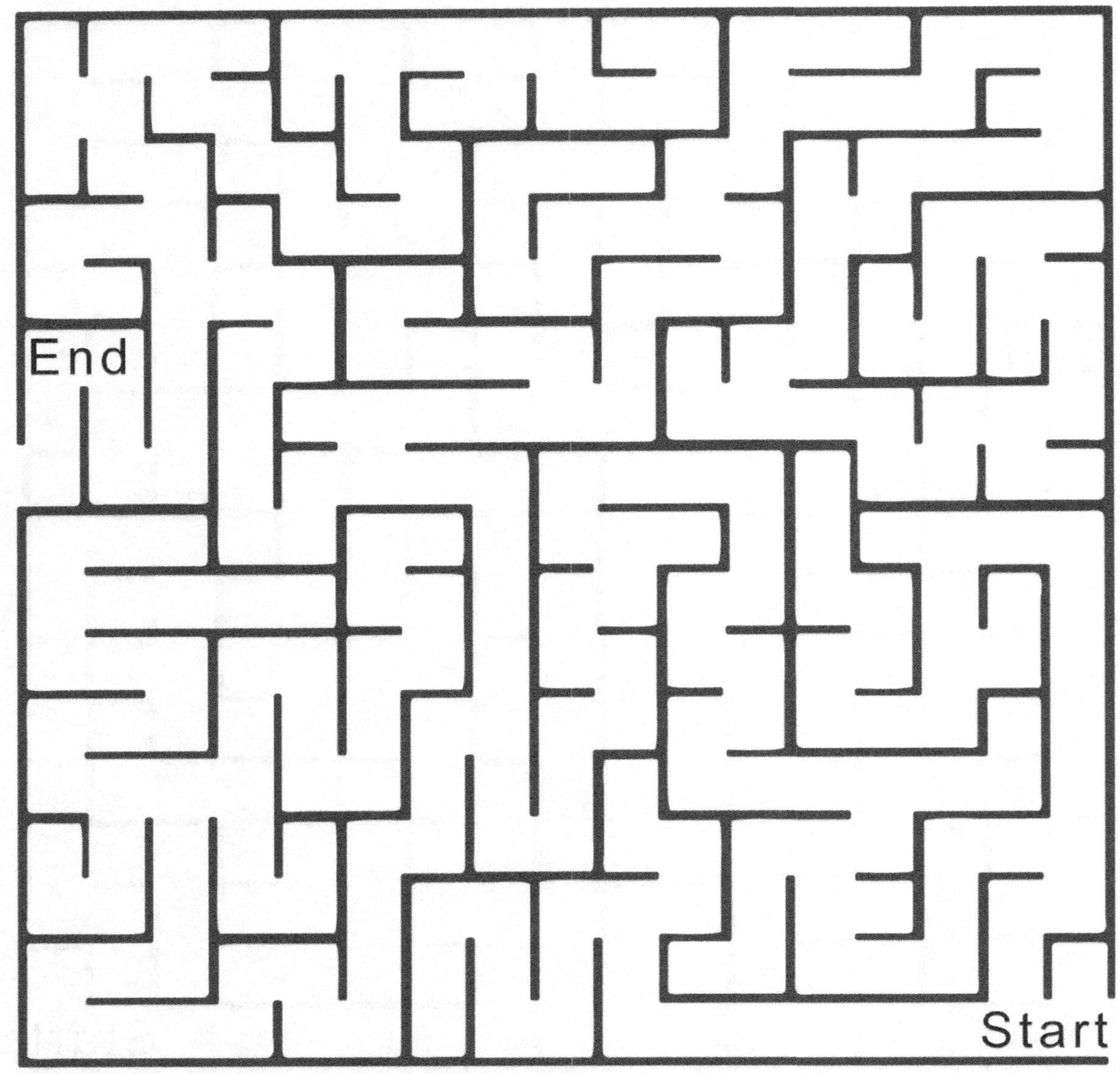

Start time: ___________ End time: ___________

Total time, maze 2: ___________

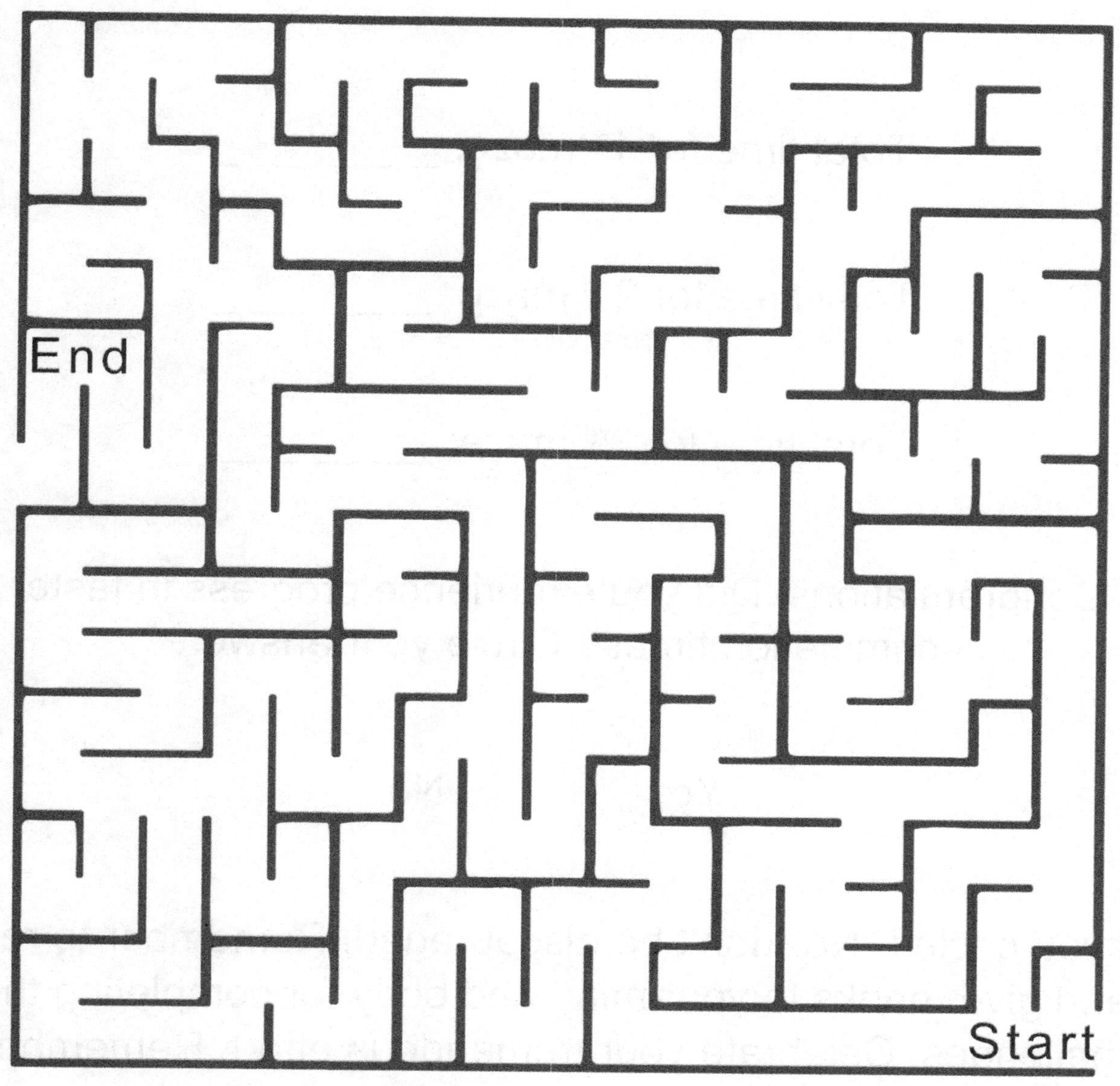

Start time: __________ End time: __________

Total time, maze 3: __________

Total time for 1st maze: __________

Total time for 2nd maze: __________

Total time for 3rd maze: __________

Congratulations! Did you experience progress in faster completion times? Circle your answer.

Yes No

If you circled "No" don't be discouraged. Remember to rest and give thanks to your mind and body for completing the challenges. Celebrate your tremendous effort. Remember, a seed doesn't turn into a tree overnight.

F.E.A.R: has two meanings: 1). Forget Everything And Run or 2). Face Everything And Rise; the choice is yours!

—Zig Ziglar

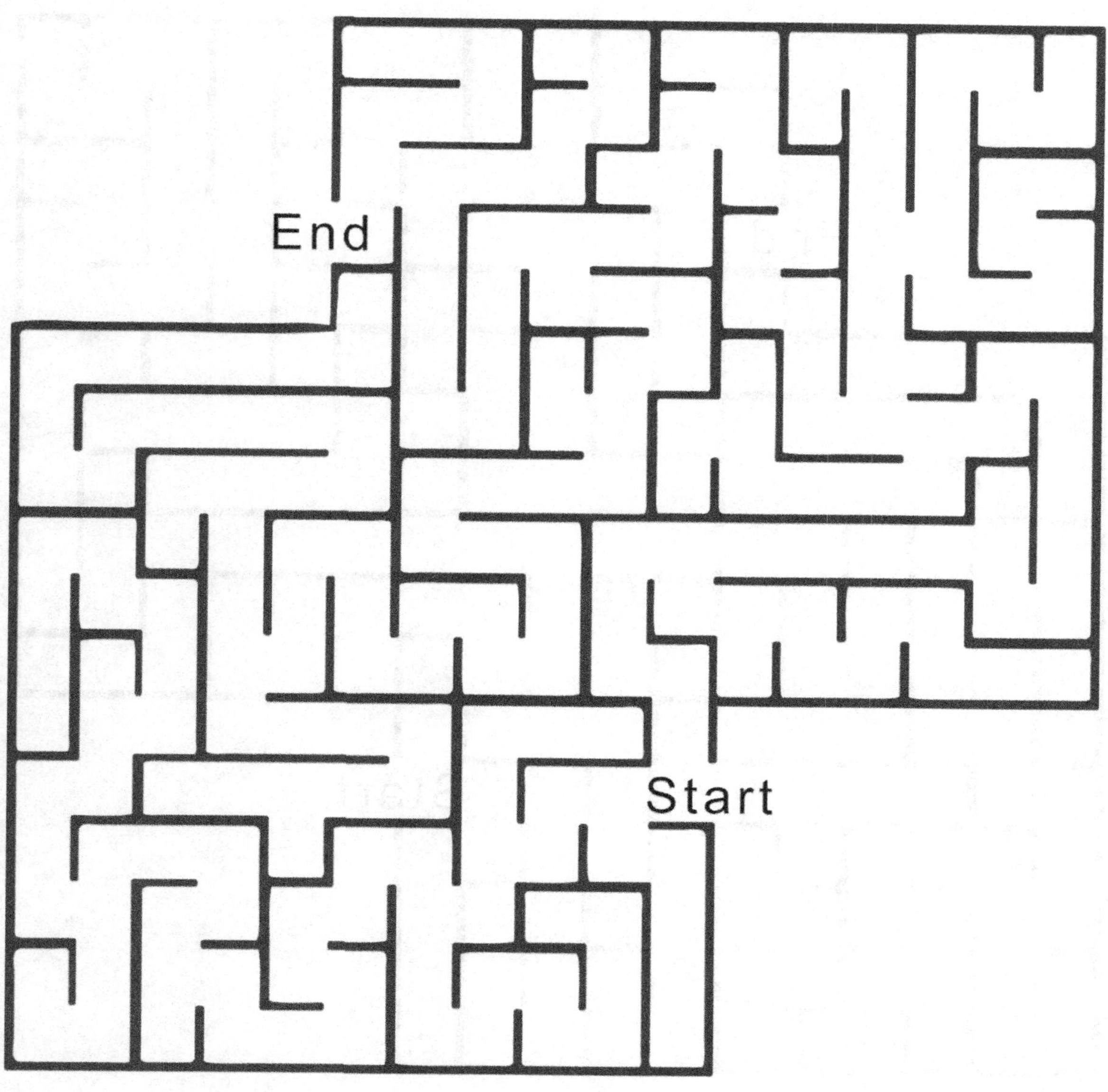

Start time: __________ End time: __________

Total time, maze 1: __________

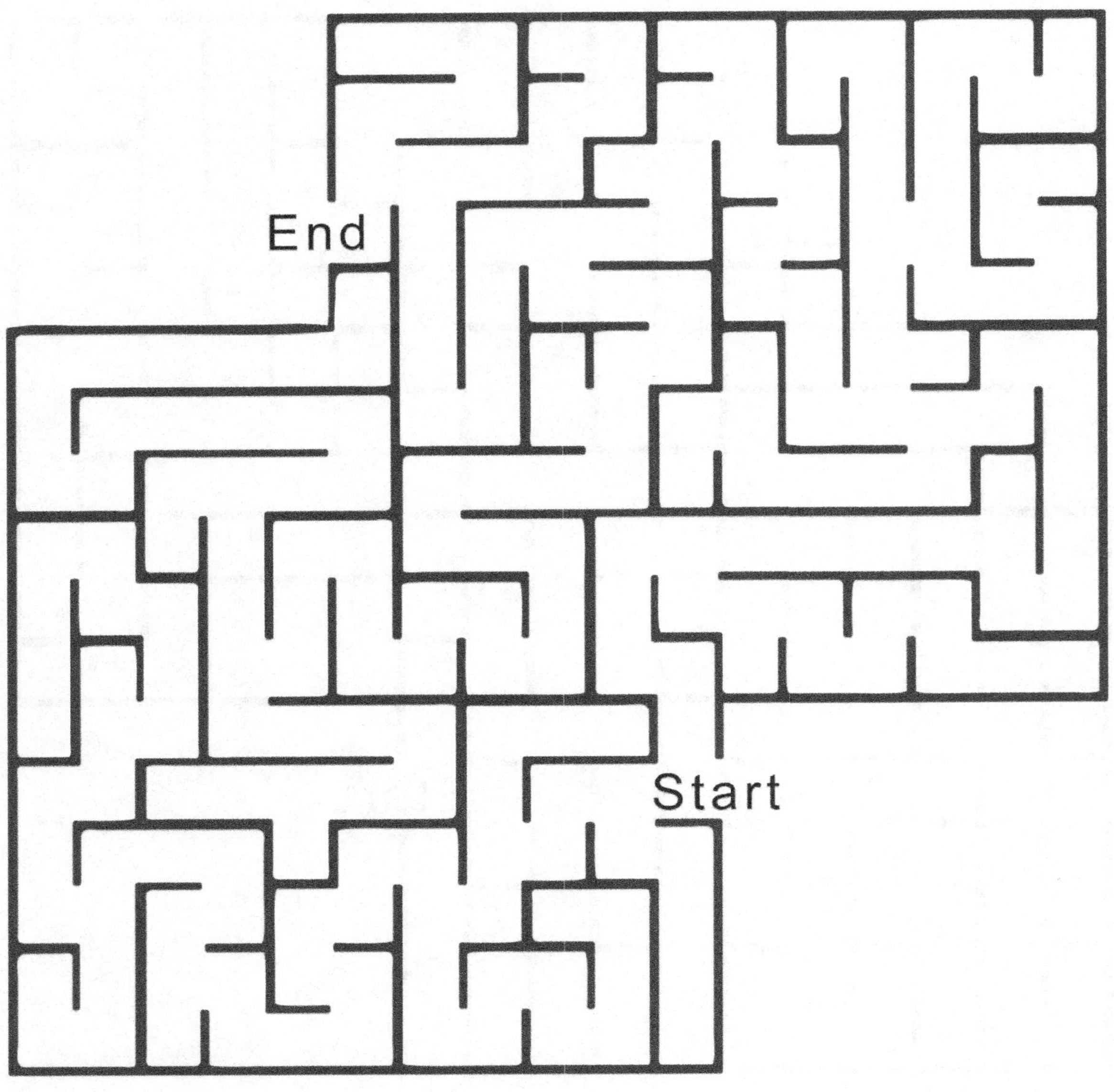

Start time: __________ End time: __________

Total time, maze 2: __________

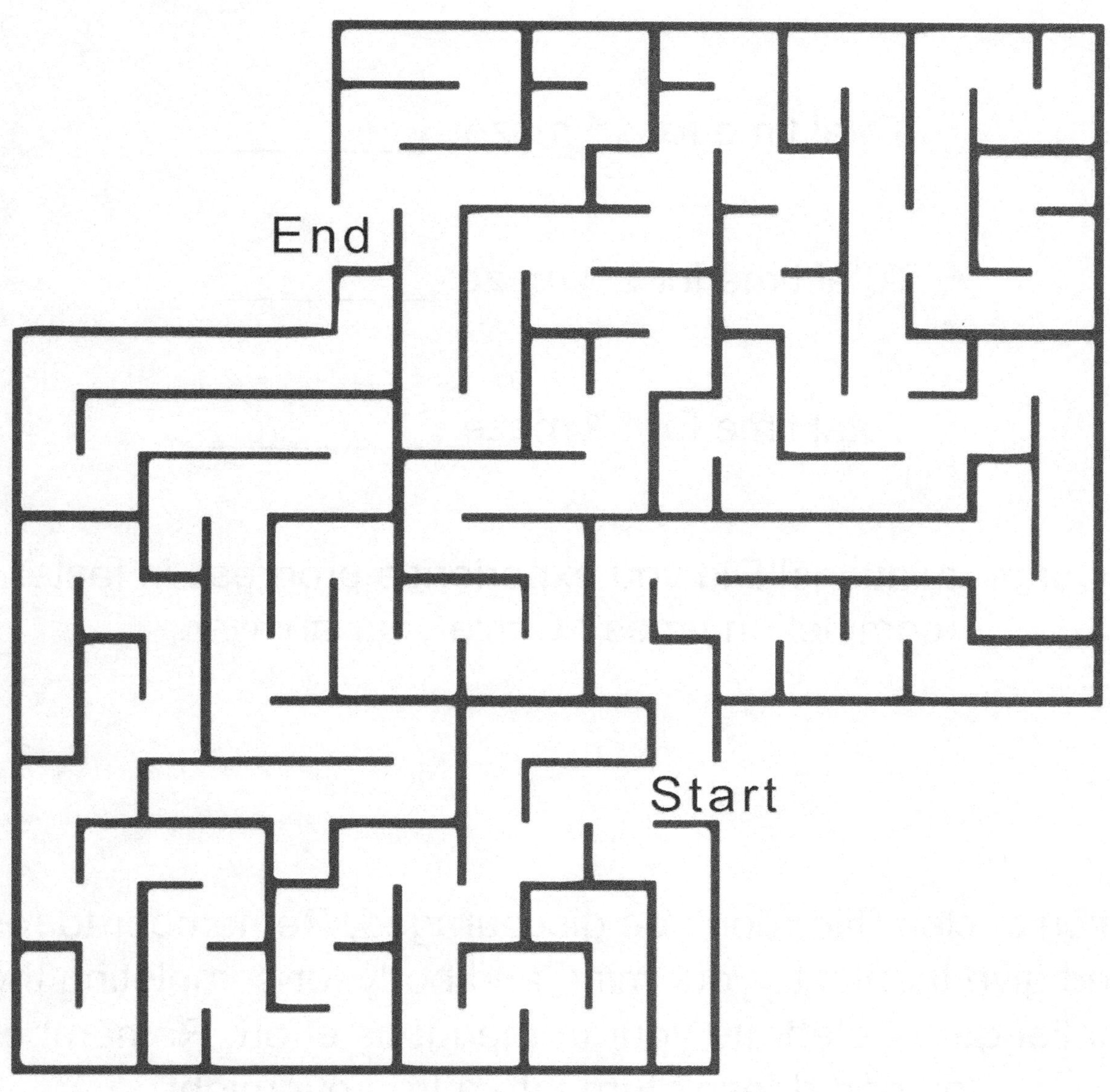

Start time: __________ End time: __________

Total time, maze 3: __________

Total time for 1st maze: __________

Total time for 2nd maze: __________

Total time for 3rd maze: __________

Congratulations! Did you experience progress in faster completion times? Circle your answer.

Yes No

If you circled “No” don’t be discouraged. Remember to rest and give thanks to your mind and body for completing the challenges. Celebrate your tremendous effort. Remember, a seed doesn’t turn into a tree overnight.

Life is like a camera… focus on what’s important, capture the good times, develop from the negatives, and if things don’t work out, take another shot.

—*Unknown*

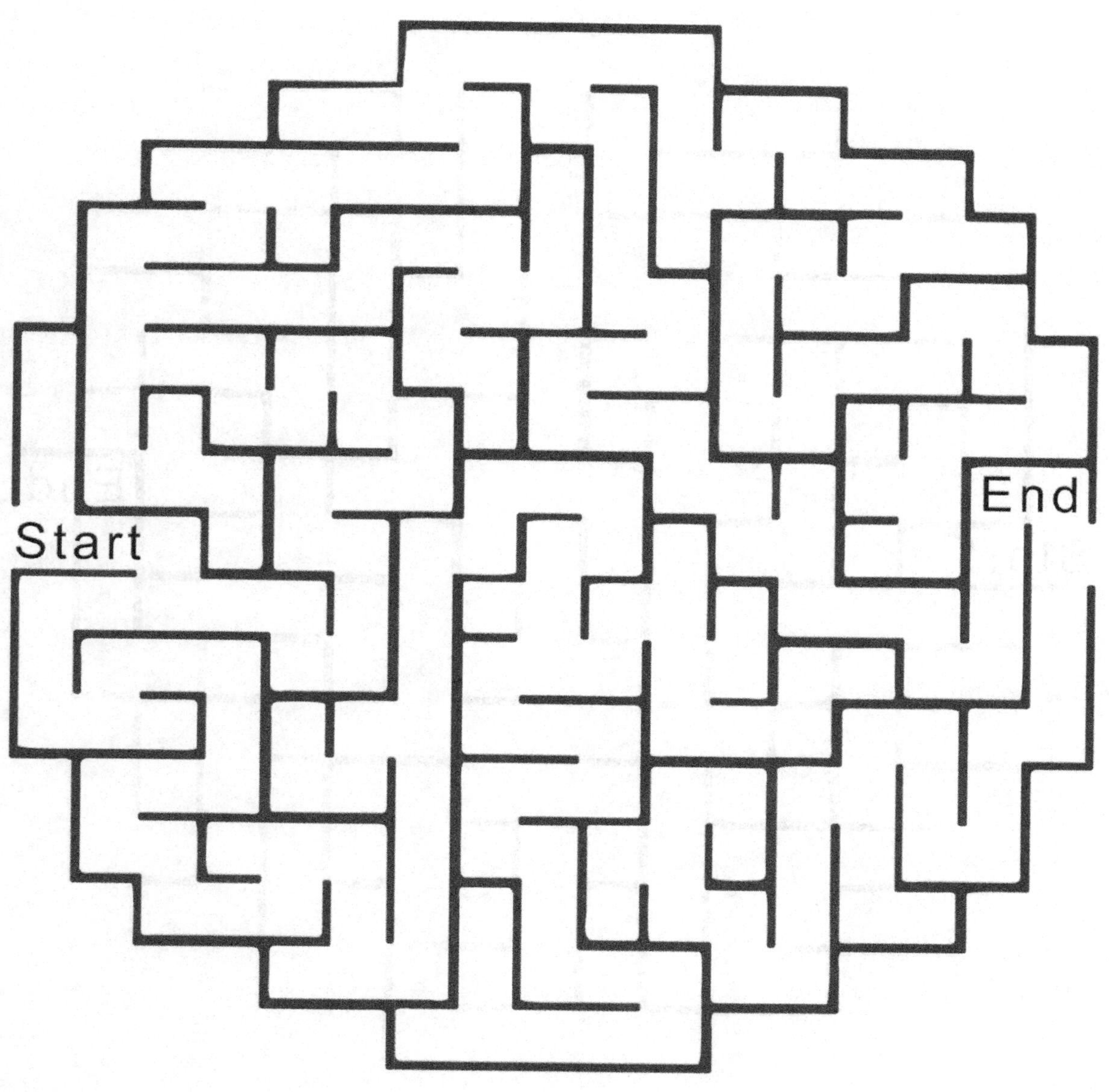

Start time: __________ End time: __________

Total time, maze 1: __________

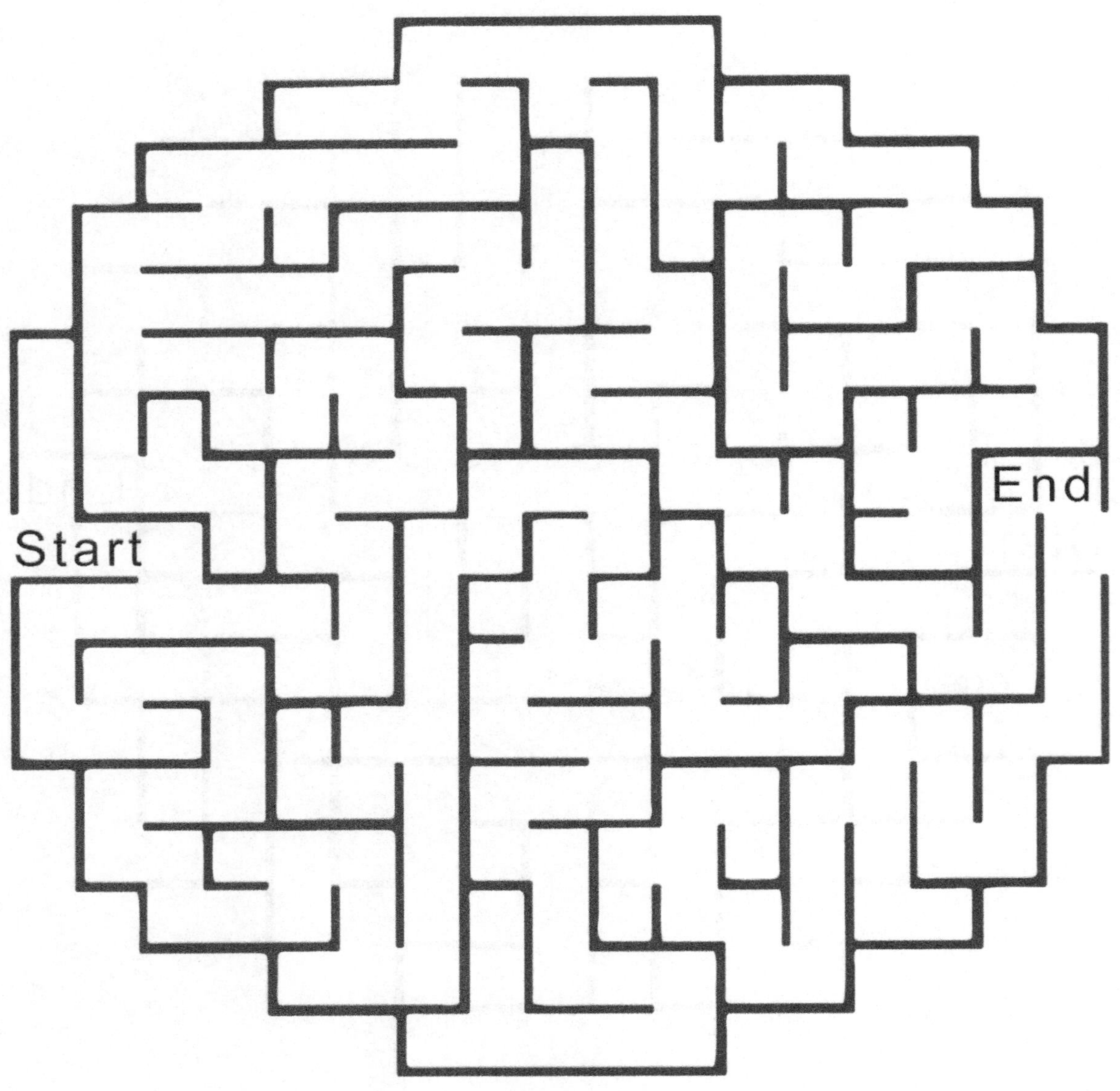

Start time: __________ End time: __________

Total time, maze 2: __________

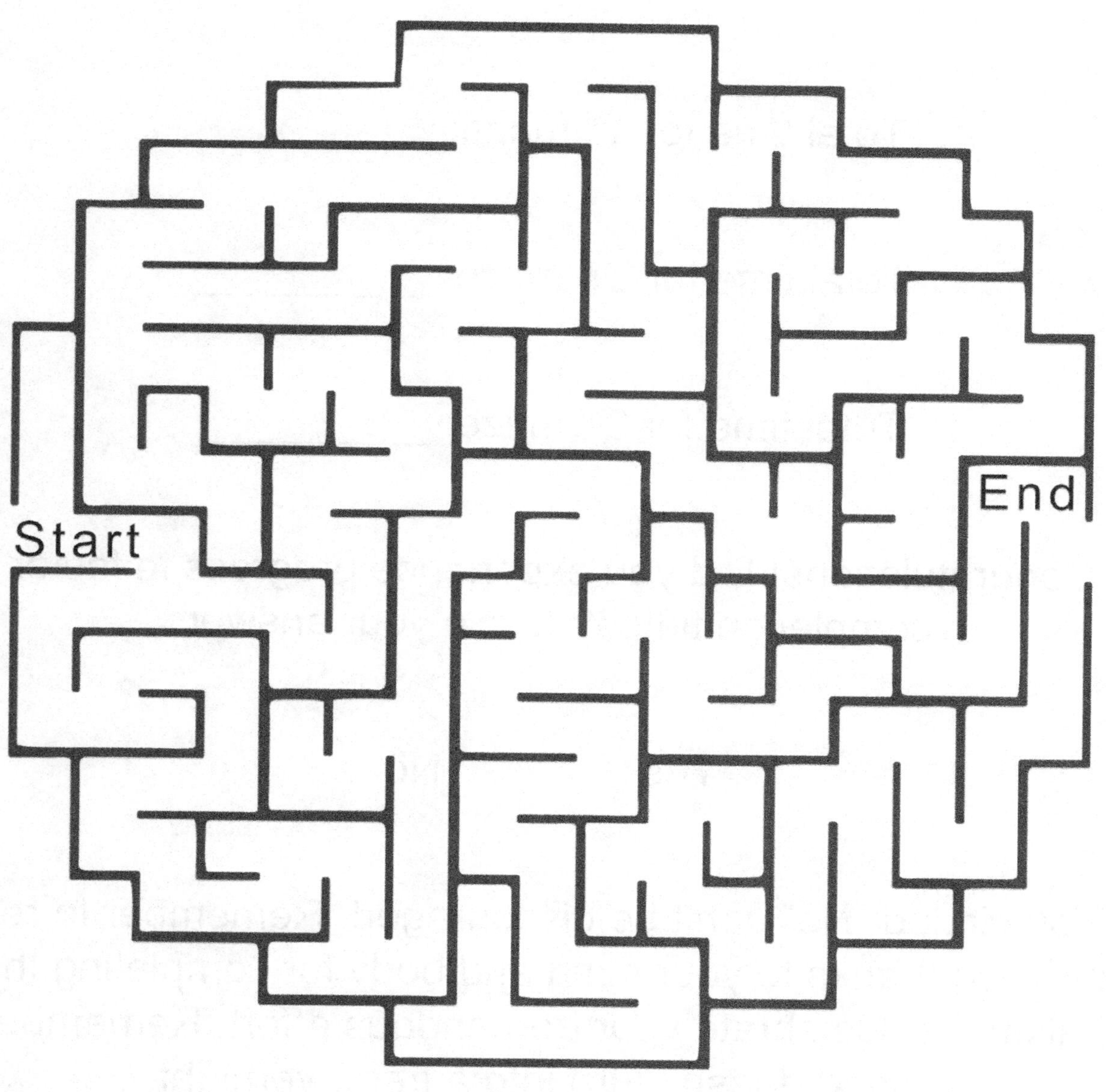

Start time: ___________ End time: ___________

Total time, maze 3: ___________

Total time for 1st maze: __________

Total time for 2nd maze: __________

Total time for 3rd maze: __________

Congratulations! Did you experience progress in faster completion times? Circle your answer.

Yes No

If you circled "No" don't be discouraged. Remember to rest and give thanks to your mind and body for completing the challenges. Celebrate your tremendous effort. Remember, a seed doesn't turn into a tree overnight.

Keep watering, keep planting, keep cultivating, and one day your garden will bloom.

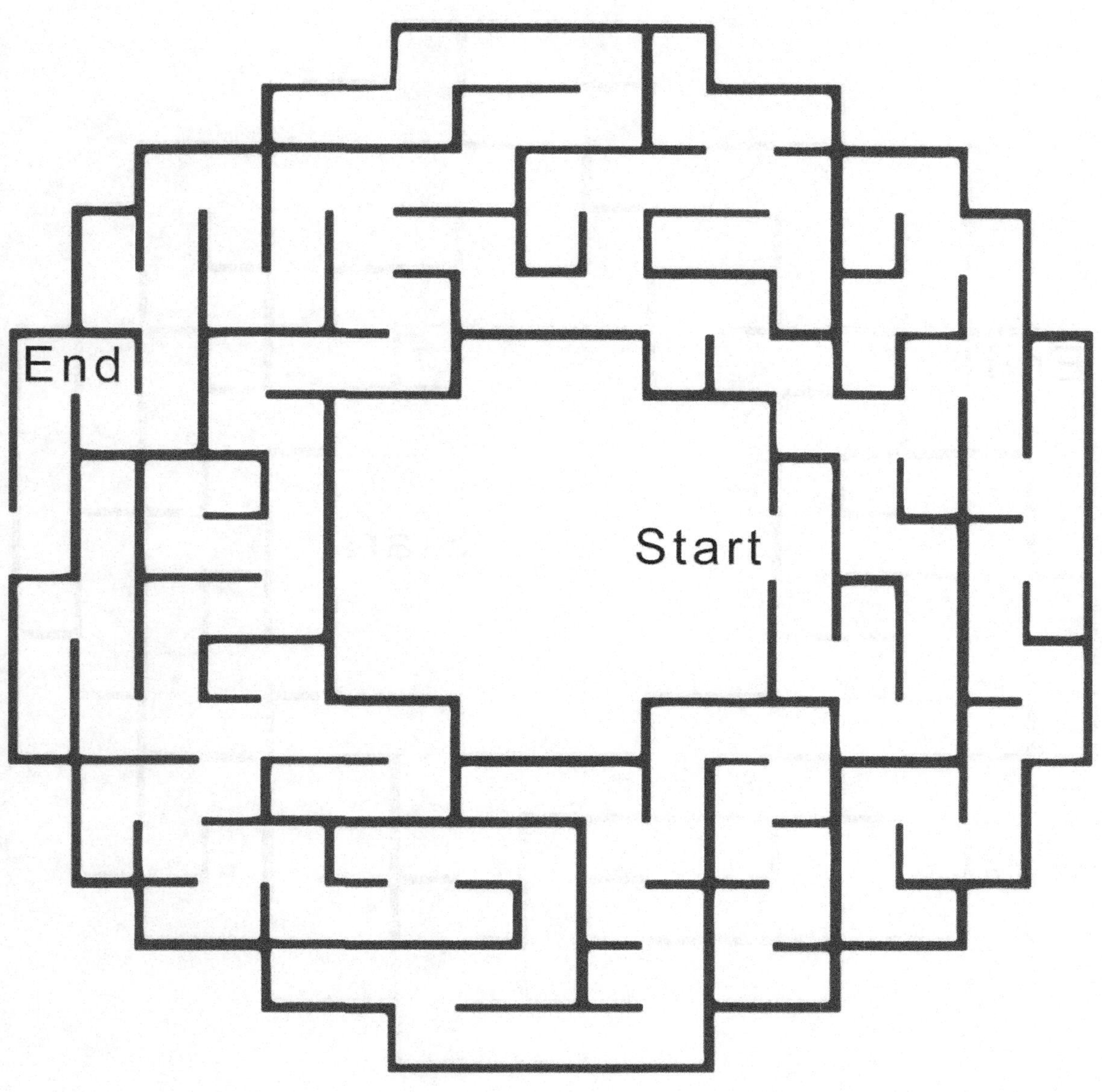

Start time: __________ End time: __________

Total time, maze 1: __________

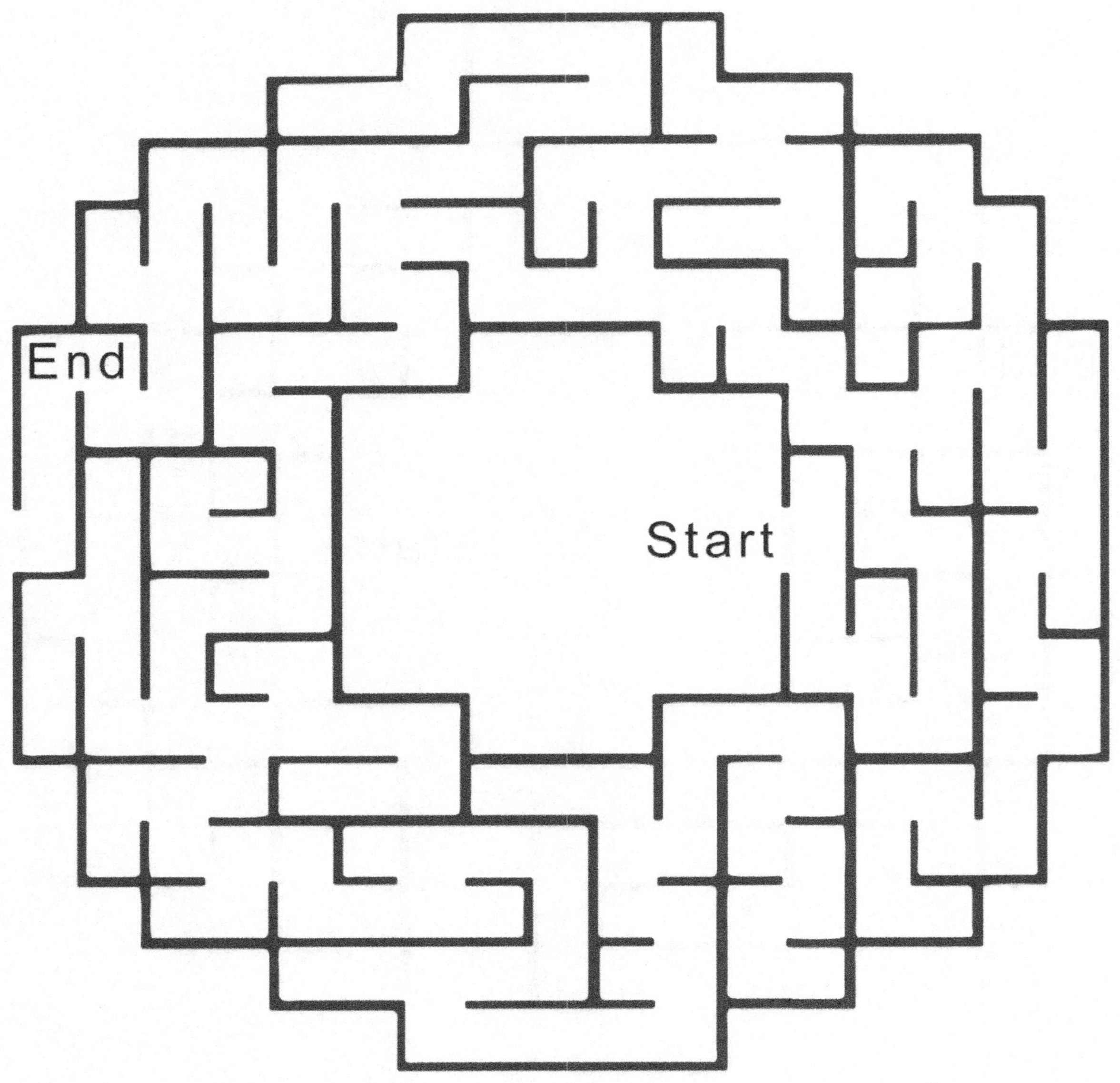

Start time: __________ End time: __________

Total time, maze 2: __________

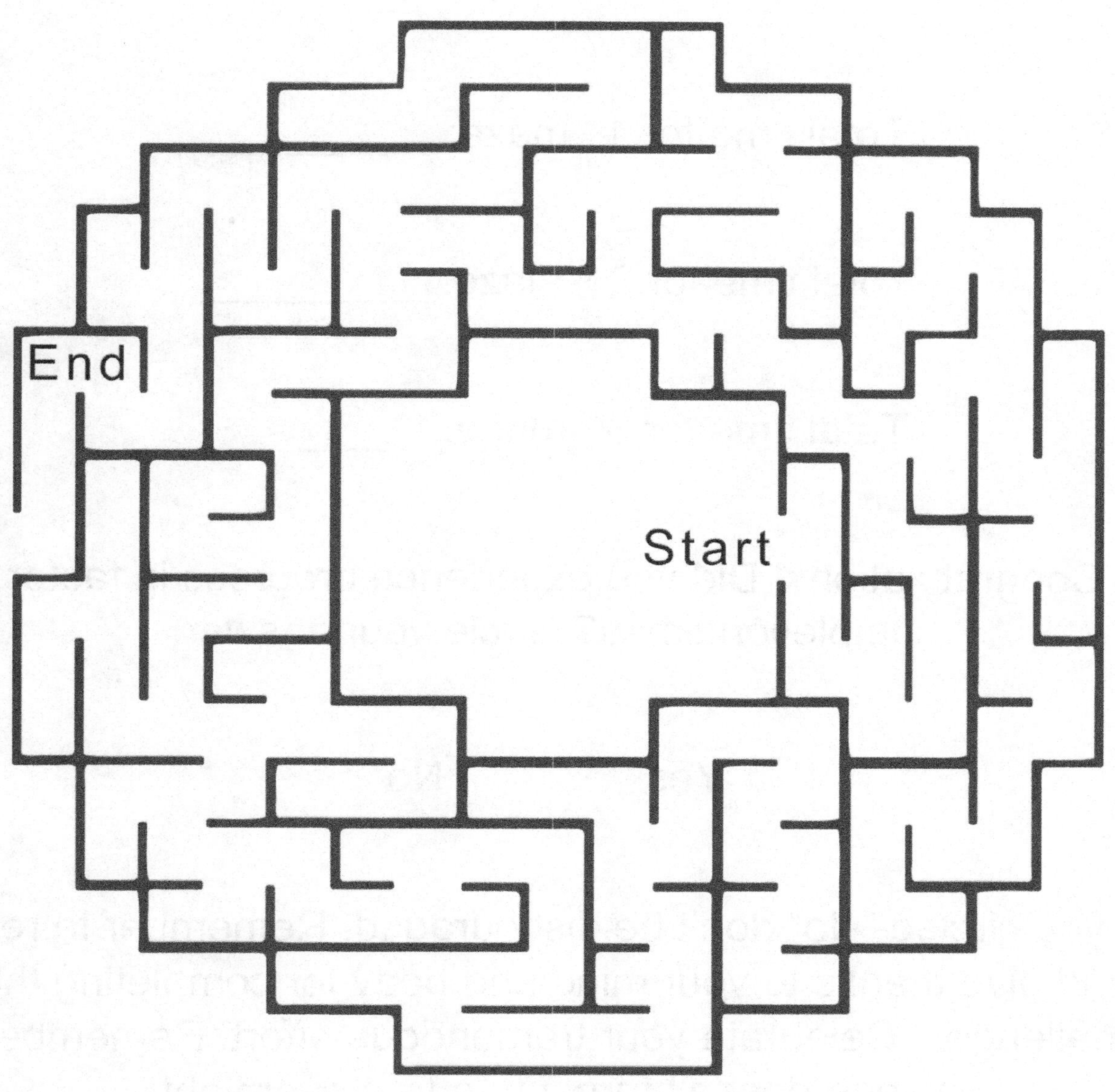

Start time: __________ End time: __________

Total time, maze 3: __________

Total time for 1st maze: __________

Total time for 2nd maze: __________

Total time for 3rd maze: __________

Congratulations! Did you experience progress in faster completion times? Circle your answer.

Yes No

If you circled "No" don't be discouraged. Remember to rest and give thanks to your mind and body for completing the challenges. Celebrate your tremendous effort. Remember, a seed doesn't turn into a tree overnight.

One of the things I learned the hard way was that it doesn't pay to get discouraged. Keeping busy and making optimism a way of life can restore your faith in yourself.

—Lucille Ball

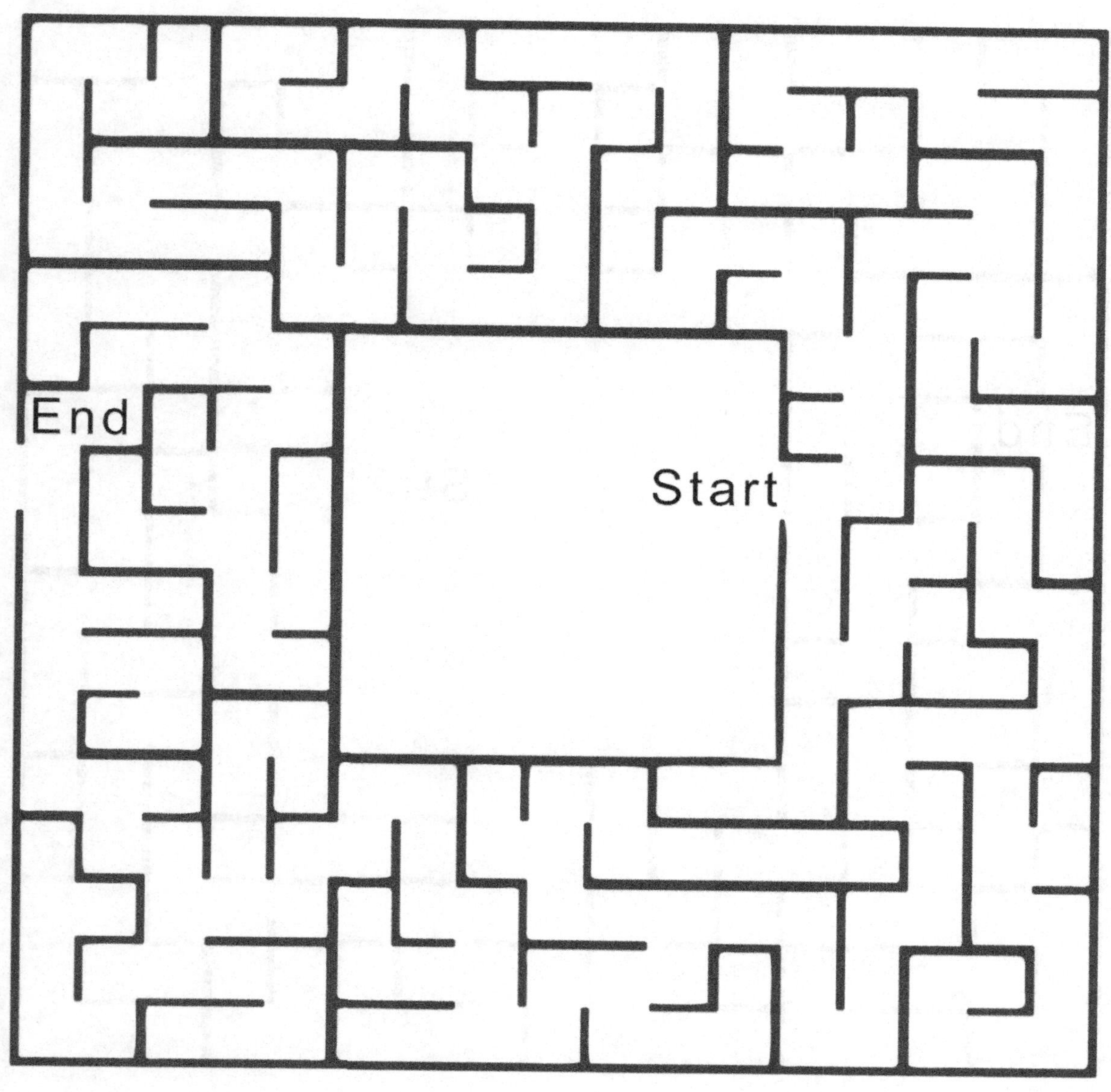

Start time: ____________ End time: ____________

Total time, maze 1: ____________

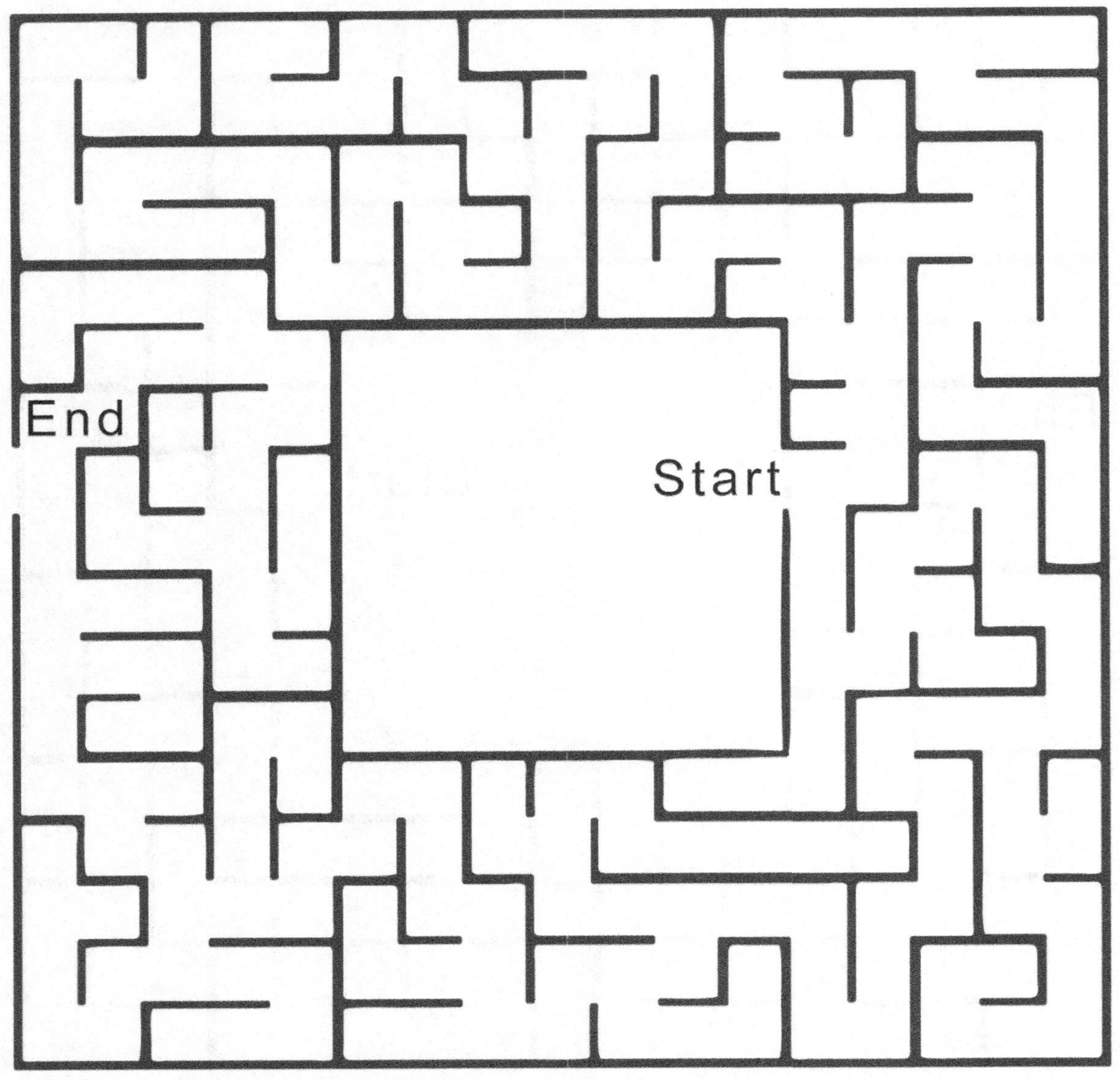

Start time: __________ End time: __________

Total time, maze 2: __________

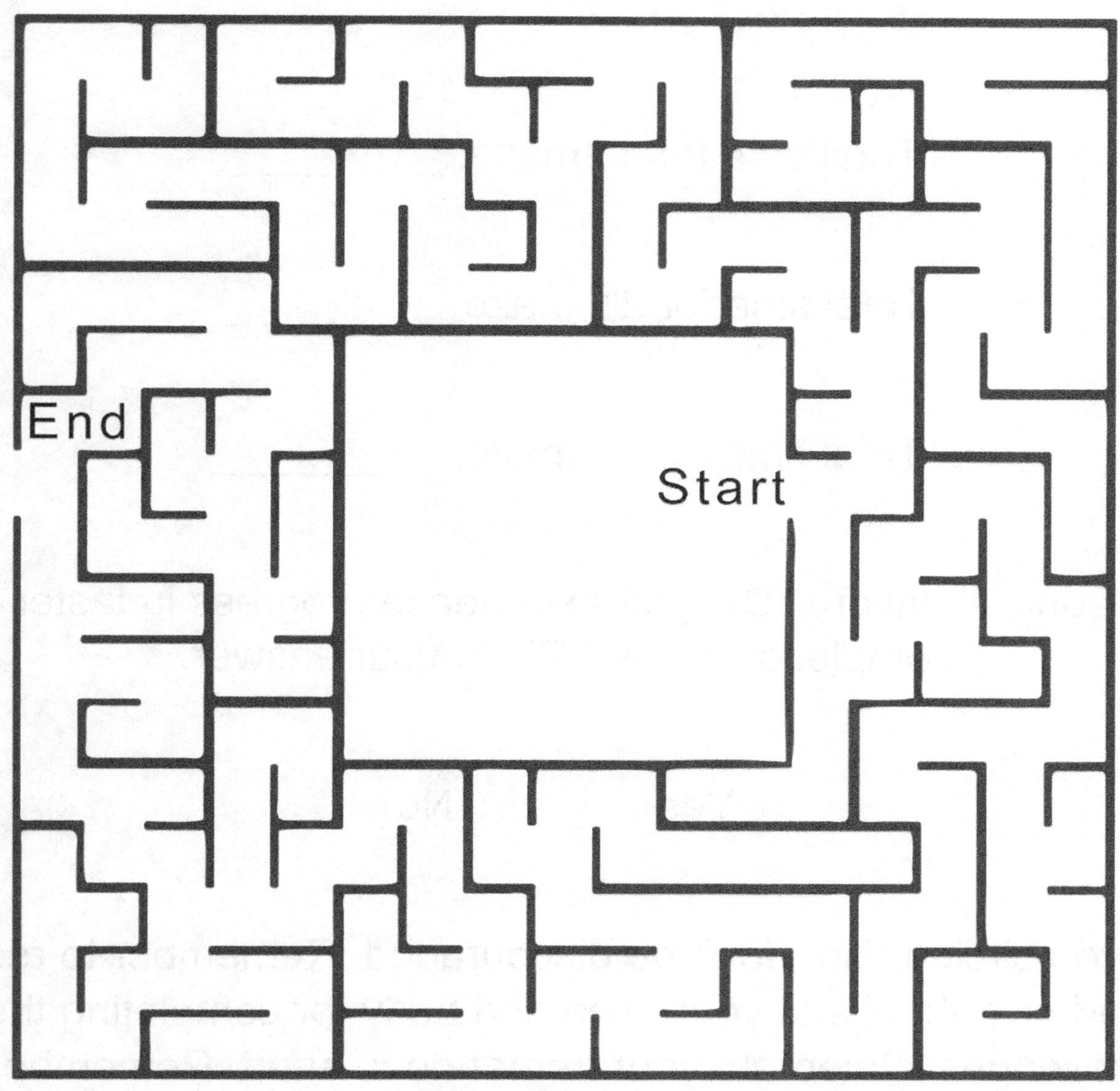

Start time: __________ End time: __________

Total time, maze 3: __________

Total time for 1st maze: __________

Total time for 2nd maze: __________

Total time for 3rd maze: __________

Congratulations! Did you experience progress in faster completion times? Circle your answer.

Yes   No

If you circled "No" don't be discouraged. Remember to rest and give thanks to your mind and body for completing the challenges. Celebrate your tremendous effort. Remember, a seed doesn't turn into a tree overnight.

Edison failed 10,000 times before he made the electric light. Do not be discouraged if you fail a few times.

—Napoleon Hill

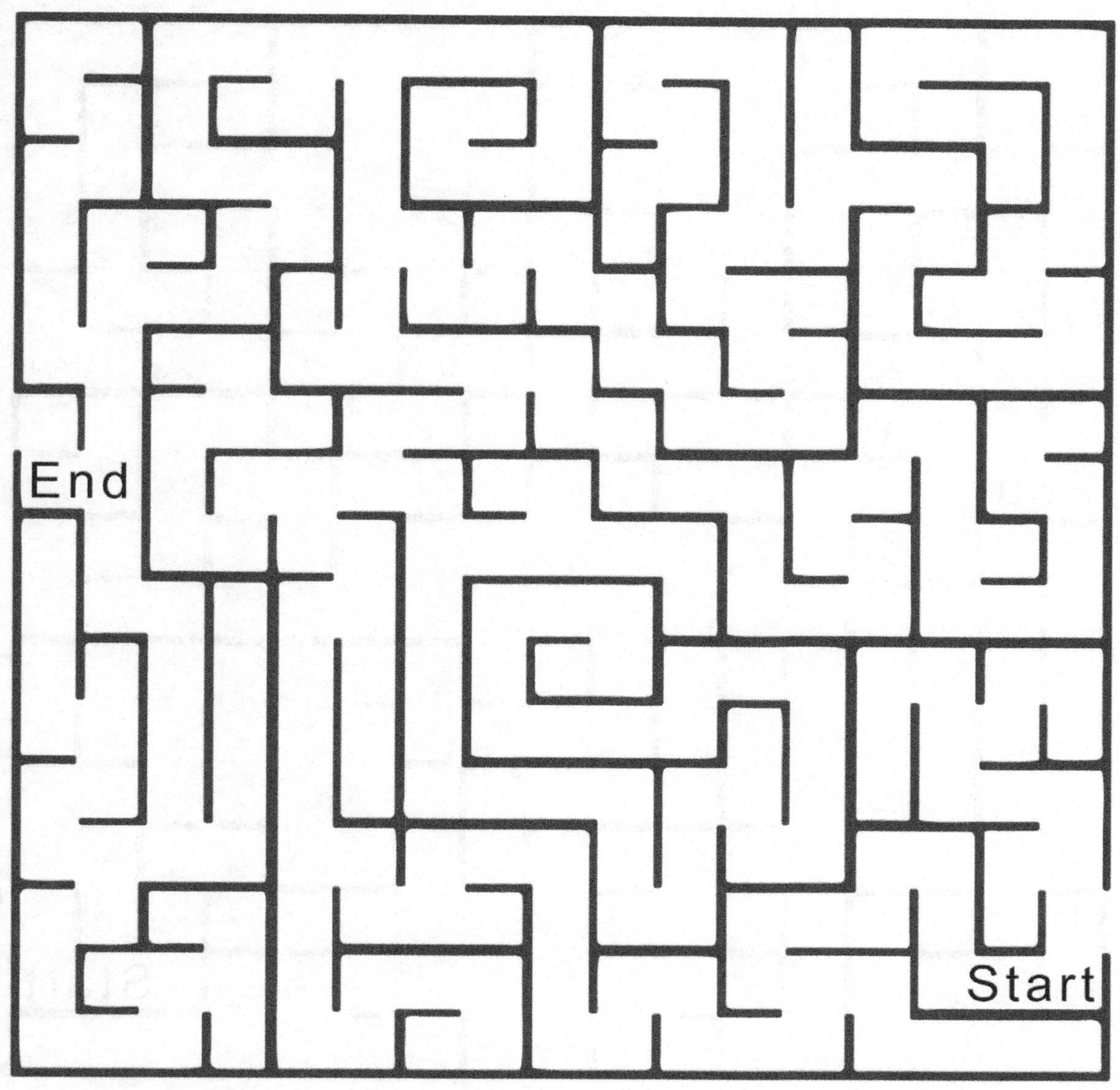

Start time: __________ End time: __________

Total time, maze 1: __________

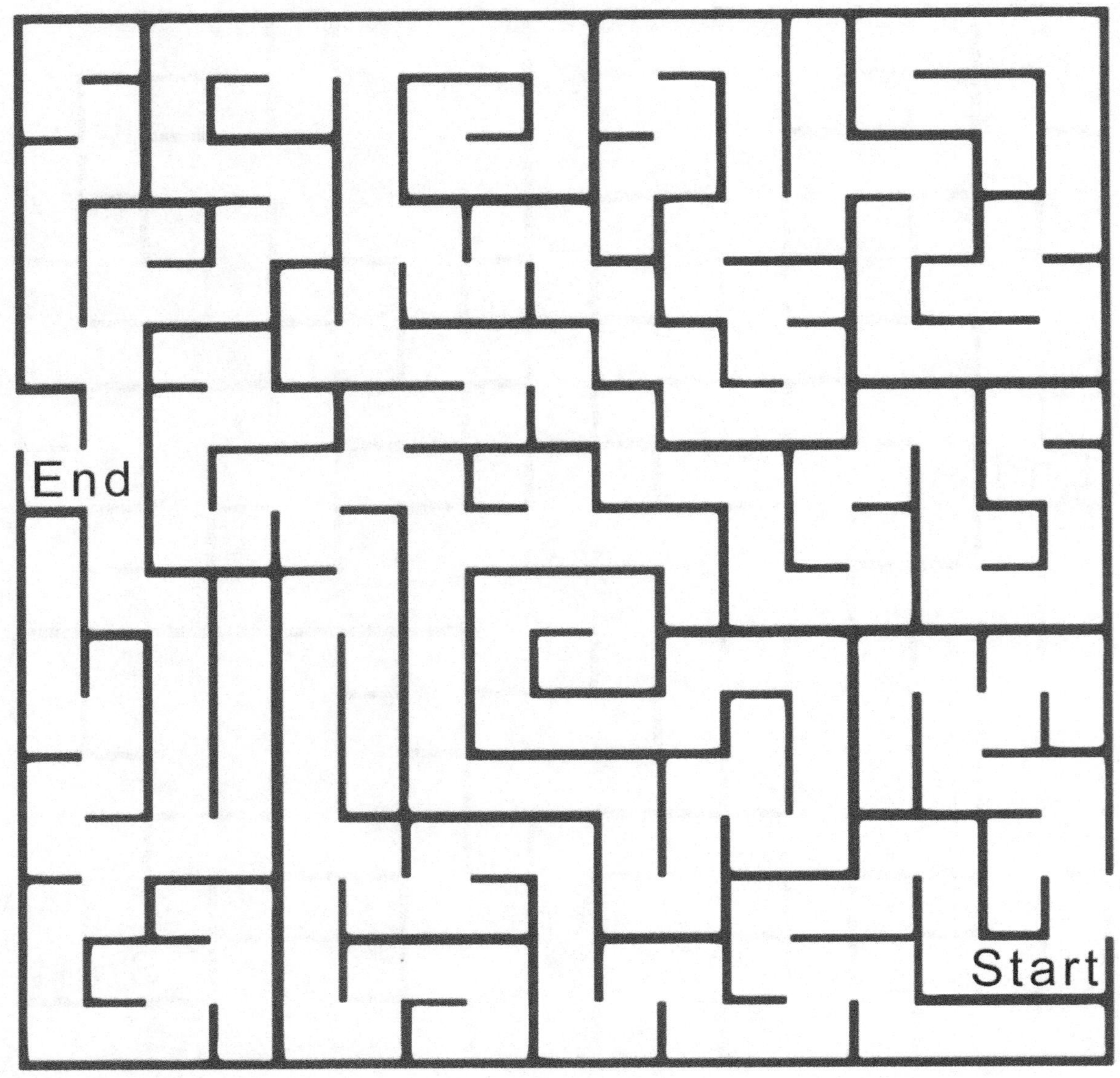

Start time: __________ End time: __________

Total time, maze 2: __________

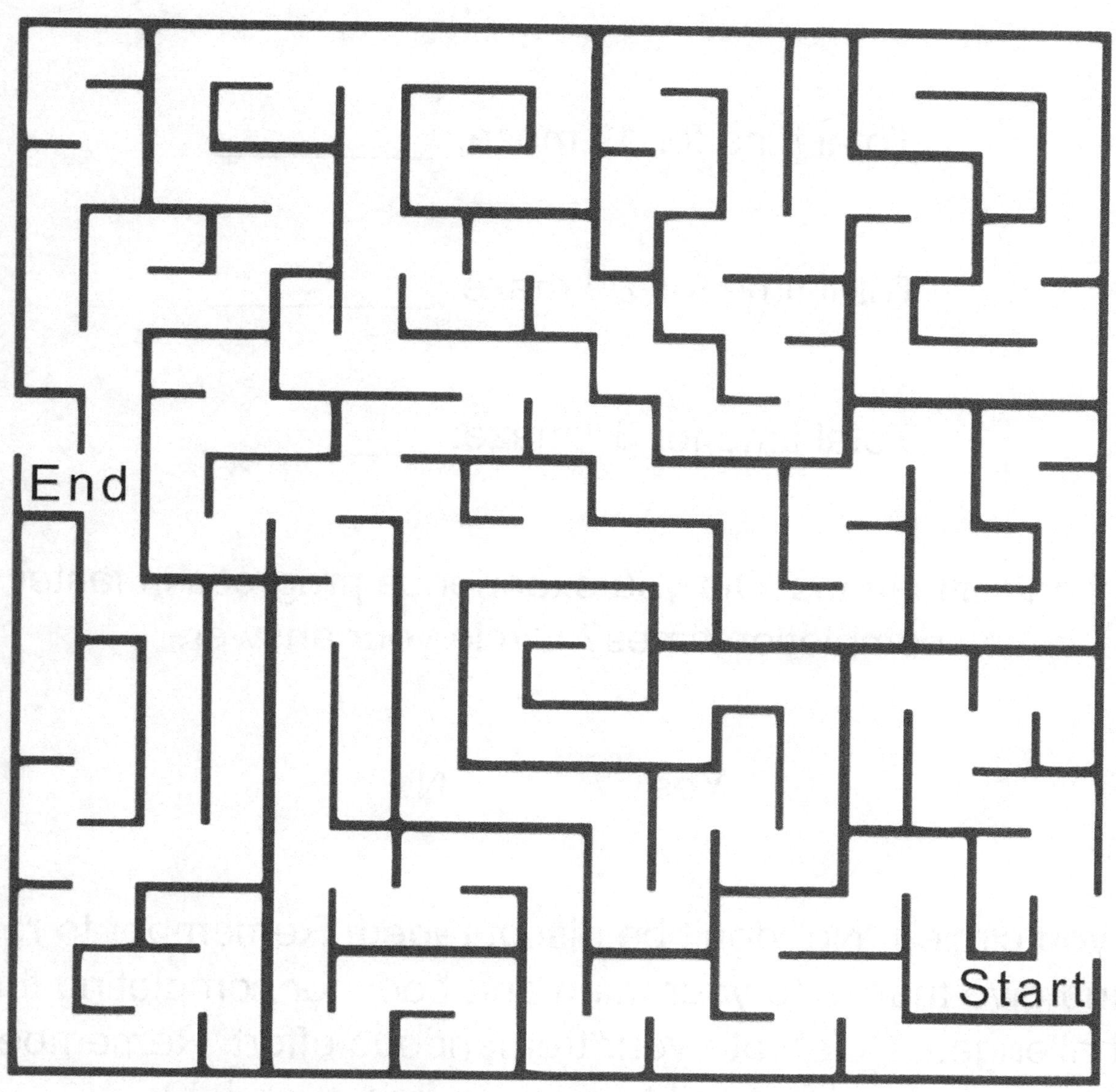

Start time: __________ End time: __________

Total time, maze 3: __________

Total time for 1st maze: __________

Total time for 2nd maze: __________

Total time for 3rd maze: __________

Congratulations! Did you experience progress in faster completion times? Circle your answer.

Yes No

If you circled "No" don't be discouraged. Remember to rest and give thanks to your mind and body for completing the challenges. Celebrate your tremendous effort. Remember, a seed doesn't turn into a tree overnight.

A man can get discouraged many times but he is not a failure until he begins to blame somebody else and stops trying.

—John Burroughs

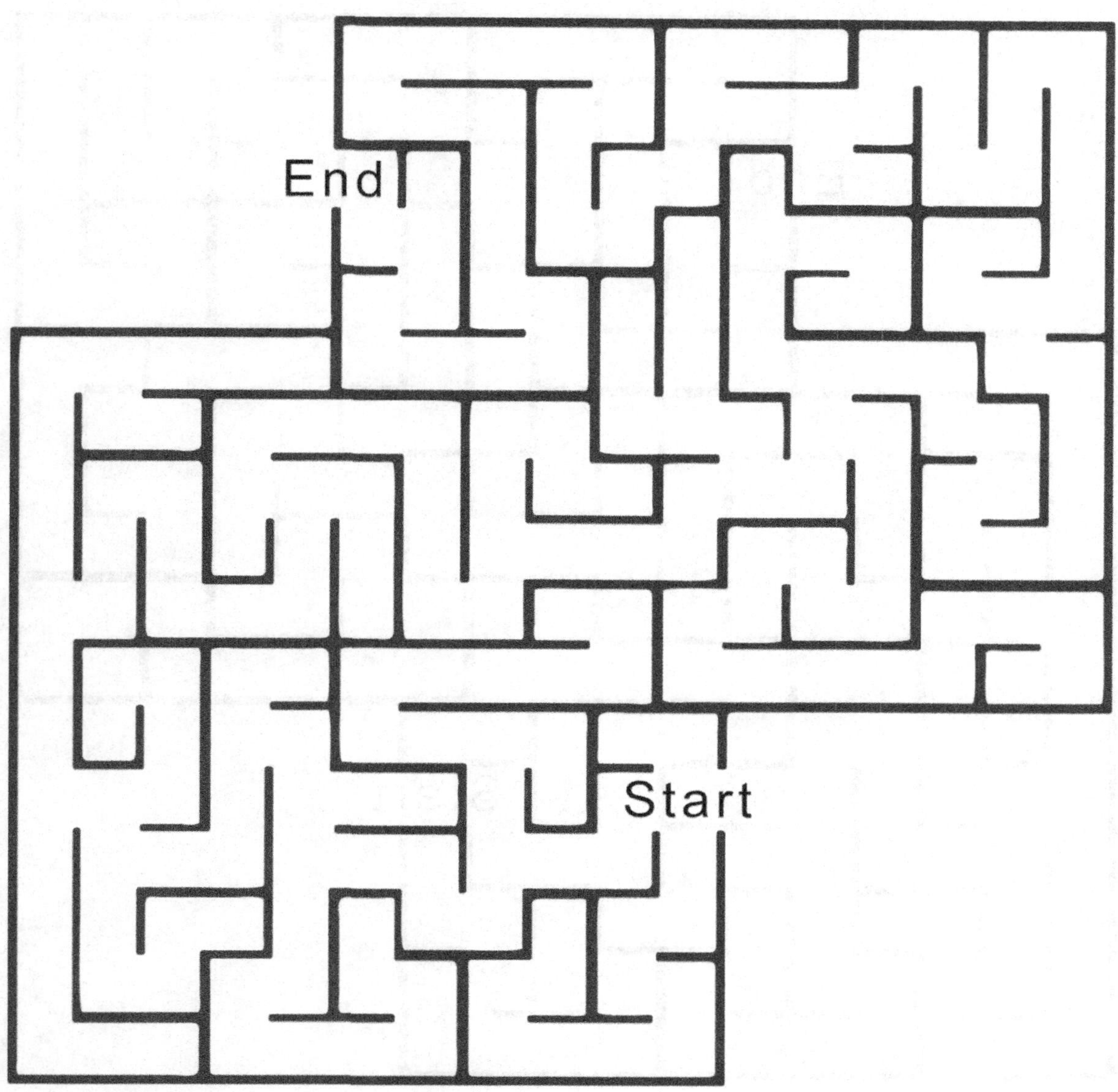

Start time: __________ End time: __________

Total time, maze 1: __________

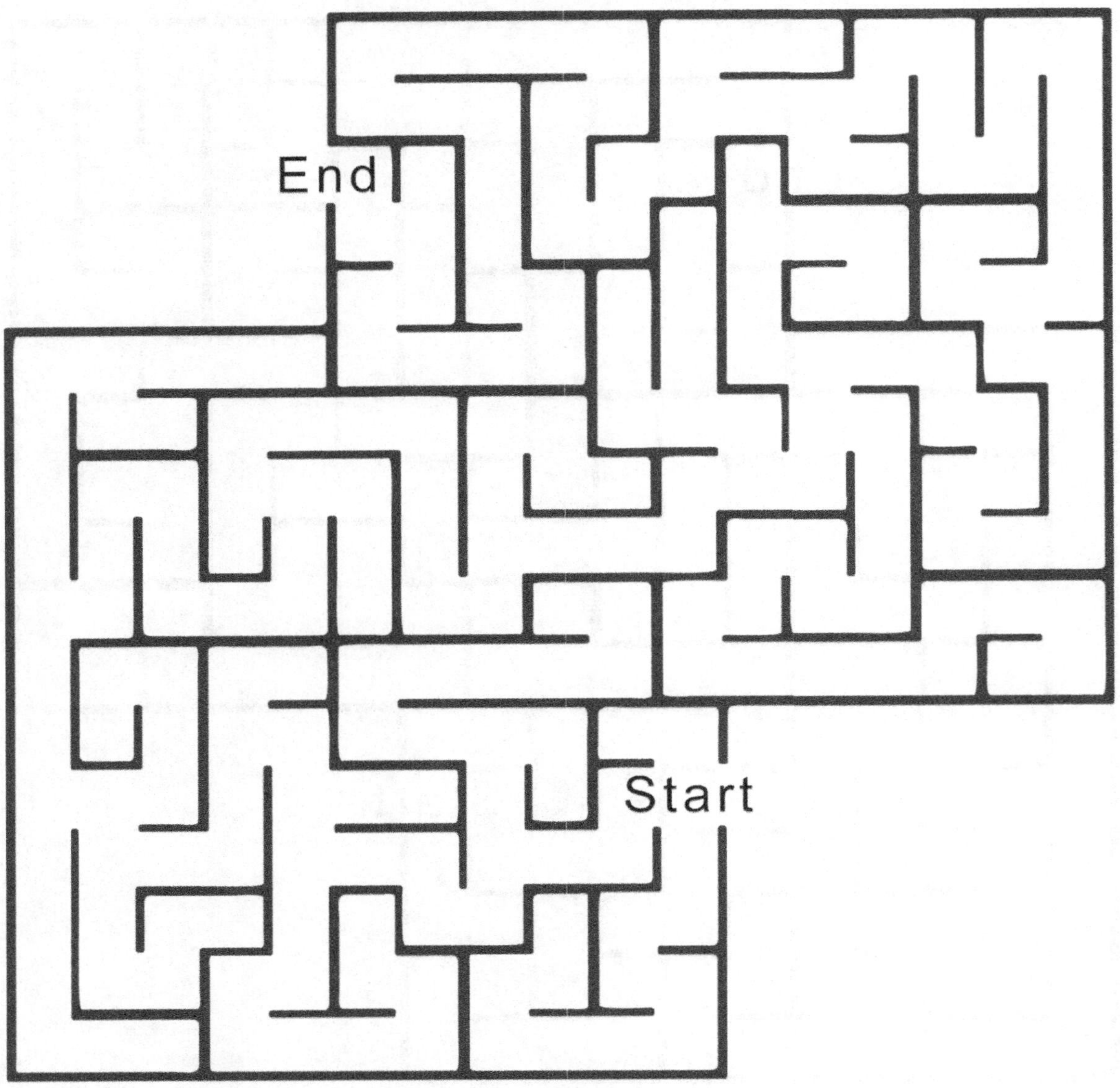

Start time: __________ End time: __________

Total time, maze 2: __________

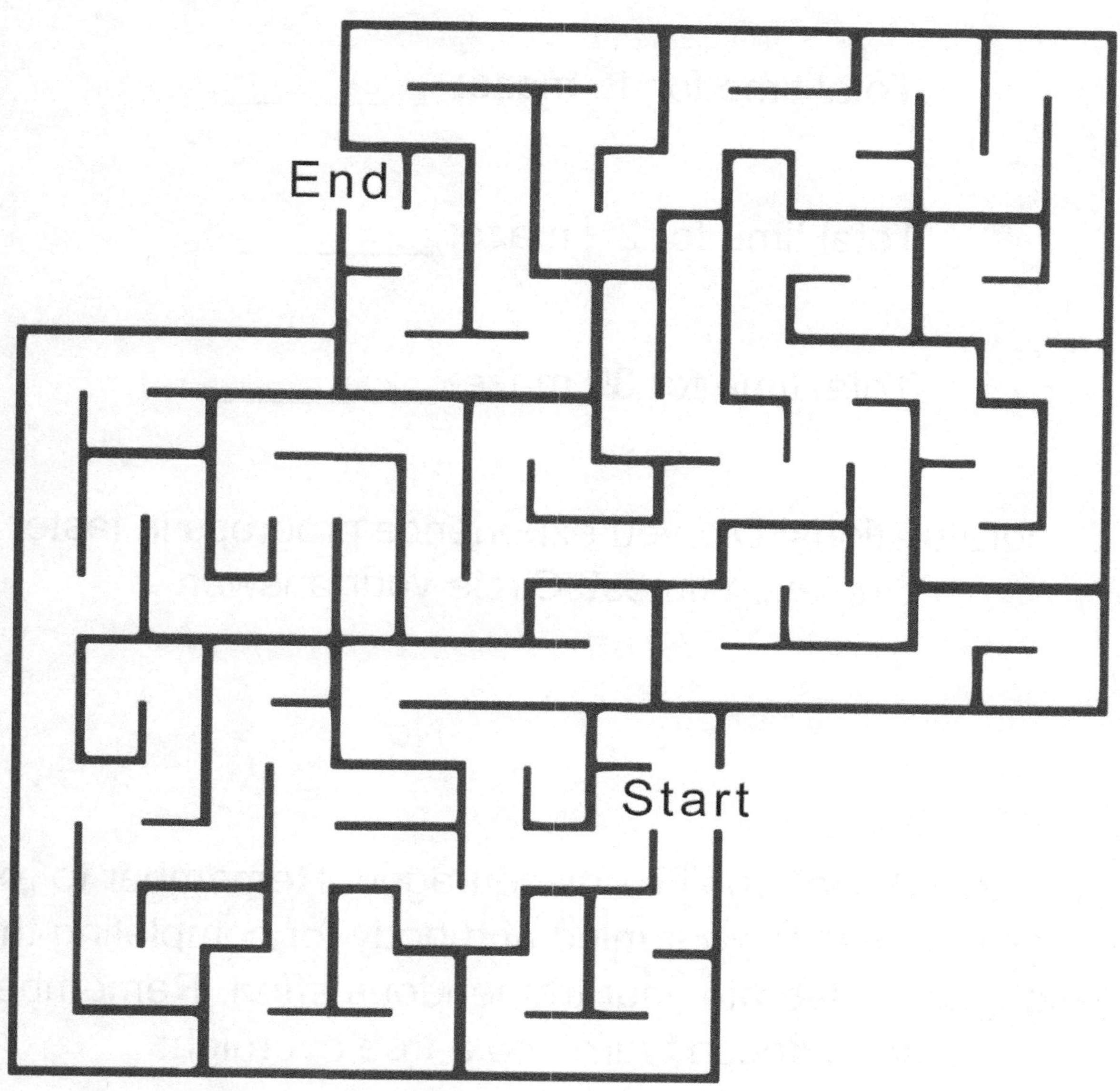

Start time: __________ End time: __________

Total time, maze 3: __________

Total time for 1st maze: __________

Total time for 2nd maze: __________

Total time for 3rd maze: __________

Congratulations! Did you experience progress in faster completion times? Circle your answer.

Yes No

If you circled "No" don't be discouraged. Remember to rest and give thanks to your mind and body for completing the challenges. Celebrate your tremendous effort. Remember, a seed doesn't turn into a tree overnight.

Continuous, unflagging effort, persistence and determination will win. Let not the man be discouraged who has these.

—*James Whitcomb Riley*

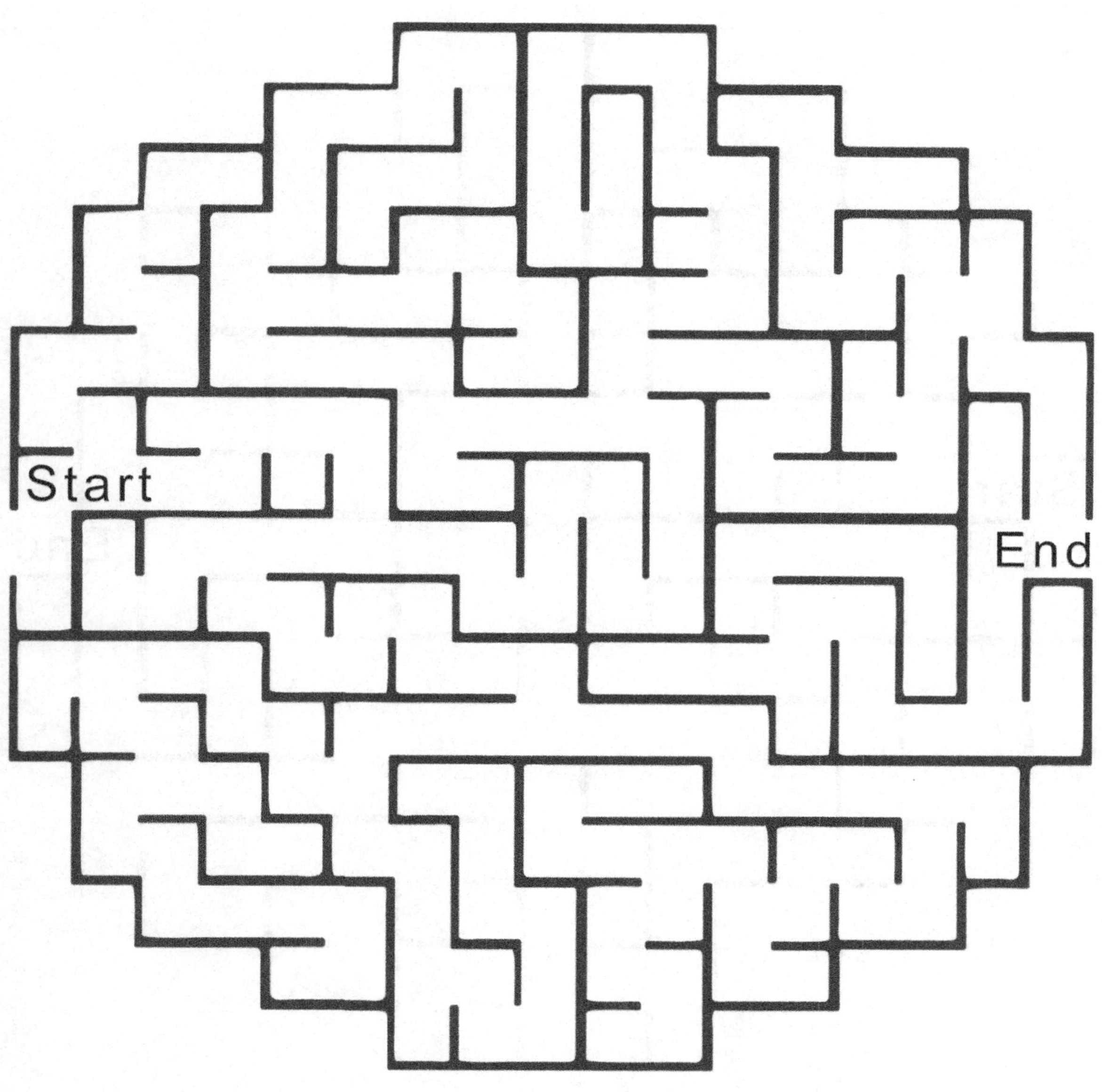

Start time: ___________ End time: ___________

Total time, maze 1: ___________

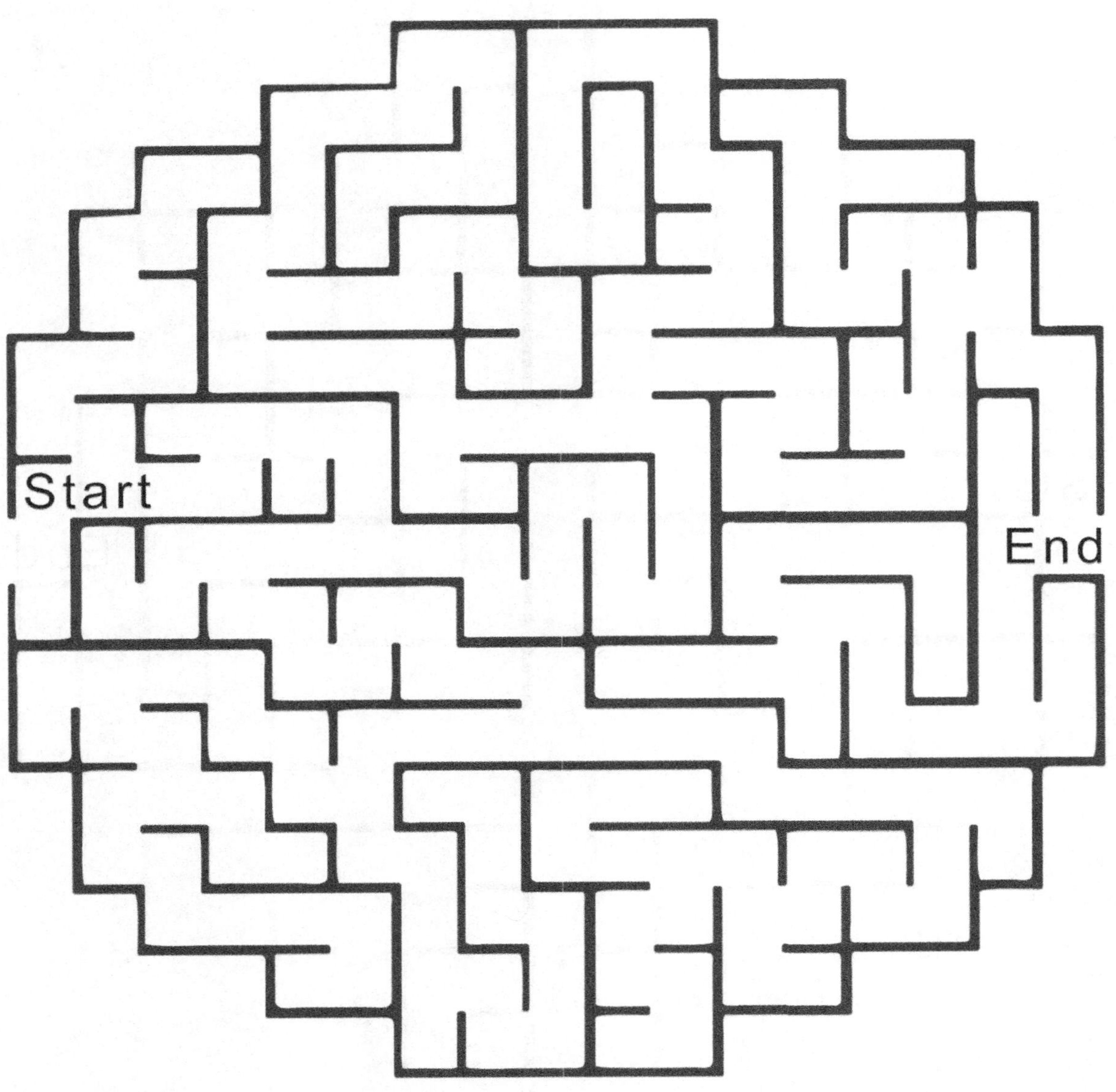

Start time: __________ End time: __________

Total time, maze 2: __________

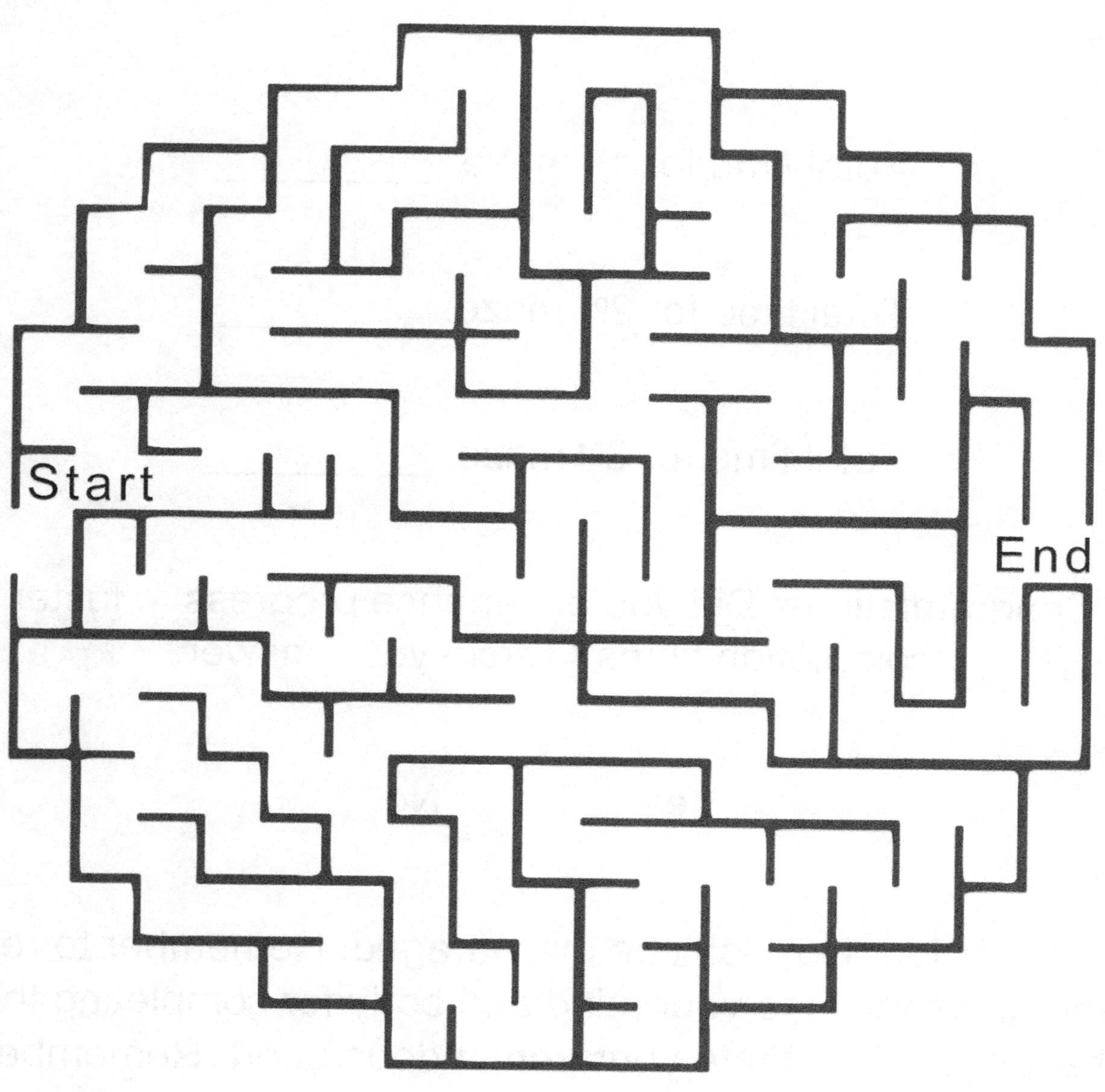

Start time: __________ End time: __________

Total time, maze 3: __________

Total time for 1st maze: __________

Total time for 2nd maze: __________

Total time for 3rd maze: __________

Congratulations! Did you experience progress in faster completion times? Circle your answer.

Yes No

If you circled "No" don't be discouraged. Remember to rest and give thanks to your mind and body for completing the challenges. Celebrate your tremendous effort. Remember, a seed doesn't turn into a tree overnight.

What is important is to believe in something so strongly that you're never discouraged.

—*Salma Hayek*

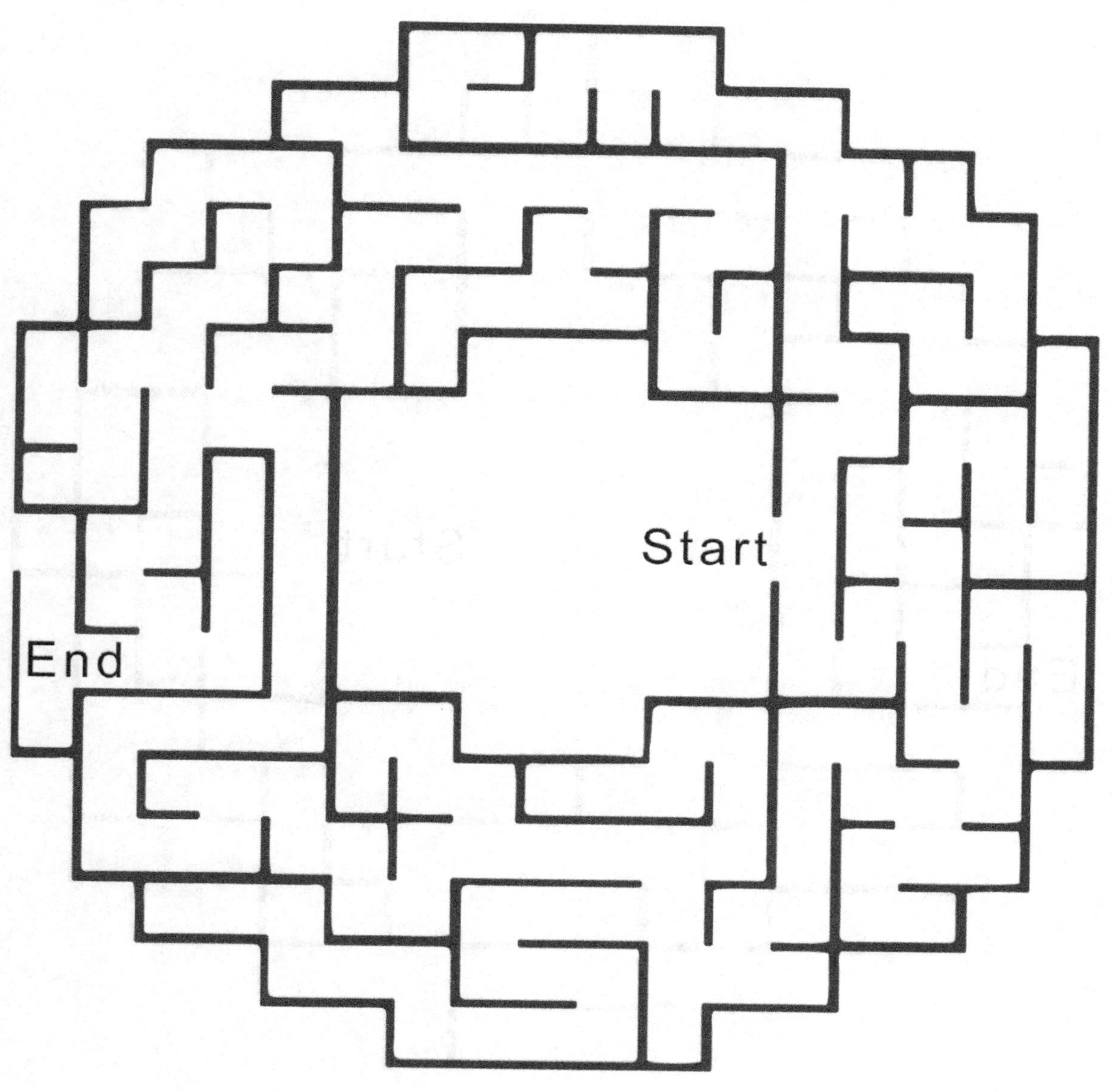

Start time: ___________ End time: ___________

Total time, maze 1: ___________

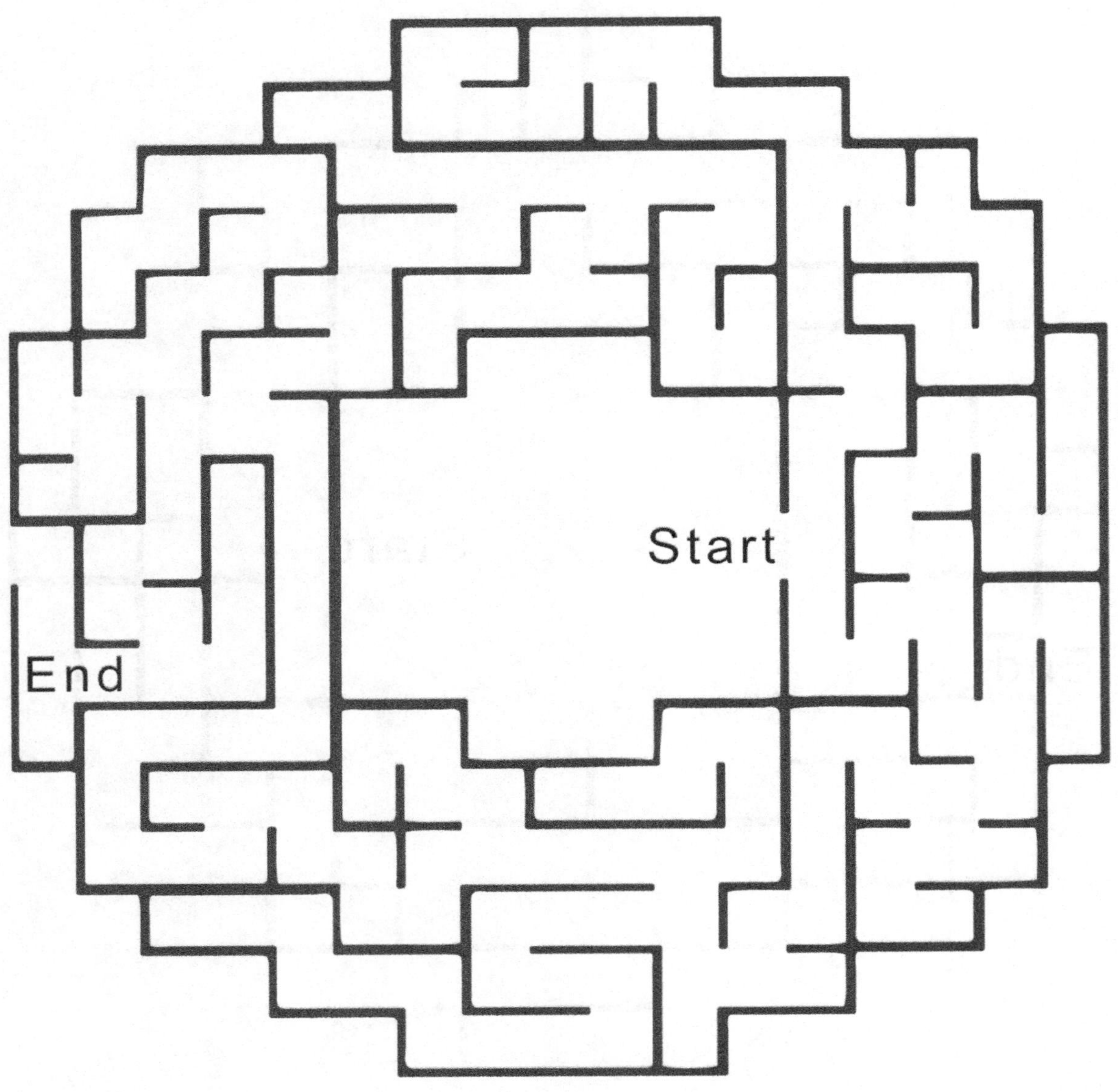

Start time: __________ End time: __________

Total time, maze 2: __________

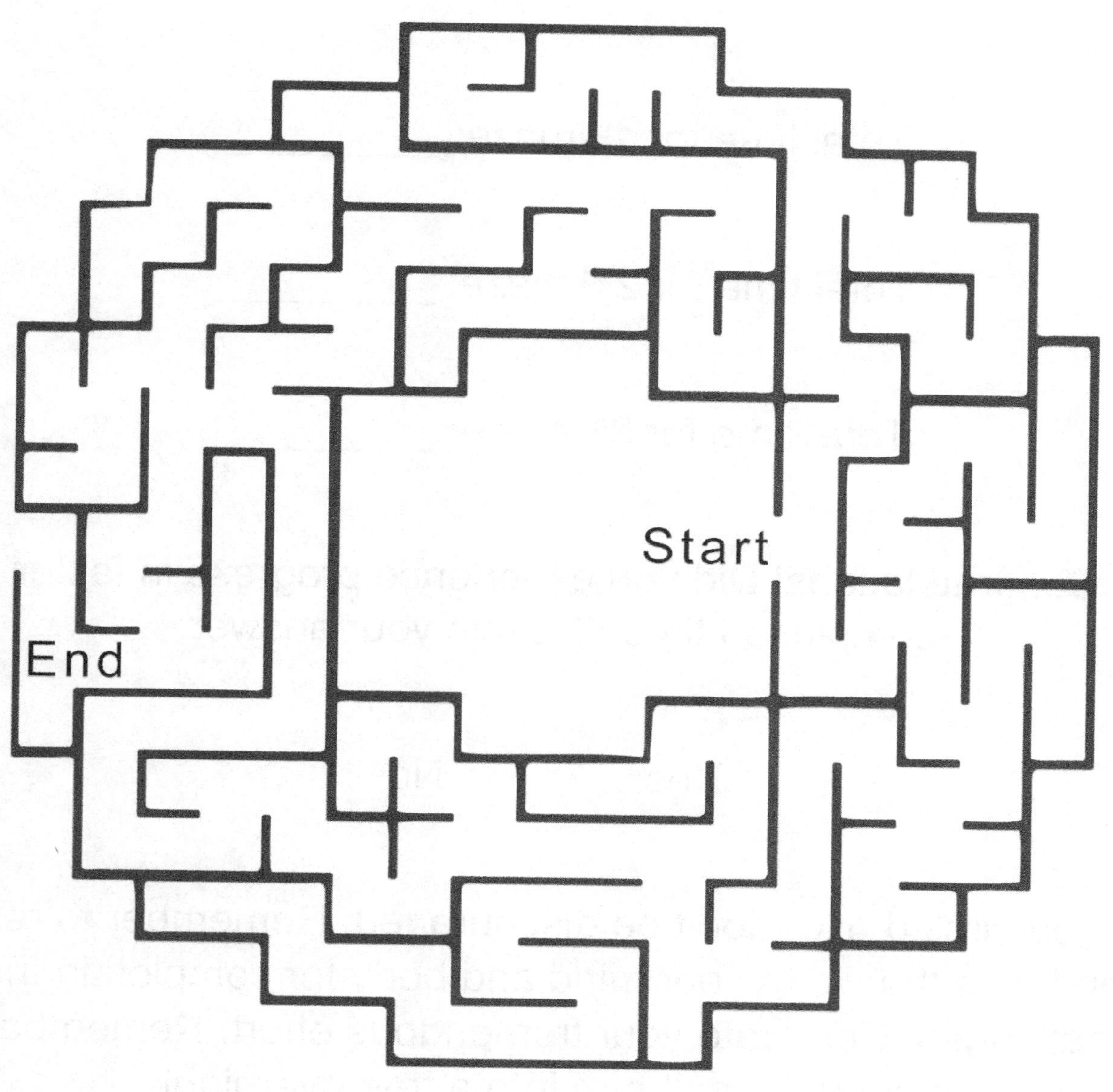

Start time: __________ End time: __________

Total time, maze 3: __________

Total time for 1st maze: __________

Total time for 2nd maze: __________

Total time for 3rd maze: __________

Congratulations! Did you experience progress in faster completion times? Circle your answer.

Yes No

If you circled "No" don't be discouraged. Remember to rest and give thanks to your mind and body for completing the challenges. Celebrate your tremendous effort. Remember, a seed doesn't turn into a tree overnight.

Stop beating yourself up. You are a work in progress - which means you get there a little at a time, not all at once.

—*Unknown*

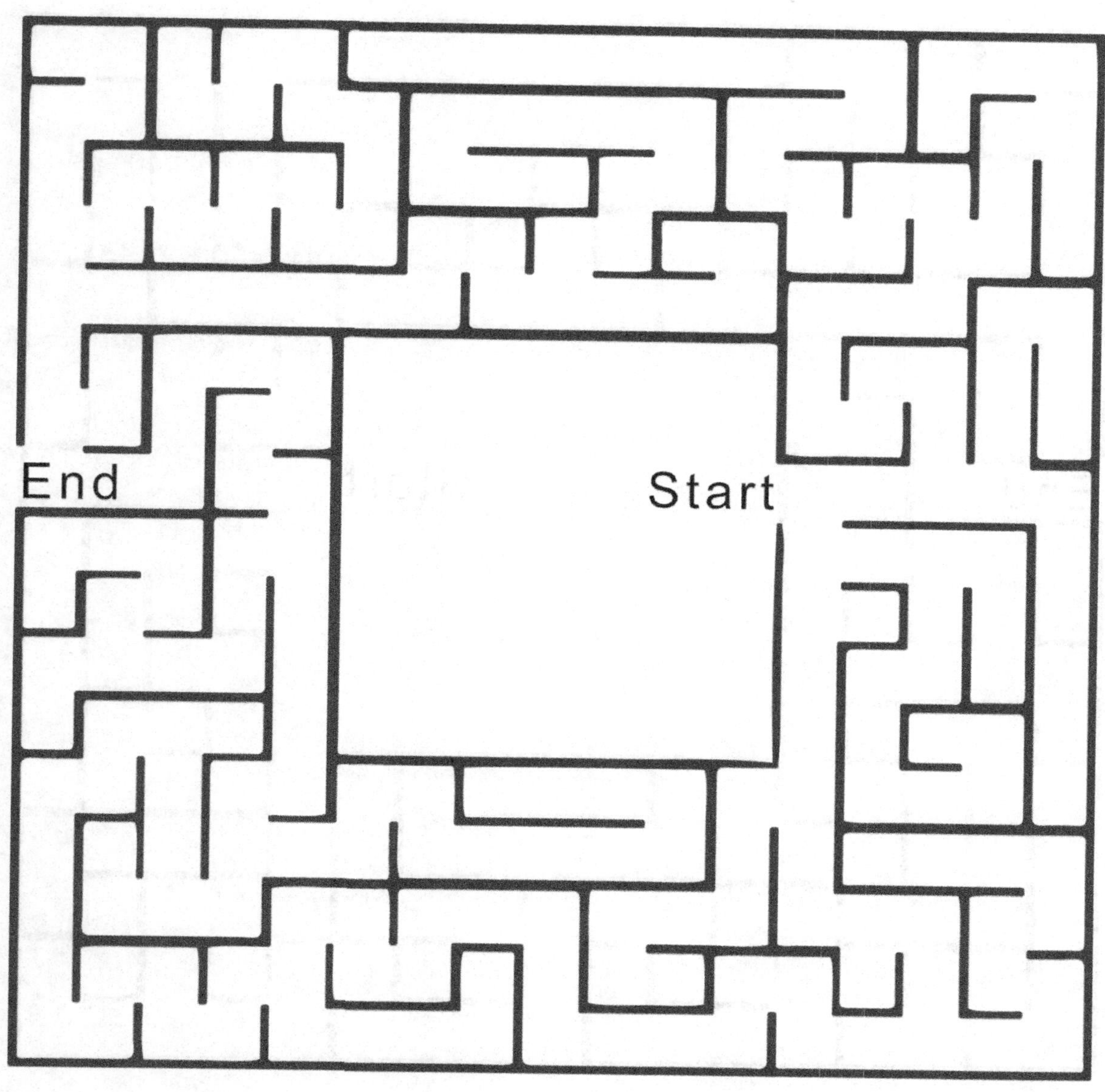

Start time: __________ End time: __________

Total time, maze 1: __________

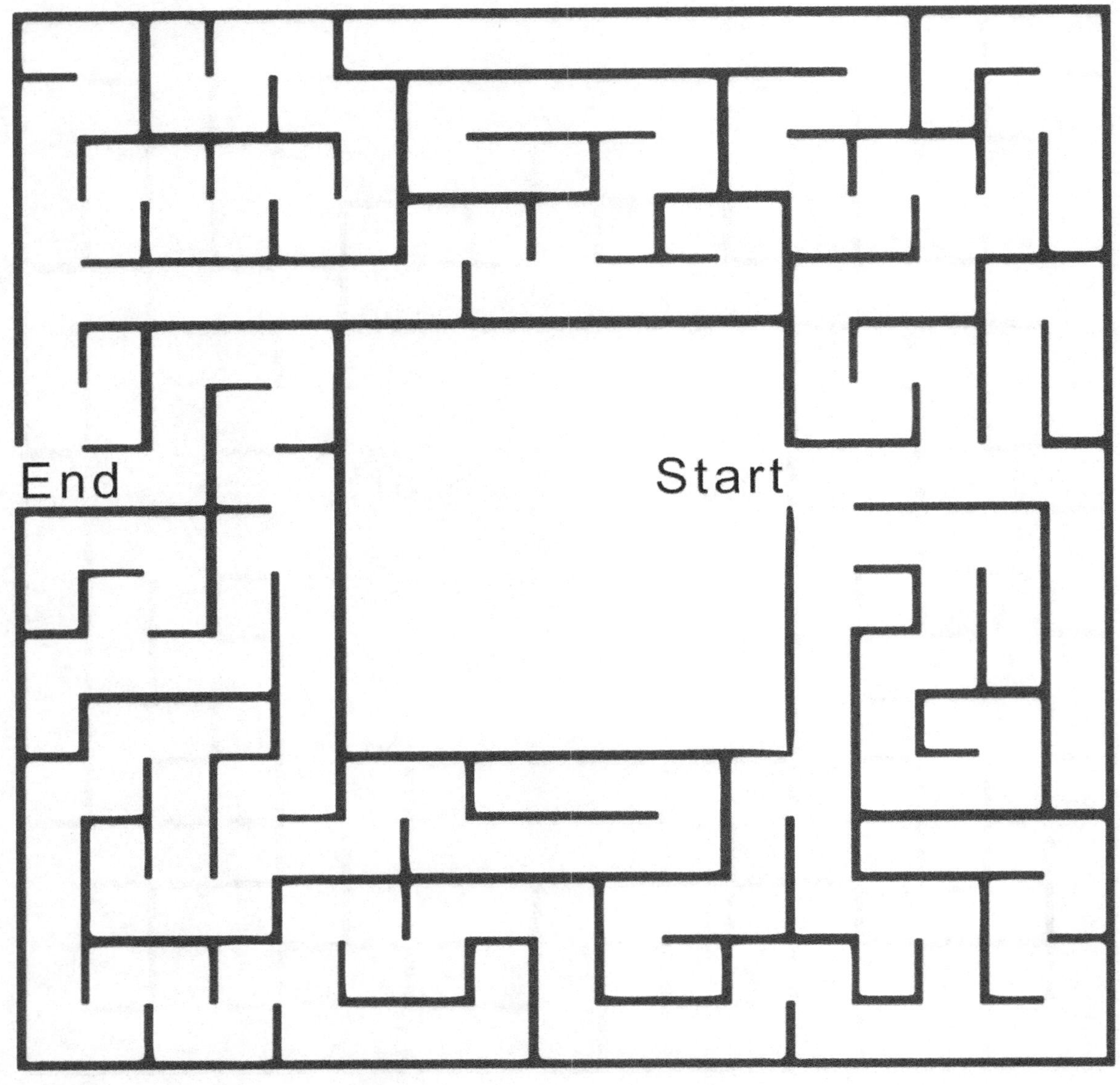

Start time: __________ End time: __________

Total time, maze 2: __________

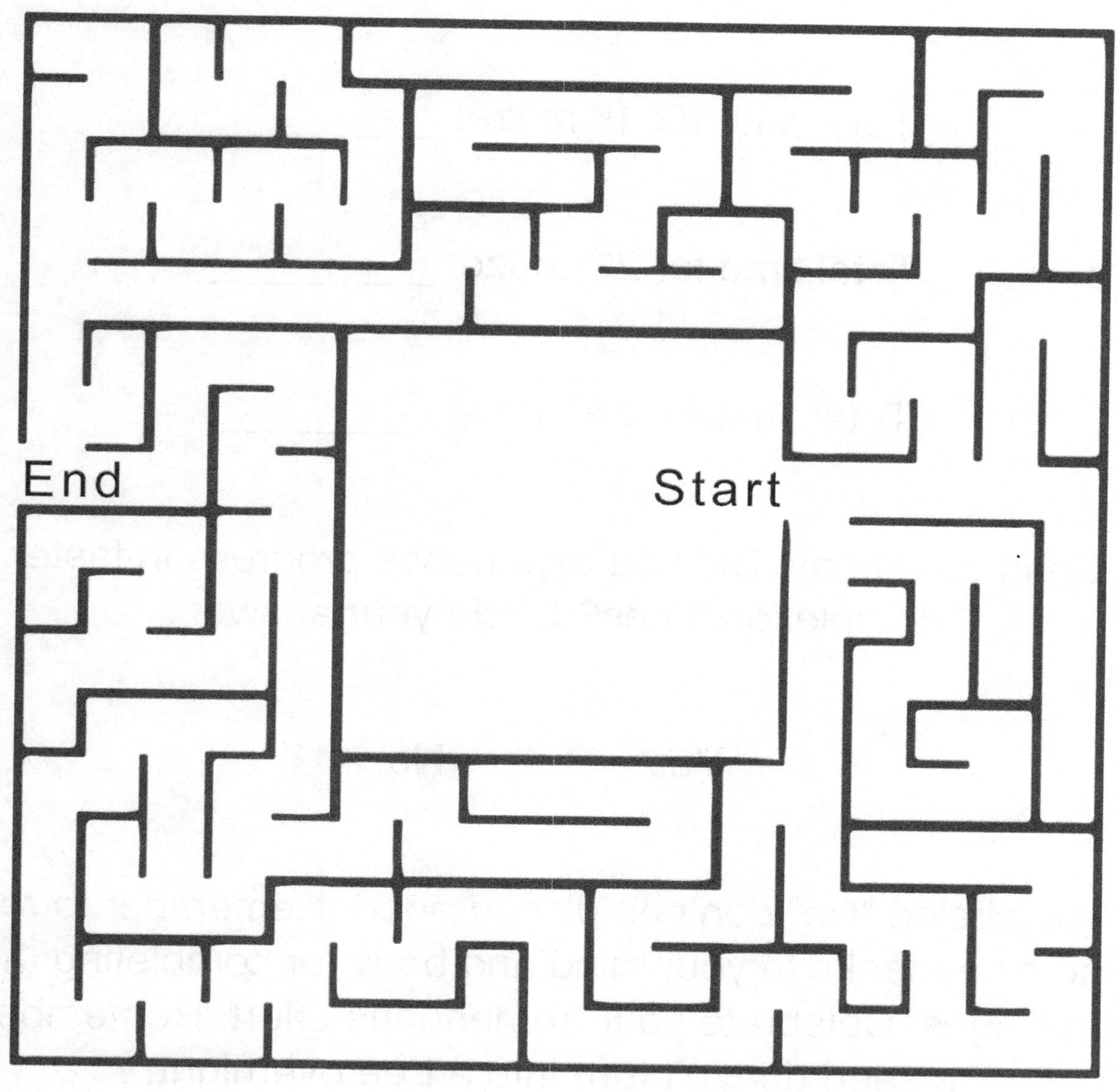

Start time: __________ End time: __________

Total time, maze 3: __________

Total time for 1st maze: __________

Total time for 2nd maze: __________

Total time for 3rd maze: __________

Congratulations! Did you experience progress in faster completion times? Circle your answer.

Yes No

If you circled "No" don't be discouraged. Remember to rest and give thanks to your mind and body for completing the challenges. Celebrate your tremendous effort. Remember, a seed doesn't turn into a tree overnight.

Yesterday I was clever so I wanted to change the world. Today I am wise, so I am changing myself.

—*Rumi*

The heartiest plants survive because they weather the storms and never stop reaching for the light.

—Robert Clancy

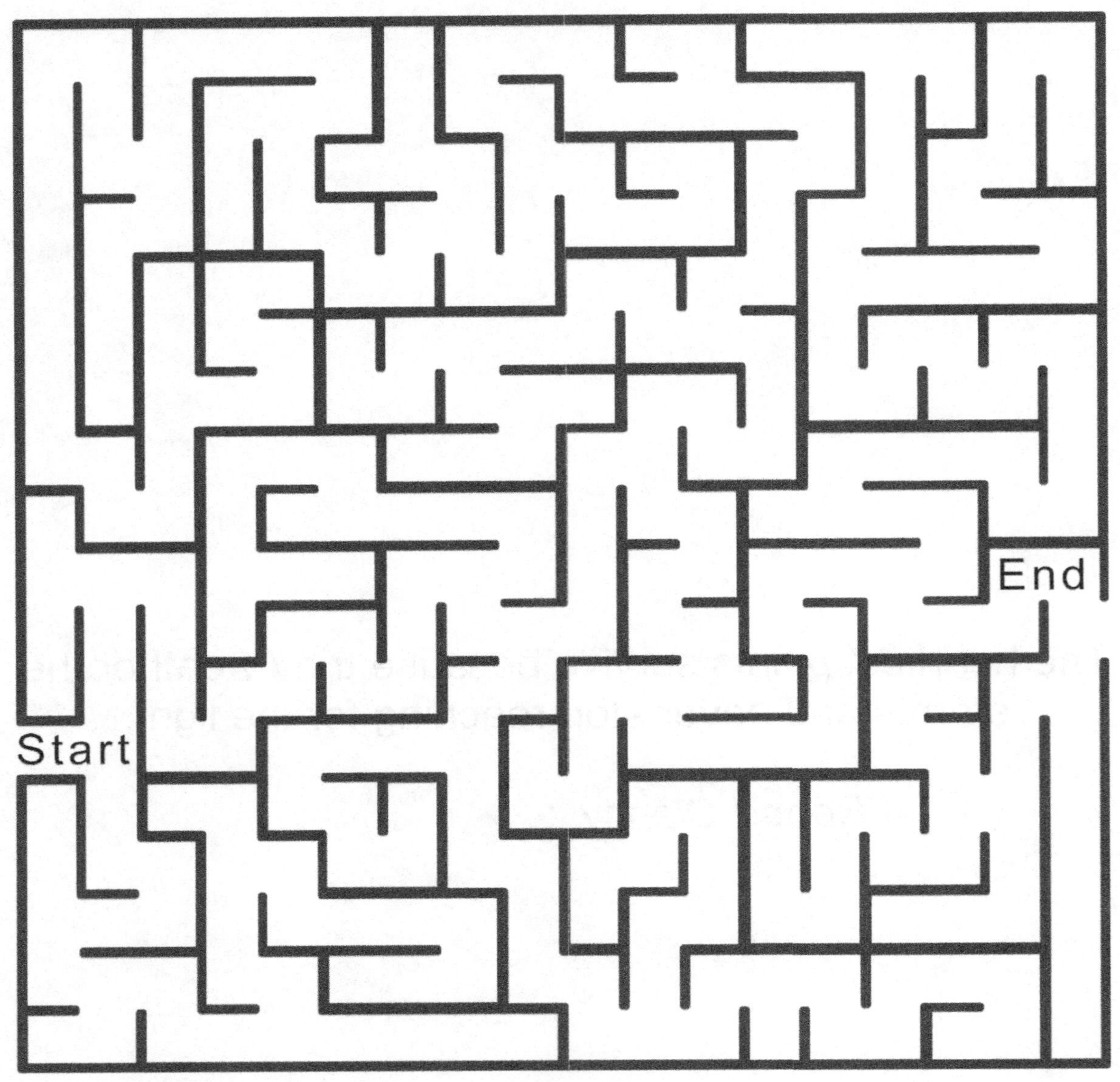

Start time: __________ End time: __________

Total time, maze 1: __________

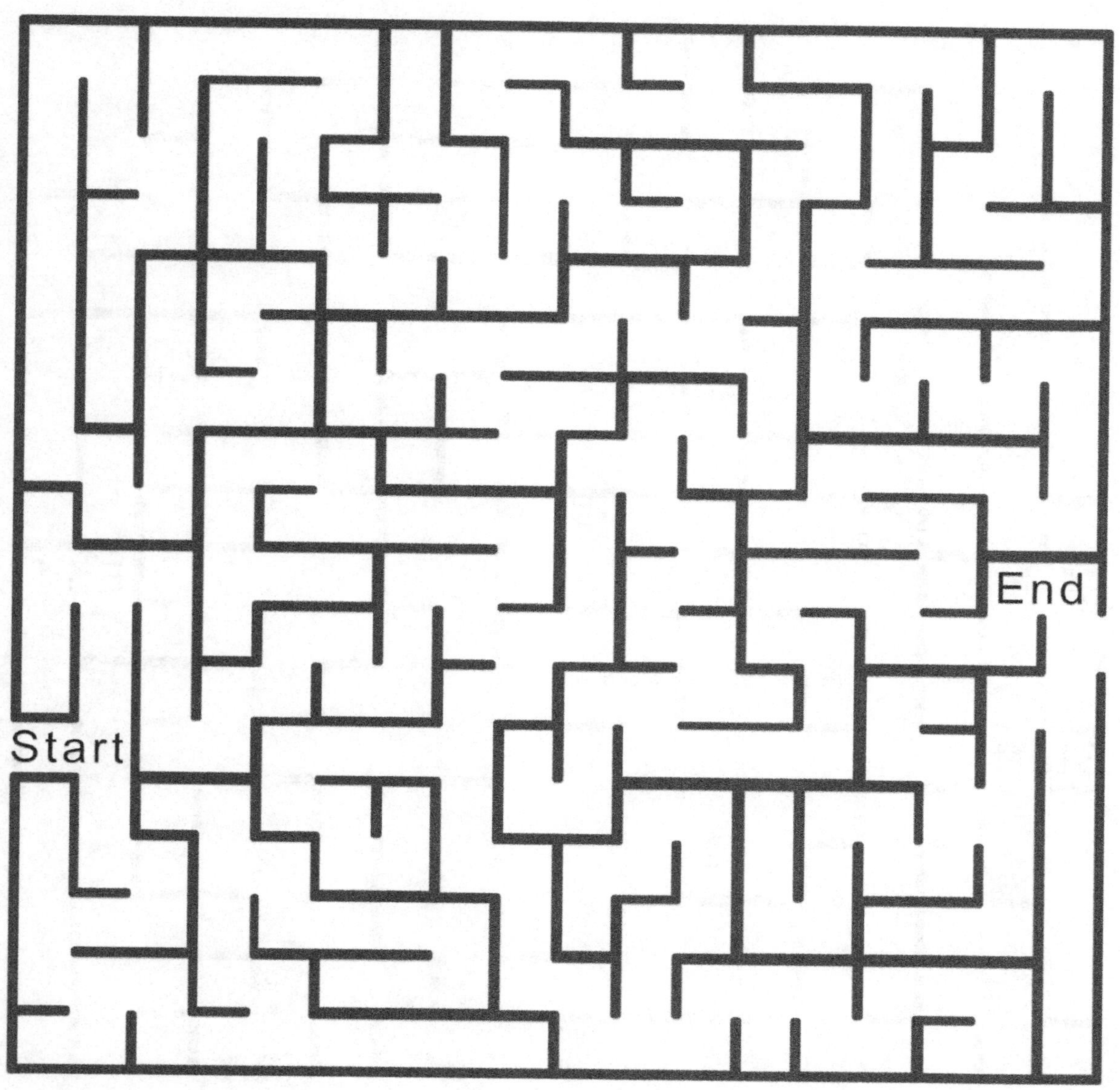

Start time: ____________ End time: ____________

Total time, maze 2: ____________

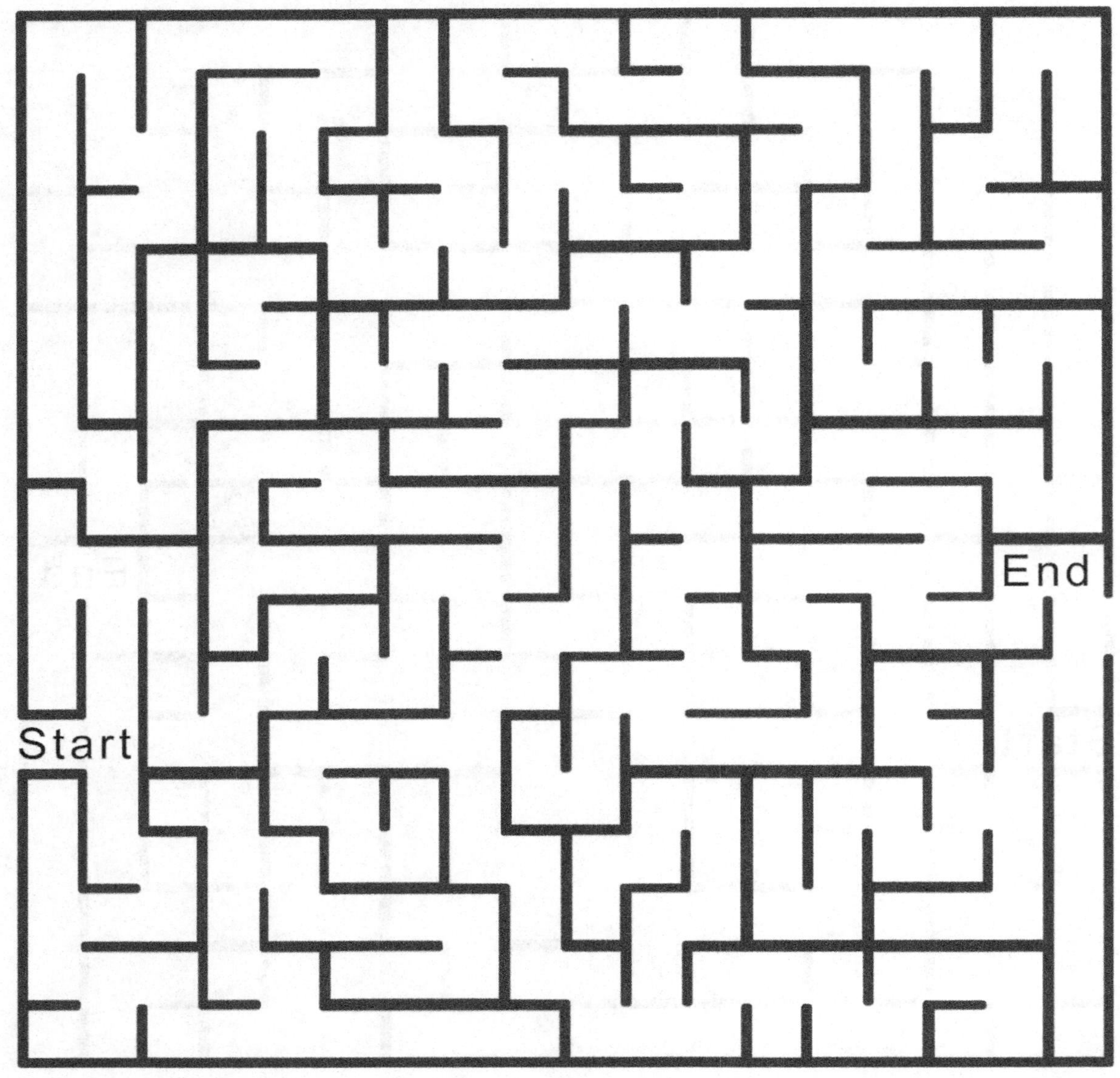

Start time: __________ End time: __________

Total time, maze 3: __________

Total time for 1st maze: __________

Total time for 2nd maze: __________

Total time for 3rd maze: __________

Congratulations! Did you experience progress in faster completion times? Circle your answer.

Yes No

If you circled "No" don't be discouraged. Remember to rest and give thanks to your mind and body for completing the challenges. Celebrate your tremendous effort. Remember, a seed doesn't turn into a tree overnight.

If you really want to do something, you'll find a way. If you don't, you'll find an excuse.

—Jim Rohn

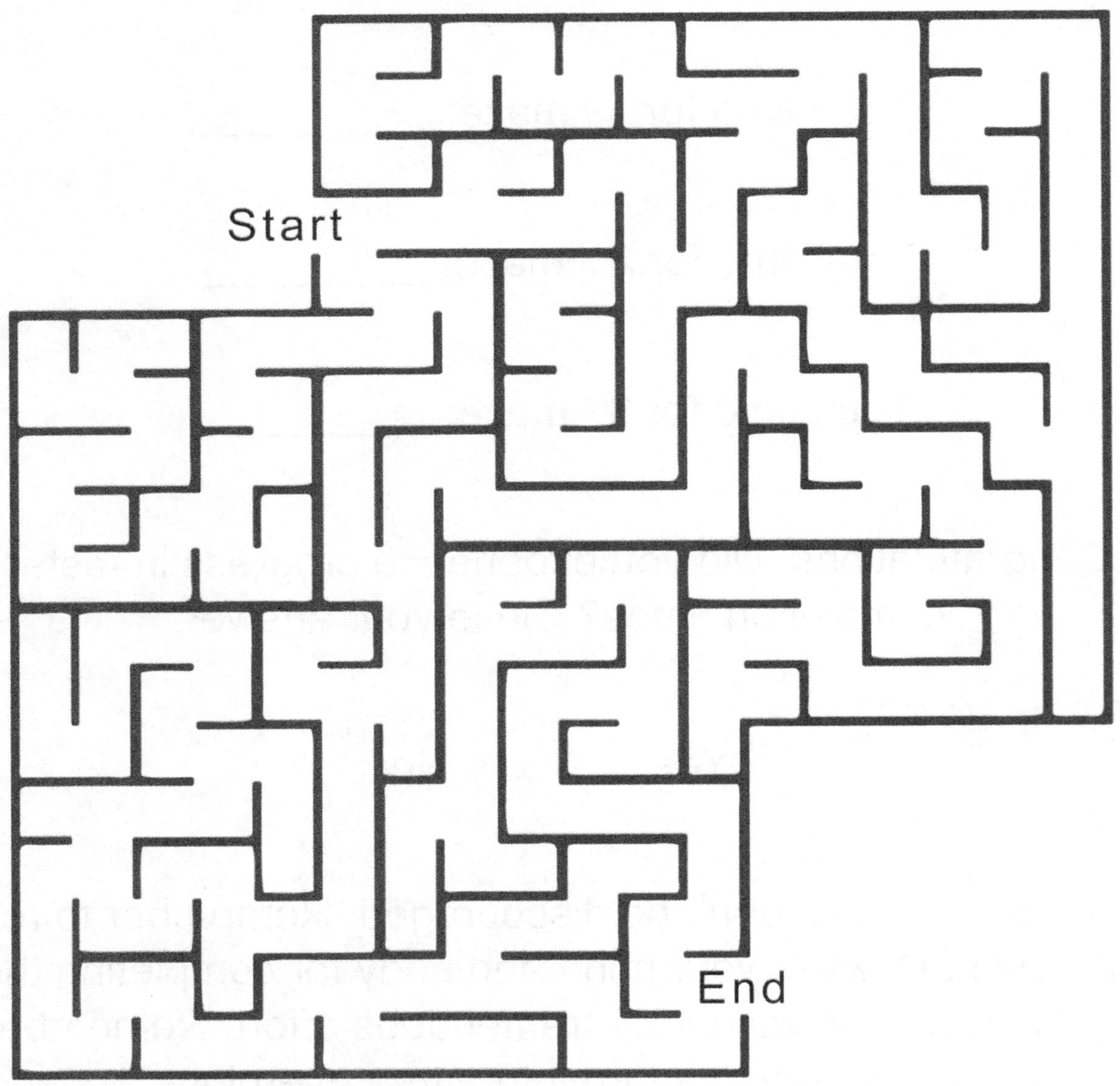

Start time: __________ End time: __________

Total time, maze 1: __________

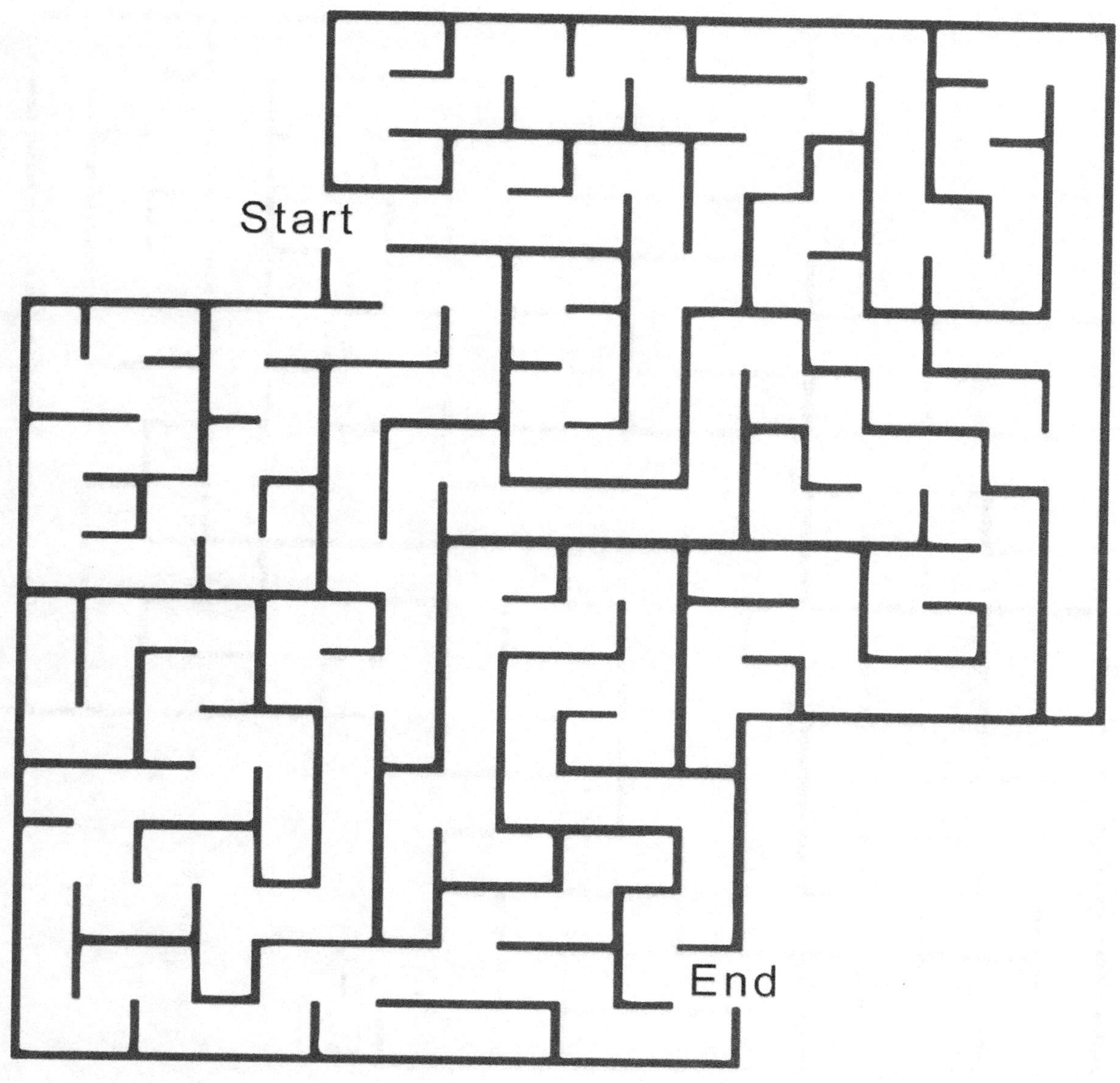

Start time: __________ End time: __________

Total time, maze 2: __________

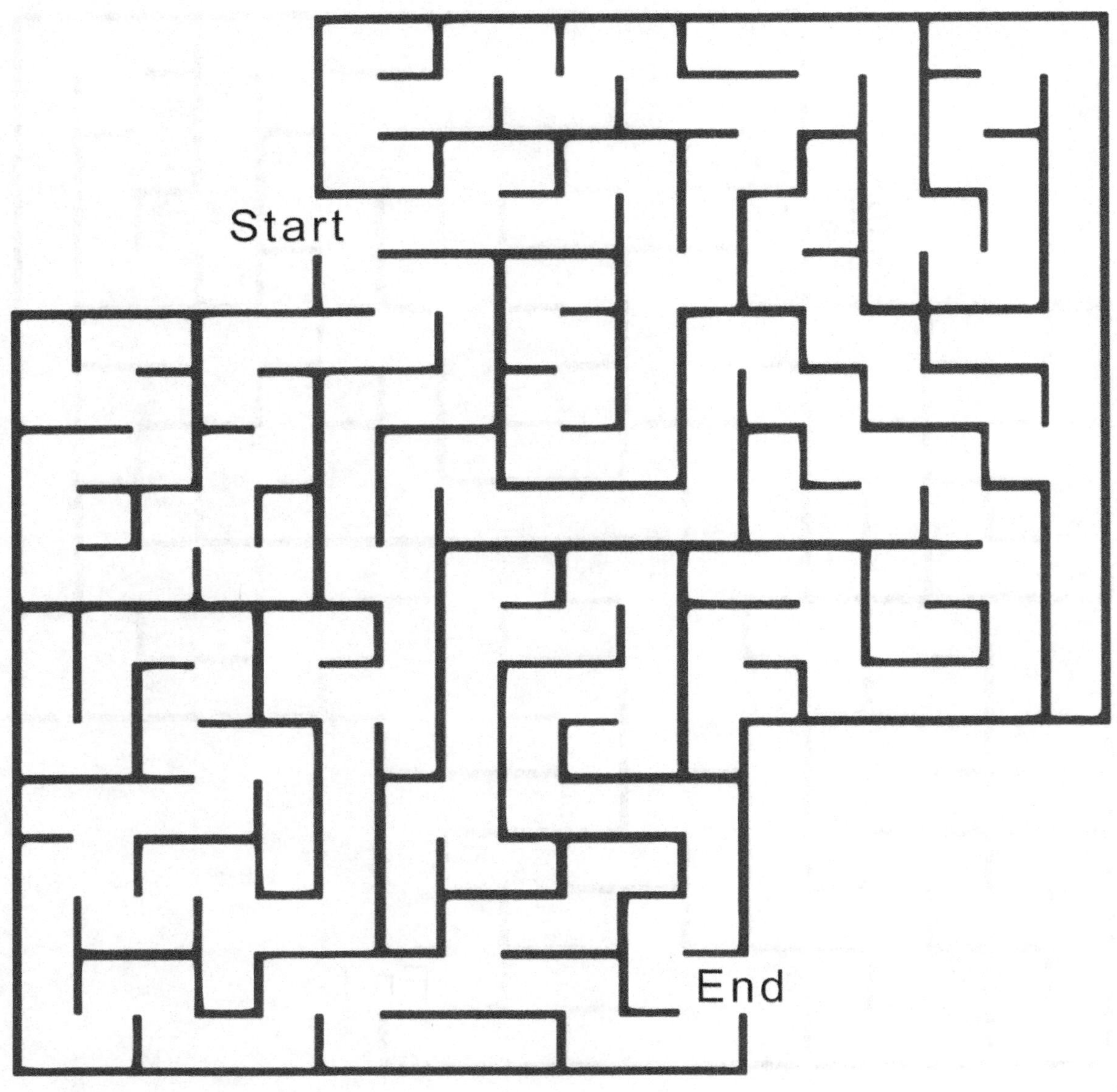

Start time: __________ End time: __________

Total time, maze 3: __________

Total time for 1st maze: __________

Total time for 2nd maze: __________

Total time for 3rd maze: __________

Congratulations! Did you experience progress in faster completion times? Circle your answer.

Yes No

If you circled "No" don't be discouraged. Remember to rest and give thanks to your mind and body for completing the challenges. Celebrate your tremendous effort. Remember, a seed doesn't turn into a tree overnight.

F.E.A.R: has two meanings: 1). Forget Everything And Run or 2). Face Everything And Rise; the choice is yours!

—Zig Ziglar

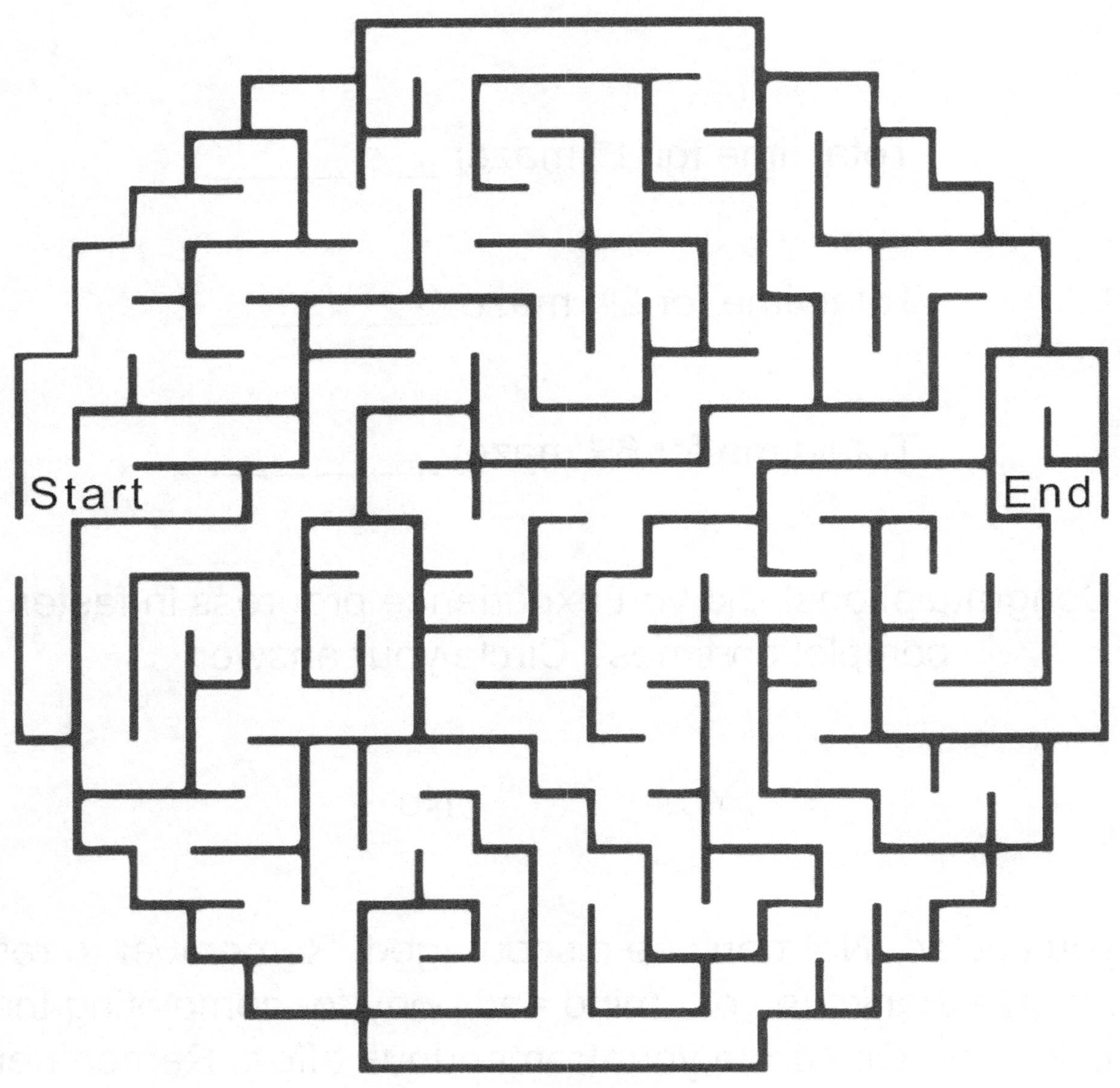

Start time: __________ End time: __________

Total time, maze 1: __________

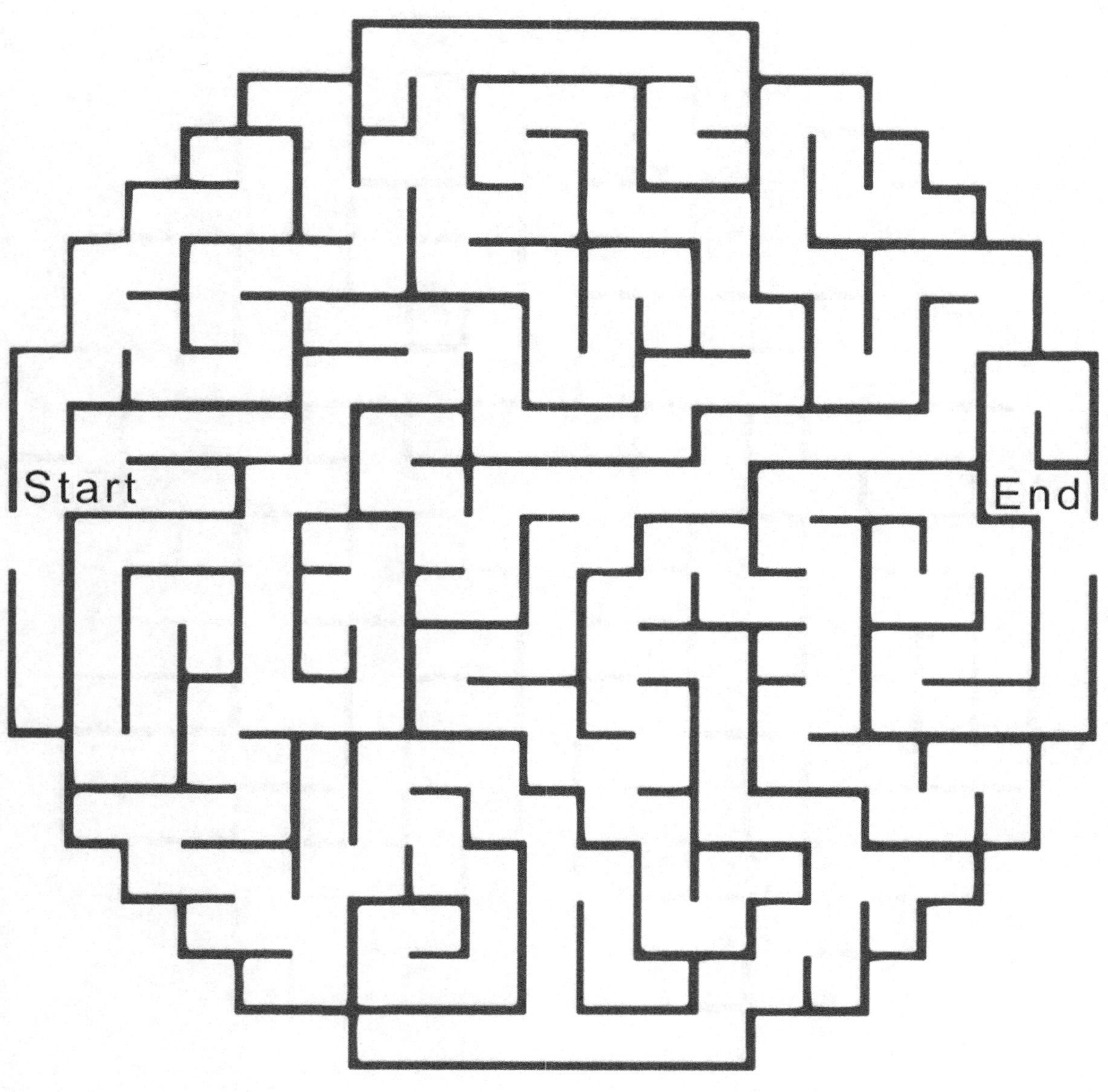

Start time: __________ End time: __________

Total time, maze 2: __________

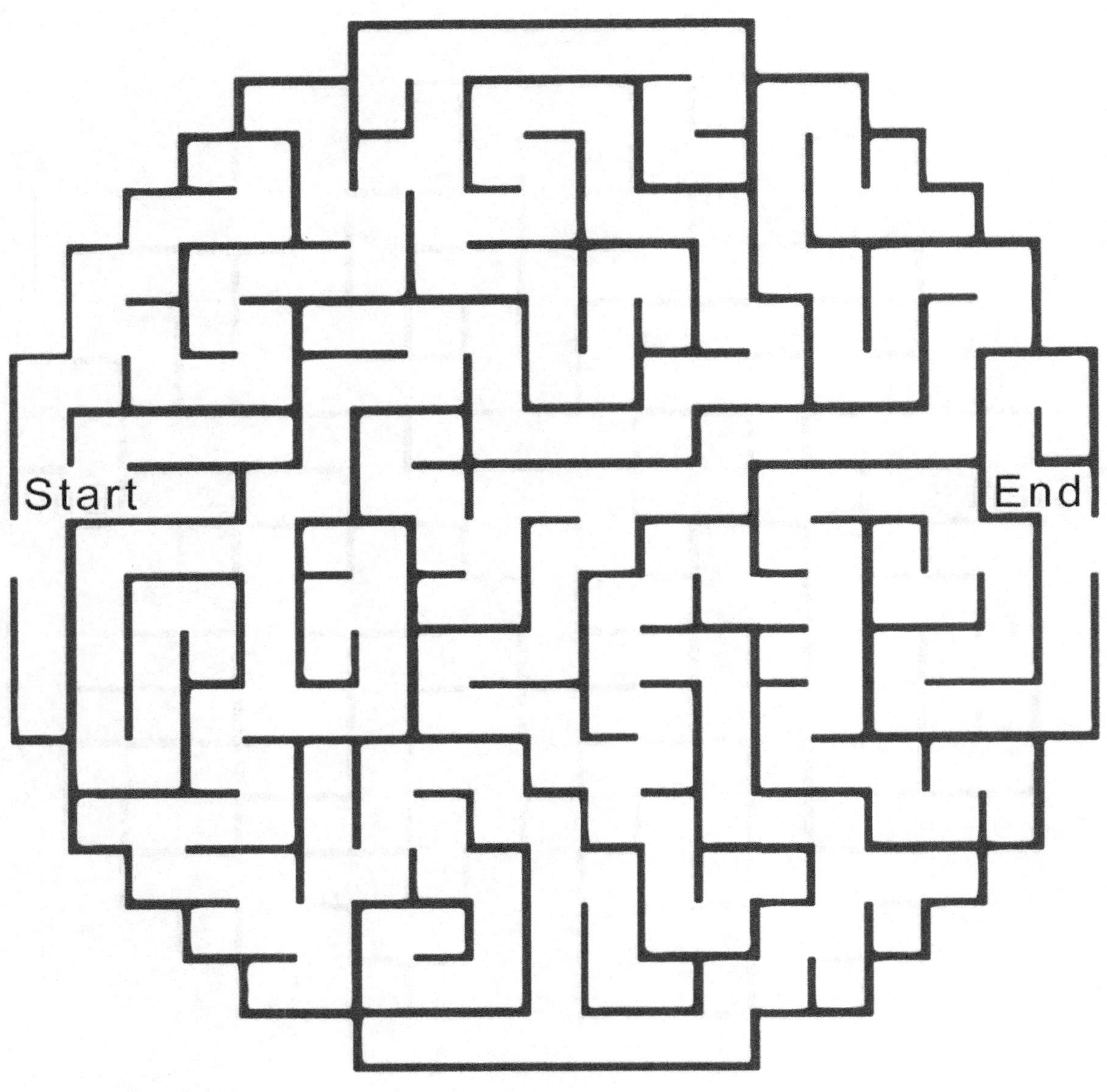

Start time: __________ End time: __________

Total time, maze 3: __________

Total time for 1st maze: __________

Total time for 2nd maze: __________

Total time for 3rd maze: __________

Congratulations! Did you experience progress in faster completion times? Circle your answer.

Yes No

If you circled "No" don't be discouraged. Remember to rest and give thanks to your mind and body for completing the challenges. Celebrate your tremendous effort. Remember, a seed doesn't turn into a tree overnight.

Life is like a camera… focus on what's important, capture the good times, develop from the negatives, and if things don't work out, take another shot.

—*Unknown*

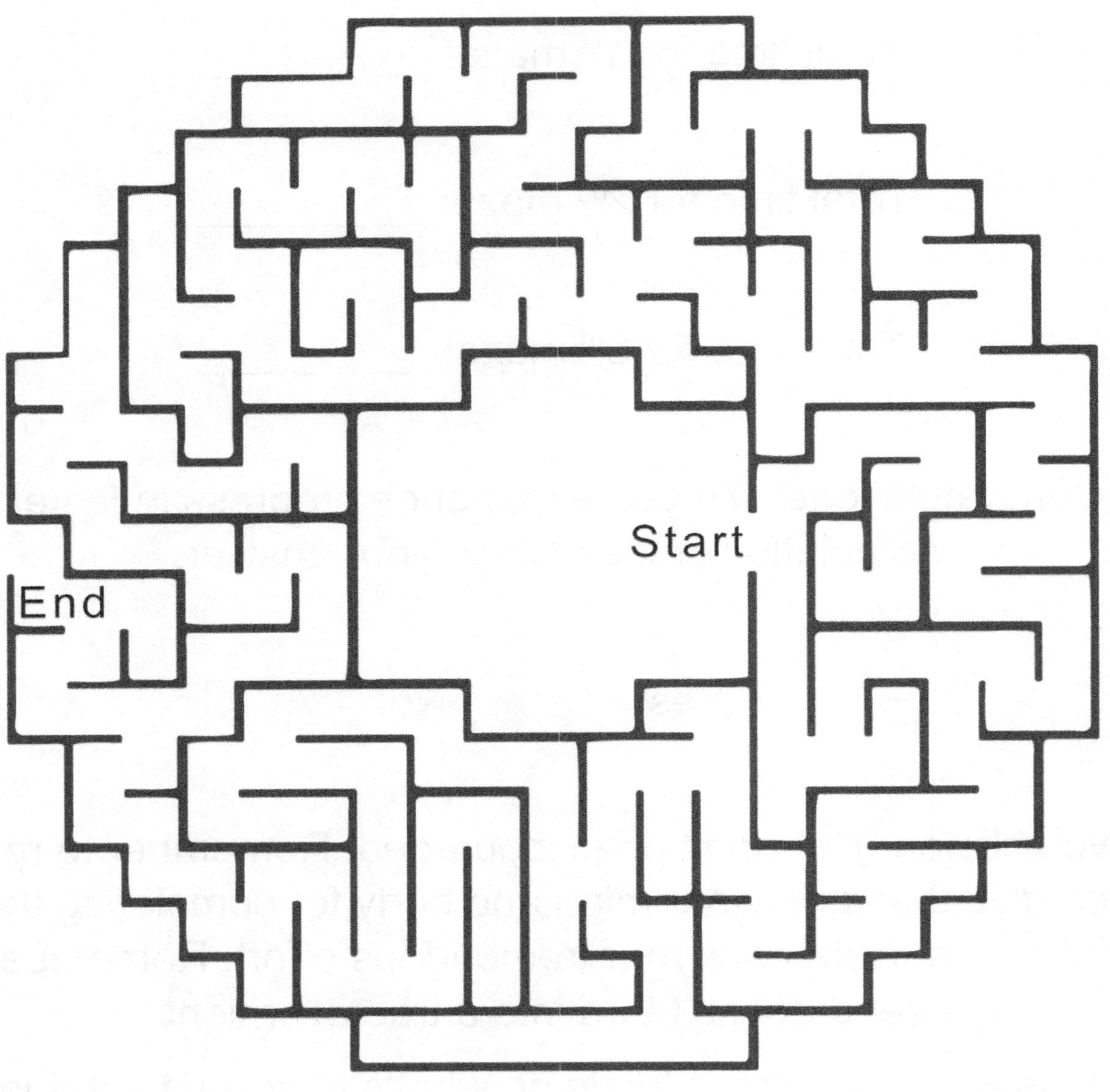

Start time: __________ End time: __________

Total time, maze 1: __________

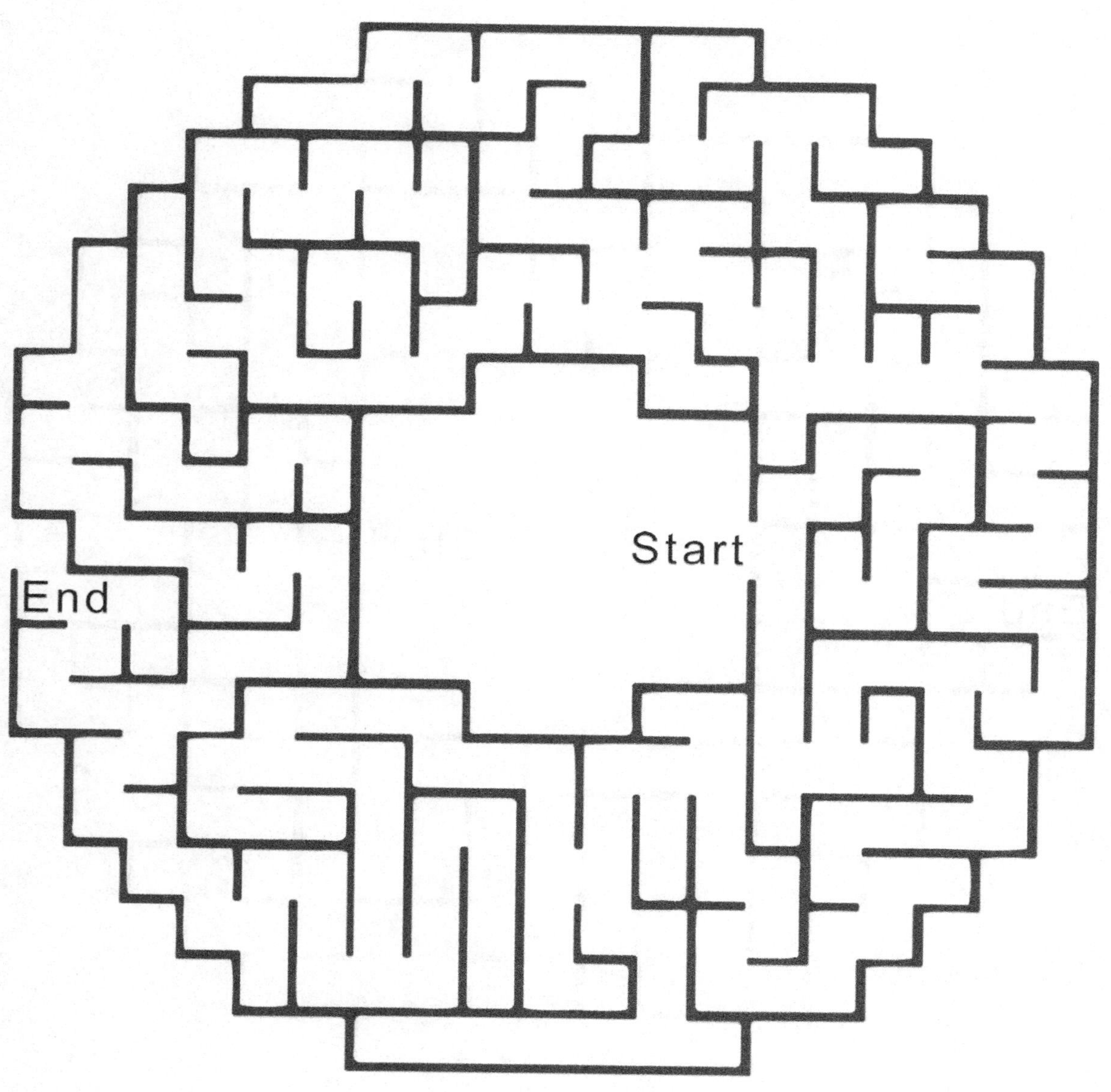

Start time: __________ End time: __________

Total time, maze 2: __________

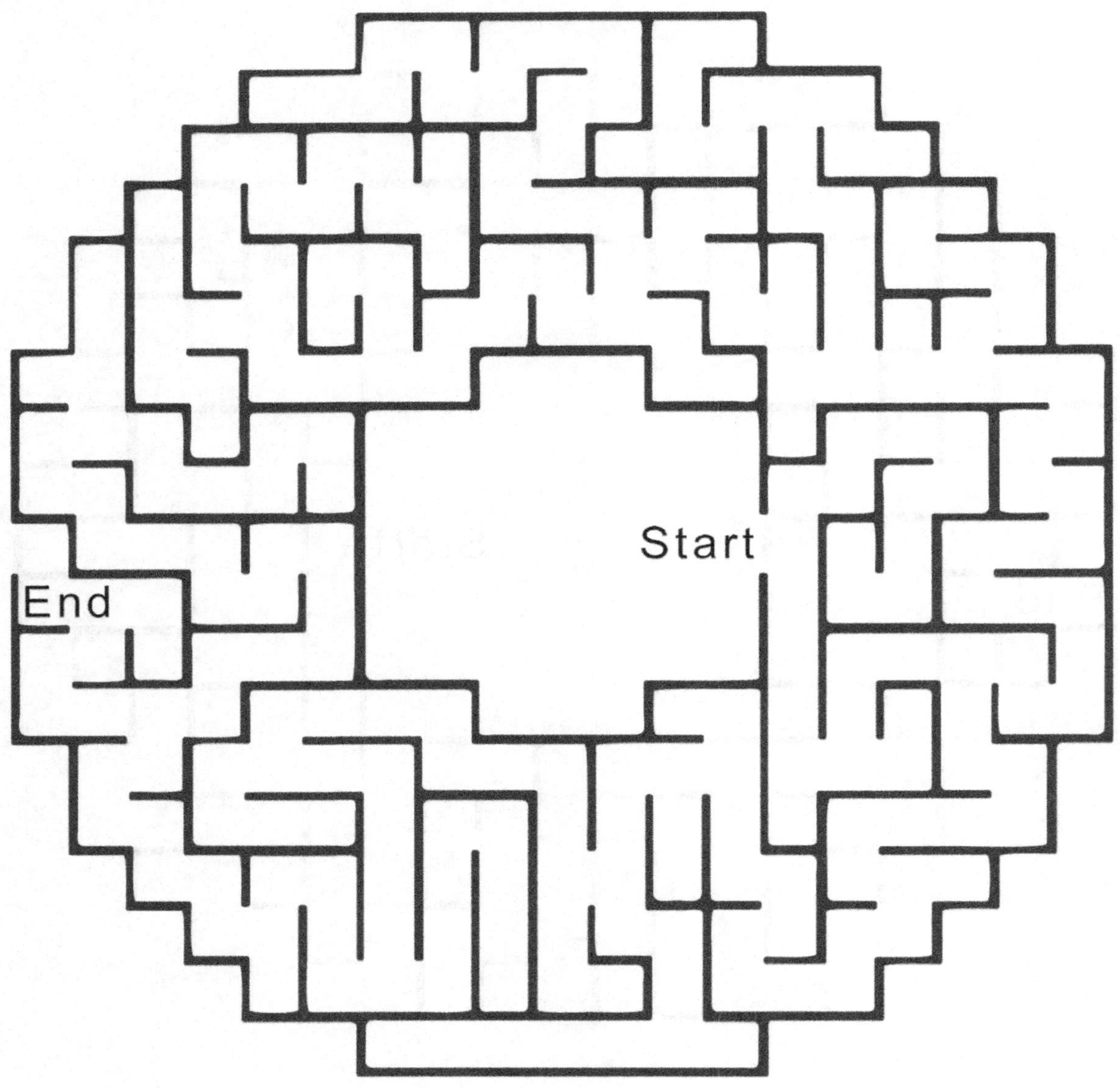

Start time: __________ End time: __________

Total time, maze 3: __________

Total time for 1st maze: ___________

Total time for 2nd maze: ___________

Total time for 3rd maze: ___________

Congratulations! Did you experience progress in faster completion times? Circle your answer.

Yes No

If you circled "No" don't be discouraged. Remember to rest and give thanks to your mind and body for completing the challenges. Celebrate your tremendous effort. Remember, a seed doesn't turn into a tree overnight.

Keep watering, keep planting, keep cultivating, and one day your garden will bloom.

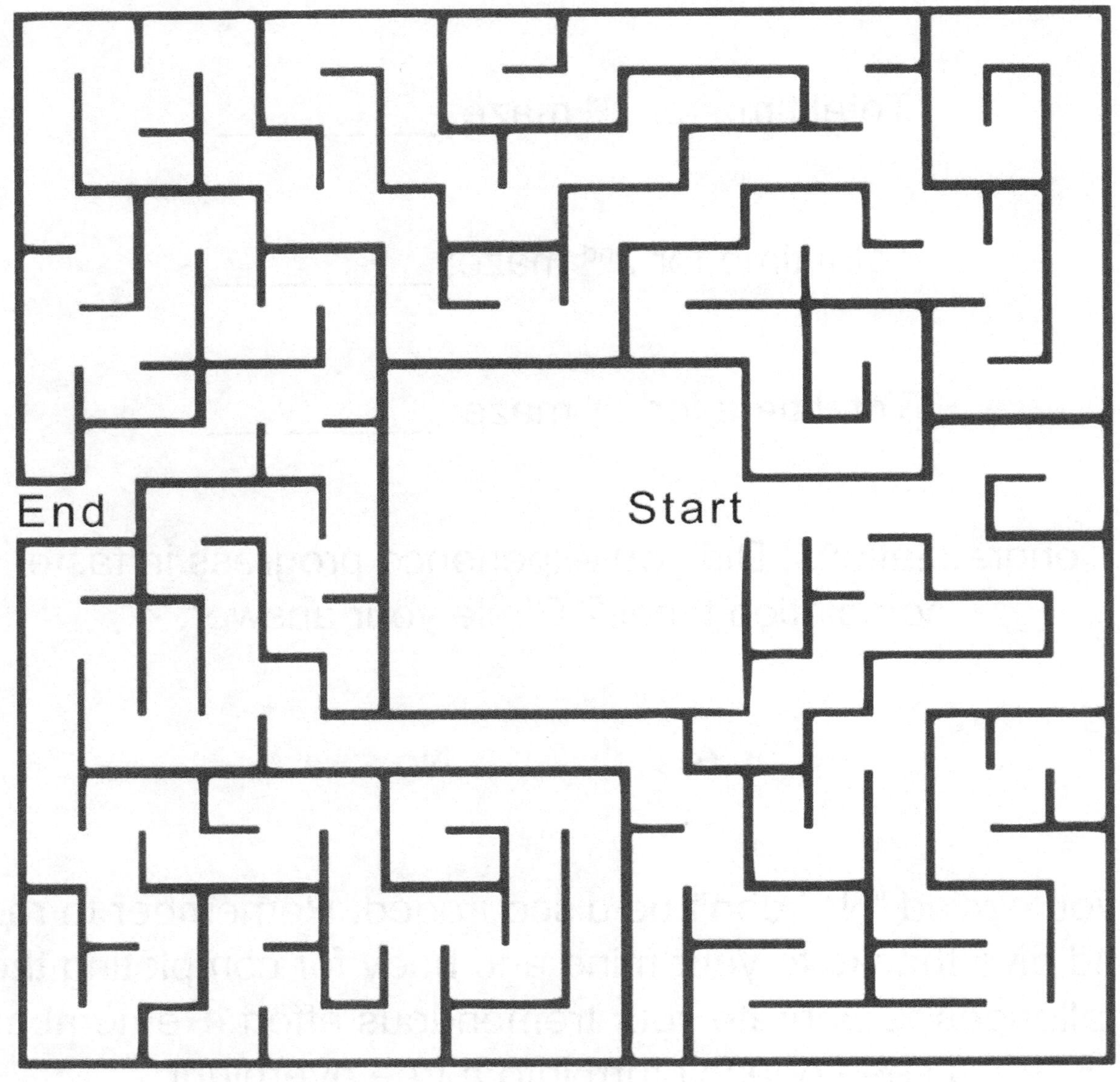

Start time: __________ End time: __________

Total time, maze 1: __________

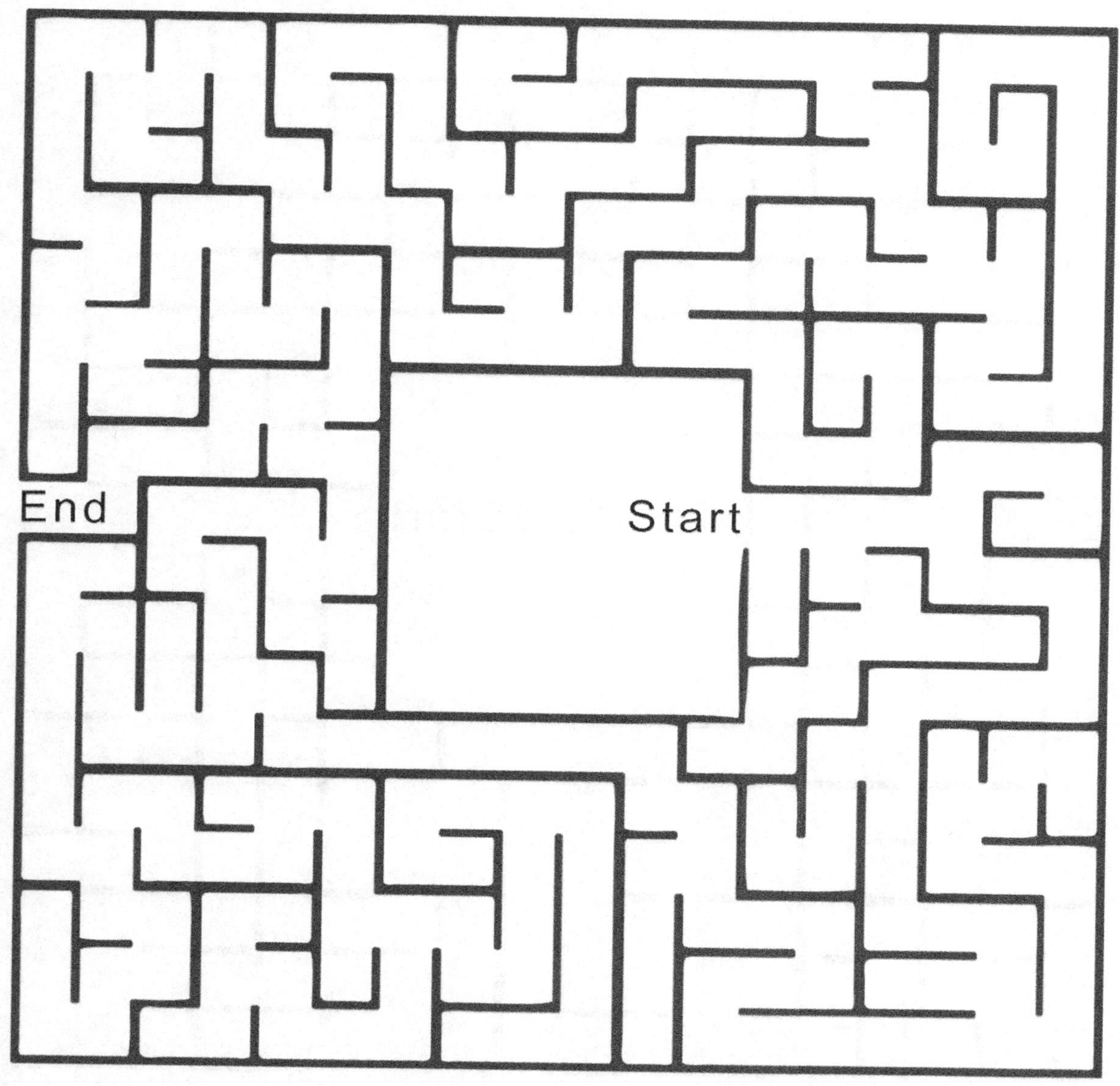

Start time: __________ End time: __________

Total time, maze 2: __________

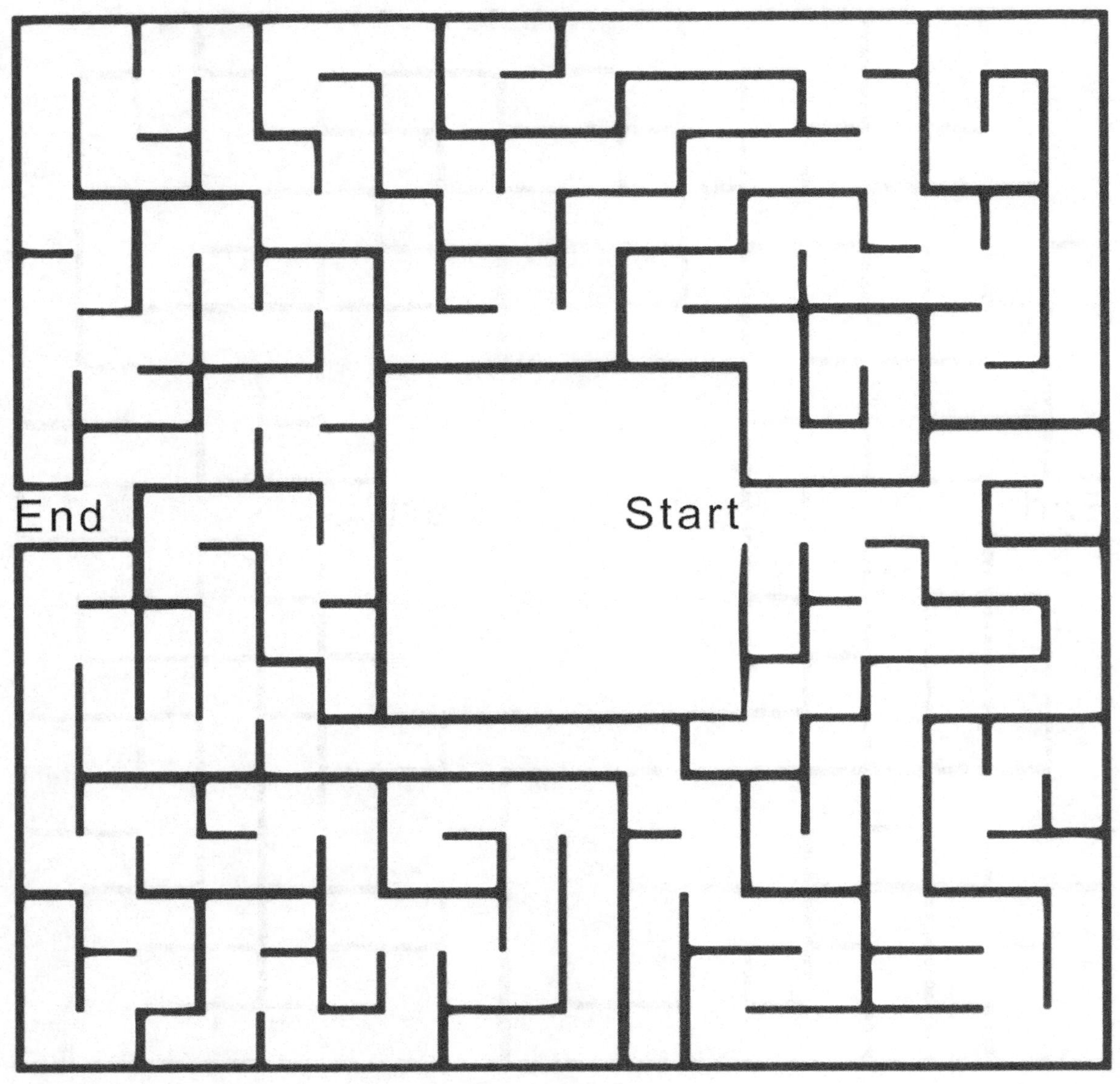

Start time: __________ End time: __________

Total time, maze 3: __________

Total time for 1st maze: __________

Total time for 2nd maze: __________

Total time for 3rd maze: __________

Congratulations! Did you experience progress in faster completion times? Circle your answer.

Yes No

If you circled “No” don’t be discouraged. Remember to rest and give thanks to your mind and body for completing the challenges. Celebrate your tremendous effort. Remember, a seed doesn’t turn into a tree overnight.

One of the things I learned the hard way was that it doesn't pay to get discouraged. Keeping busy and making optimism a way of life can restore your faith in yourself.

—Lucille Ball

Chapter 2.

25 INTERMEDIATE PUZZLES (in Triplicate to Track your Progress)

Courage in the Wake of Loss Affirmation

I savor each moment, because I do not know
exactly when a heavy gust or breeze might blow.
Should it be today, I'll shed my sorrow in a tear
while my courage battles the uncertainty I fear.

Dreadful emotions, for which I can't prepare,
will likely taunt me with sporadic dispair,
but I'll be patient amid the highs and lows
for that is the process by which grieving goes.

I will accept my fate in spite of the stress and strain,
ignoring should'ves, could'ves, would'ves to rid my pain;
as will the sun's radiance on my thirsty skin
restore in good time my contented grin.

—*Maria C. Dawson*

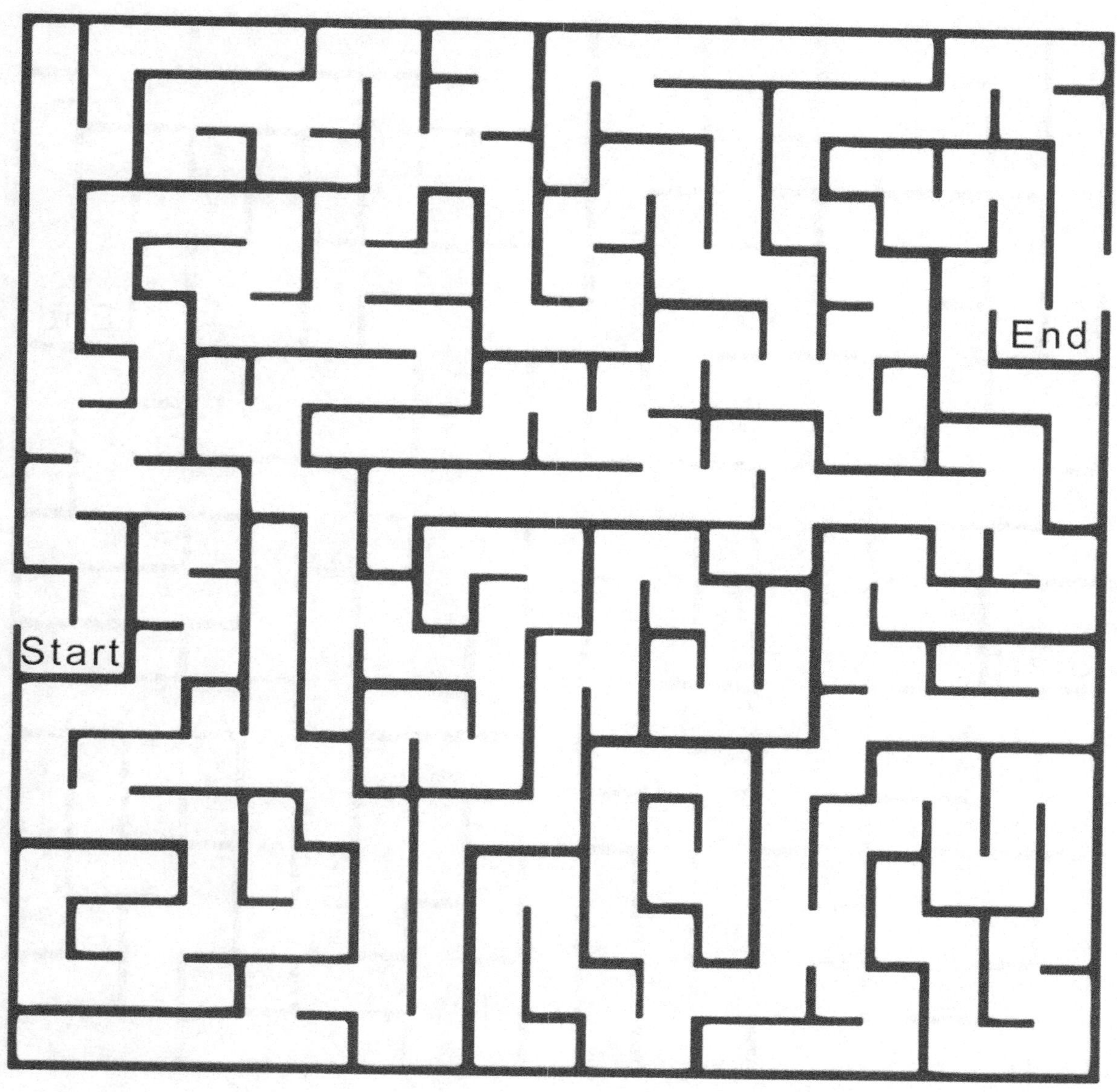

Start time: __________ End time: __________

Total time, maze 1: __________

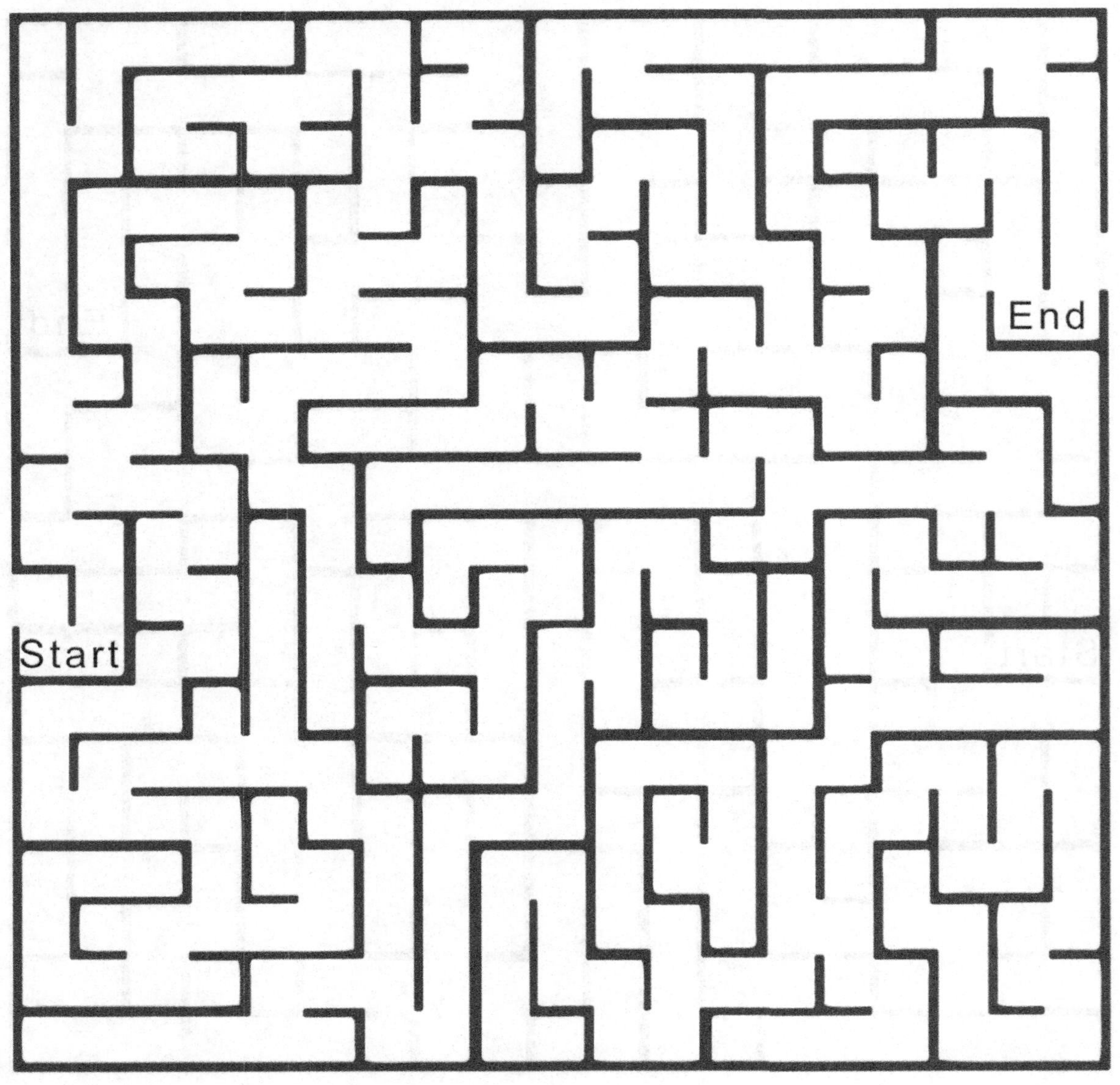

Start time: __________ End time: __________

Total time, maze 2: __________

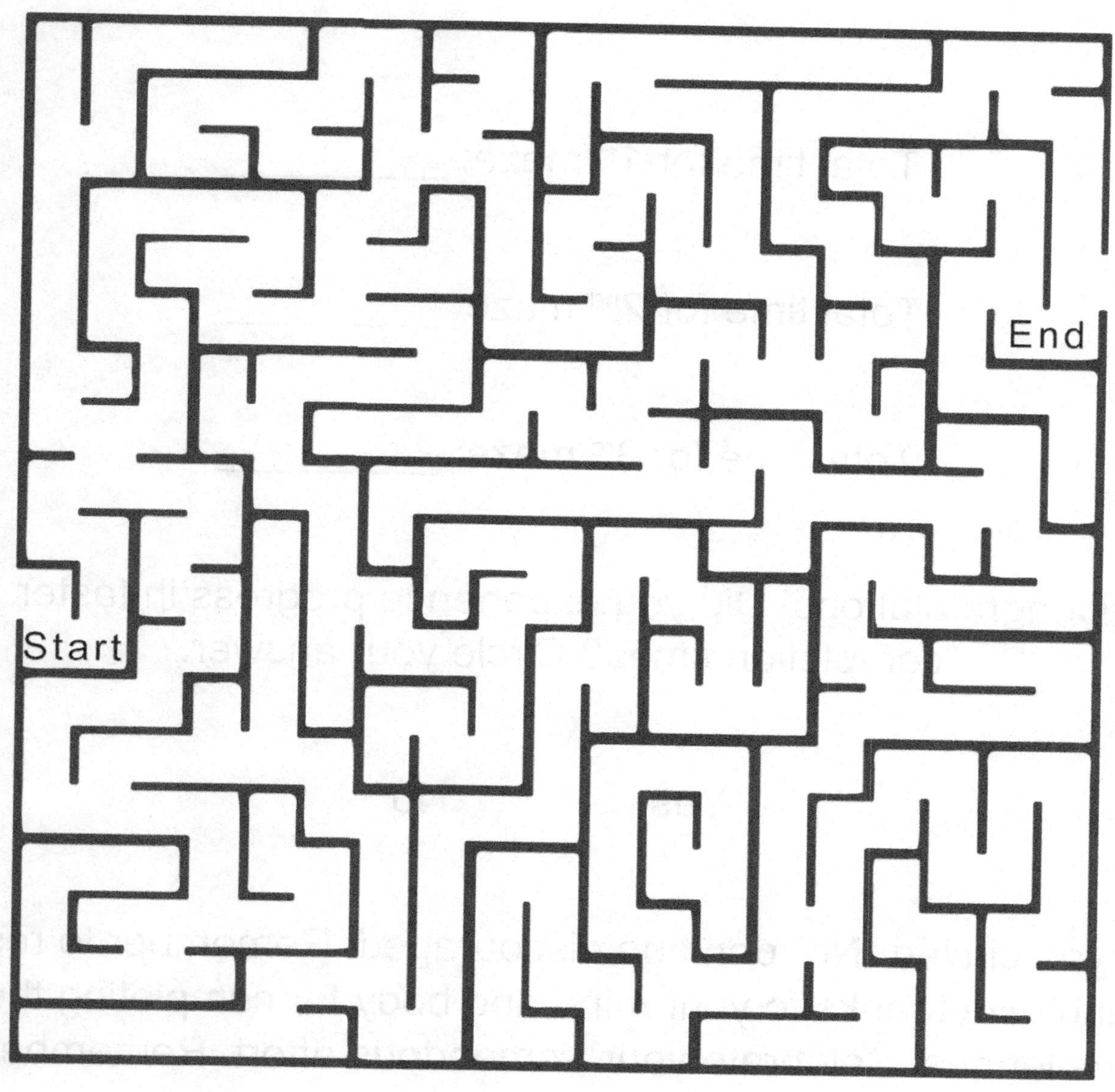

Start time: __________ End time: __________

Total time, maze 3: __________

Total time for 1st maze: __________

Total time for 2nd maze: __________

Total time for 3rd maze: __________

Congratulations! Did you experience progress in faster completion times? Circle your answer.

Yes No

If you circled "No" don't be discouraged. Remember to rest and give thanks to your mind and body for completing the challenges. Celebrate your tremendous effort. Remember, a seed doesn't turn into a tree overnight.

Edison failed 10,000 times before he made the electric light. Do not be discouraged if you fail a few times.

—Napoleon Hill

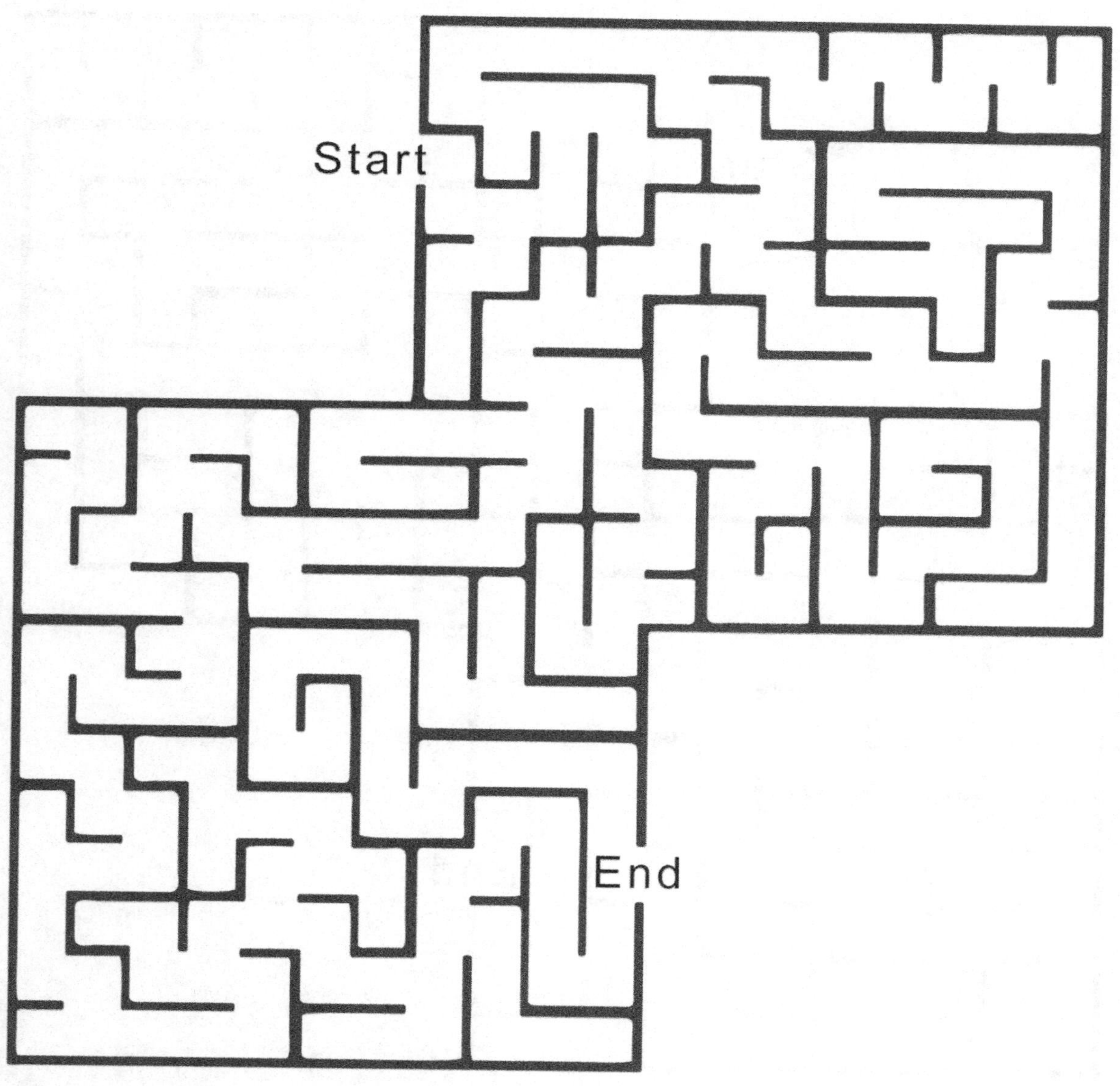

Start time: ___________ End time: ___________

Total time, maze 1: ___________

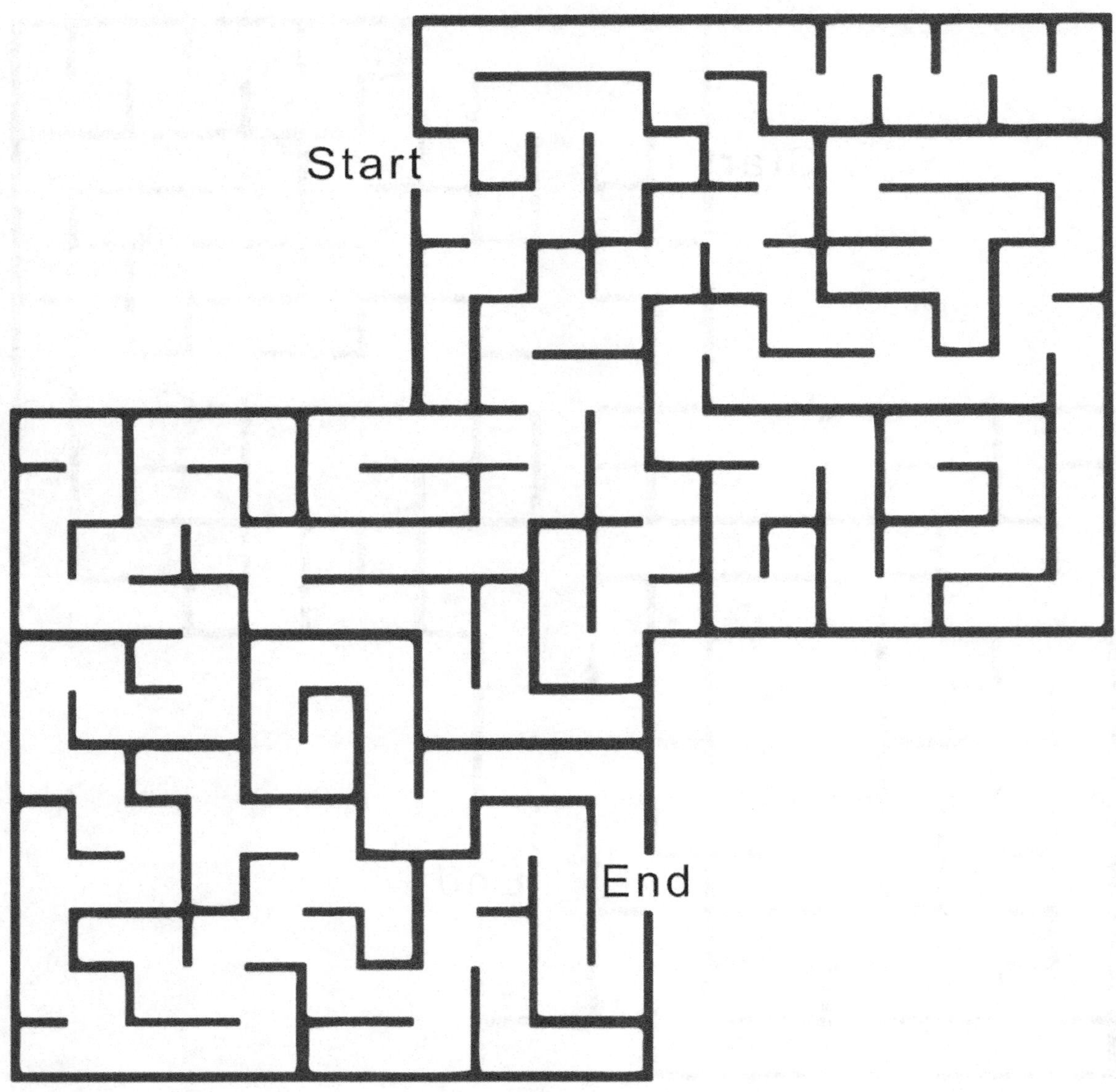

Start time: __________ End time: __________

Total time, maze 2: __________

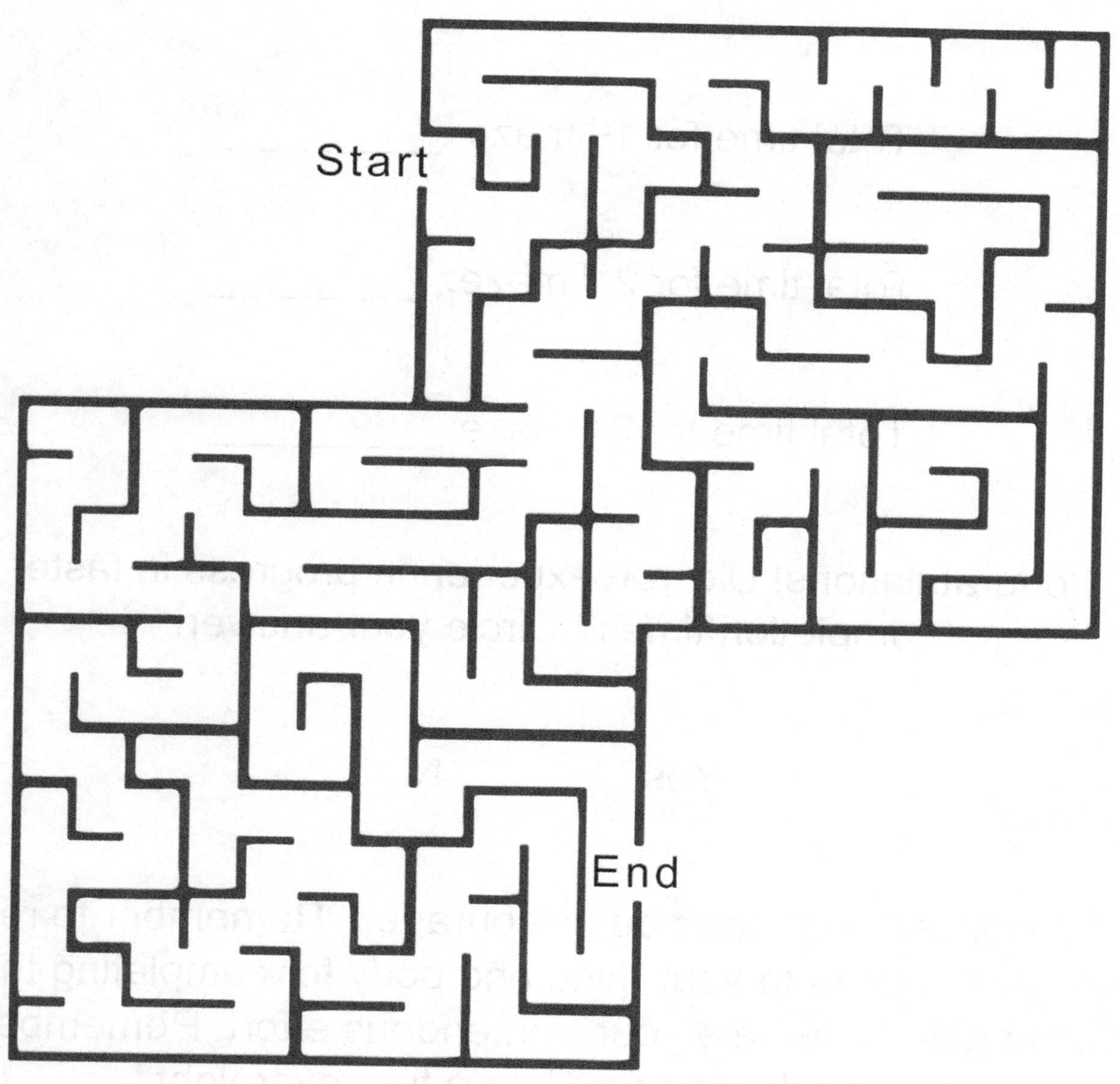

Start time: __________ End time: __________

Total time, maze 3: __________

Total time for 1st maze: __________

Total time for 2nd maze: __________

Total time for 3rd maze: __________

Congratulations! Did you experience progress in faster completion times? Circle your answer.

Yes No

If you circled "No" don't be discouraged. Remember to rest and give thanks to your mind and body for completing the challenges. Celebrate your tremendous effort. Remember, a seed doesn't turn into a tree overnight.

A man can get discouraged many times but he is not a failure until he begins to blame somebody else and stops trying.

—*John Burroughs*

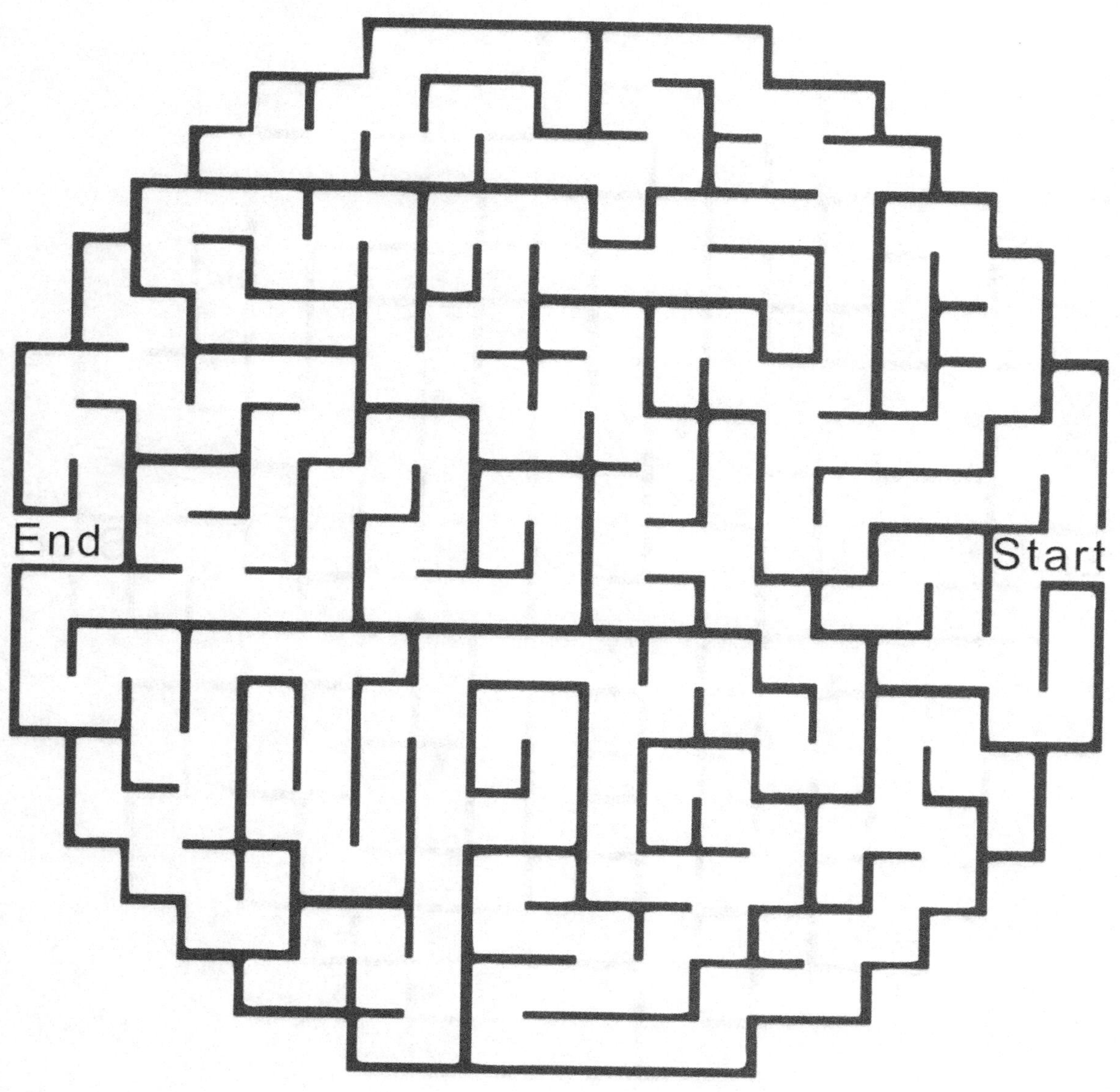

Start time: ___________ End time: ___________

Total time, maze 1: ___________

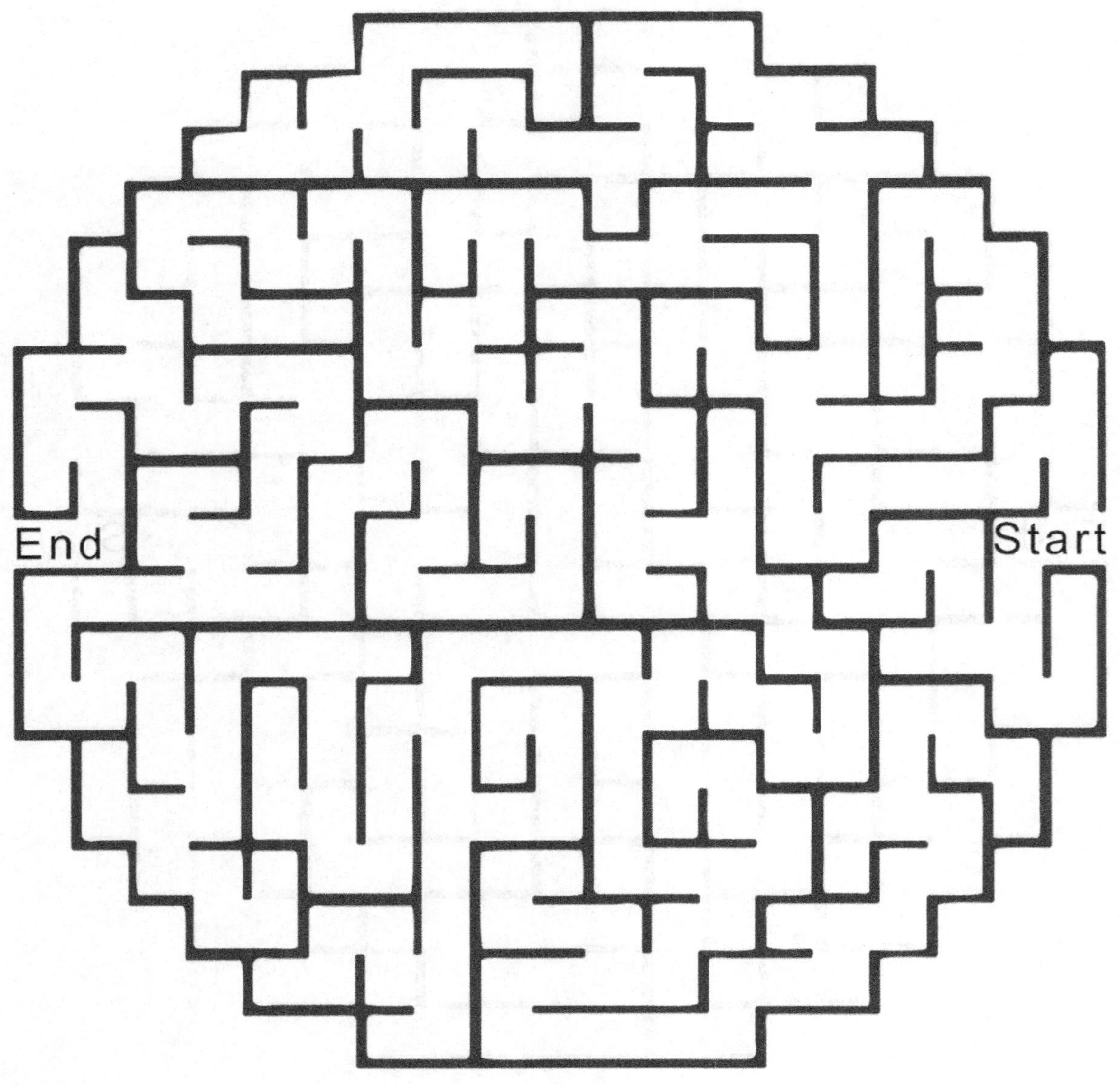

Start time: __________ End time: __________

Total time, maze 2: __________

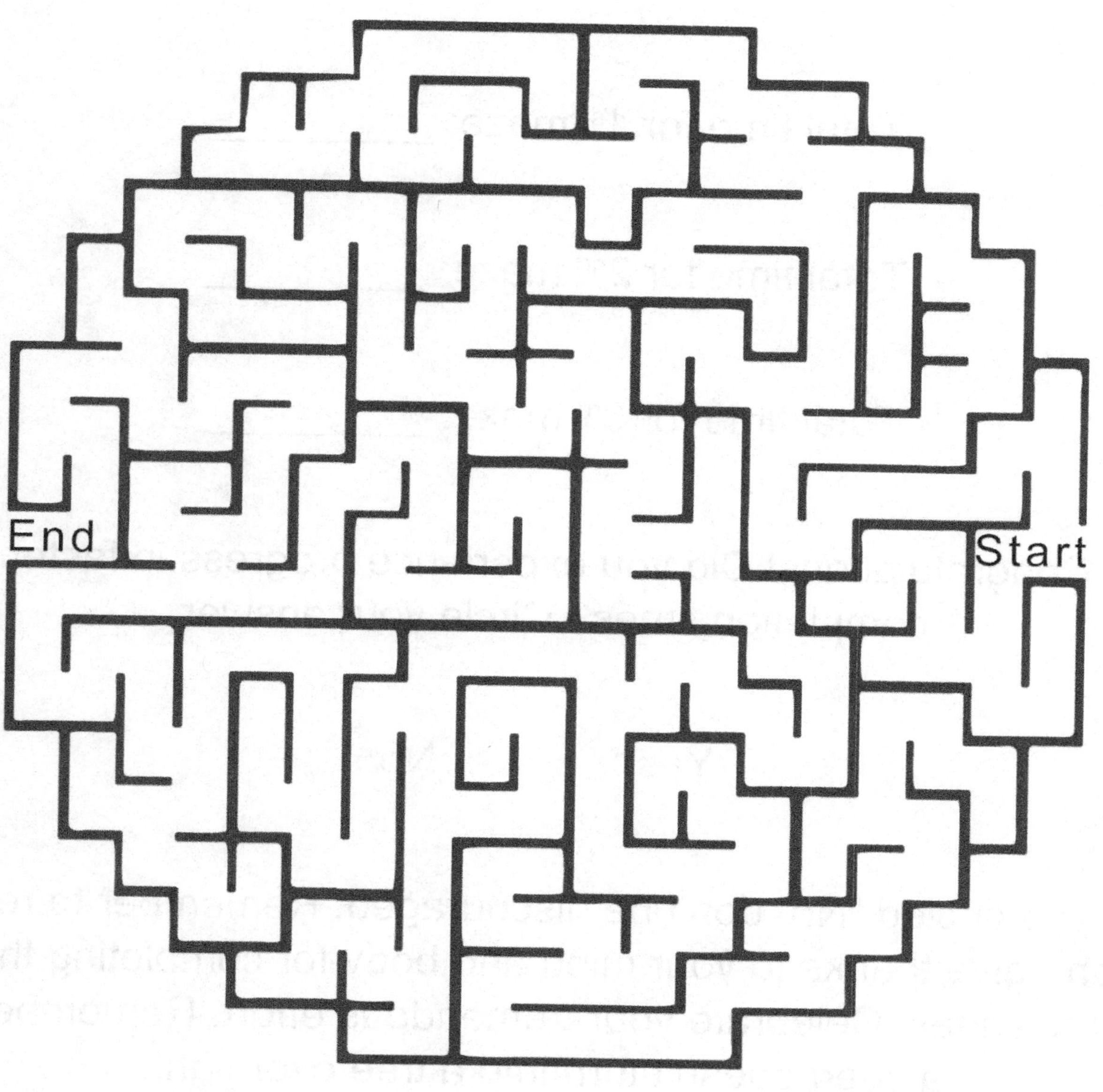

Start time: __________ End time: __________

Total time, maze 3: __________

Total time for 1st maze: __________

Total time for 2nd maze: __________

Total time for 3rd maze: __________

Congratulations! Did you experience progress in faster completion times? Circle your answer.

Yes No

If you circled “No” don’t be discouraged. Remember to rest and give thanks to your mind and body for completing the challenges. Celebrate your tremendous effort. Remember, a seed doesn’t turn into a tree overnight.

Continuous, unflagging effort, persistence and determination will win. Let not the man be discouraged who has these.

—James Whitcomb Riley

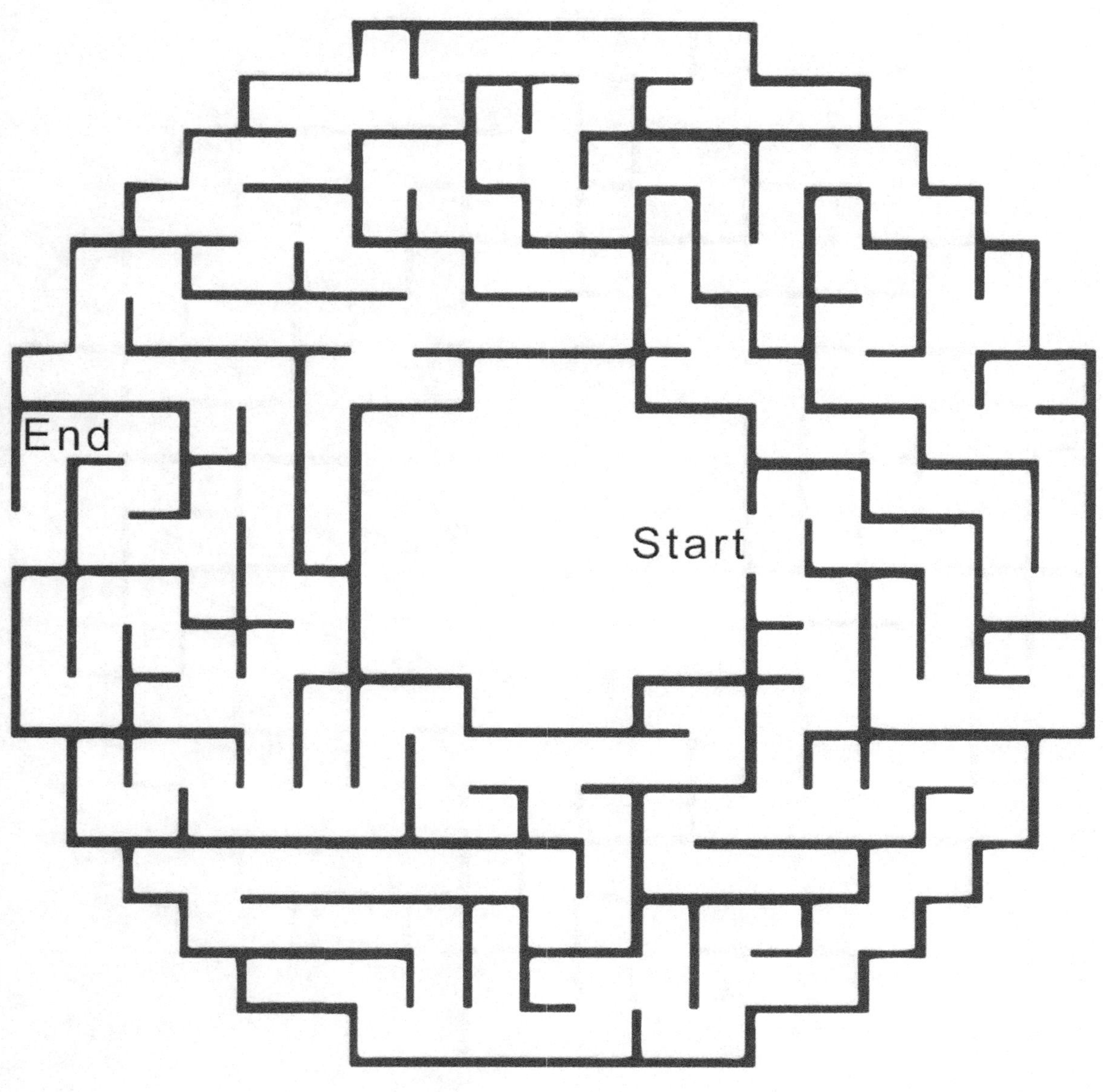

Start time: __________ End time: __________

Total time, maze 1: __________

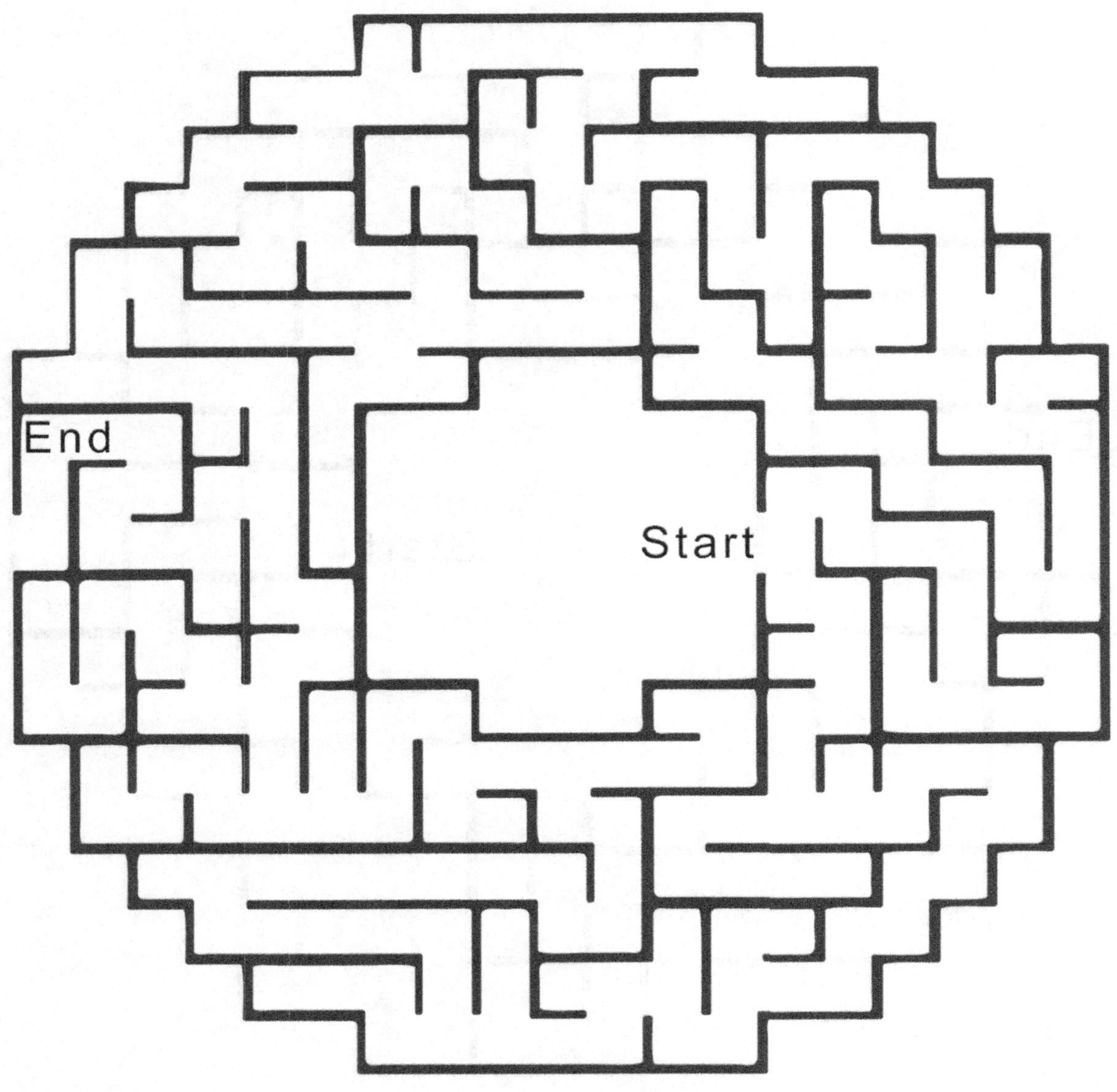

Start time: __________ End time: __________

Total time, maze 2: __________

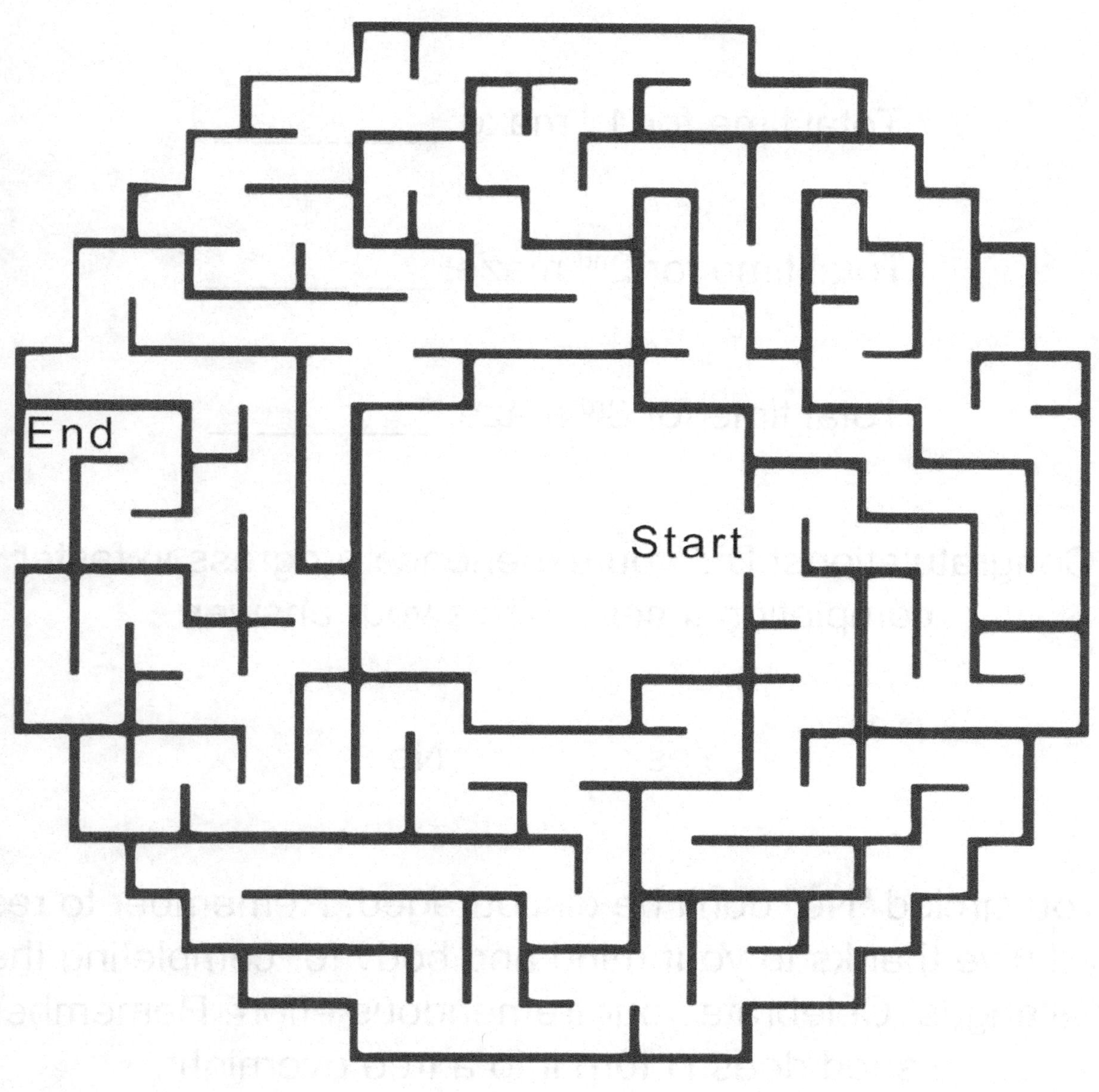

Start time: __________ End time: __________

Total time, maze 3: __________

Total time for 1st maze: __________

Total time for 2nd maze: __________

Total time for 3rd maze: __________

Congratulations! Did you experience progress in faster completion times? Circle your answer.

Yes No

If you circled “No” don’t be discouraged. Remember to rest and give thanks to your mind and body for completing the challenges. Celebrate your tremendous effort. Remember, a seed doesn’t turn into a tree overnight.

What is important is to believe in something so strongly that you're never discouraged.

—Salma Hayek

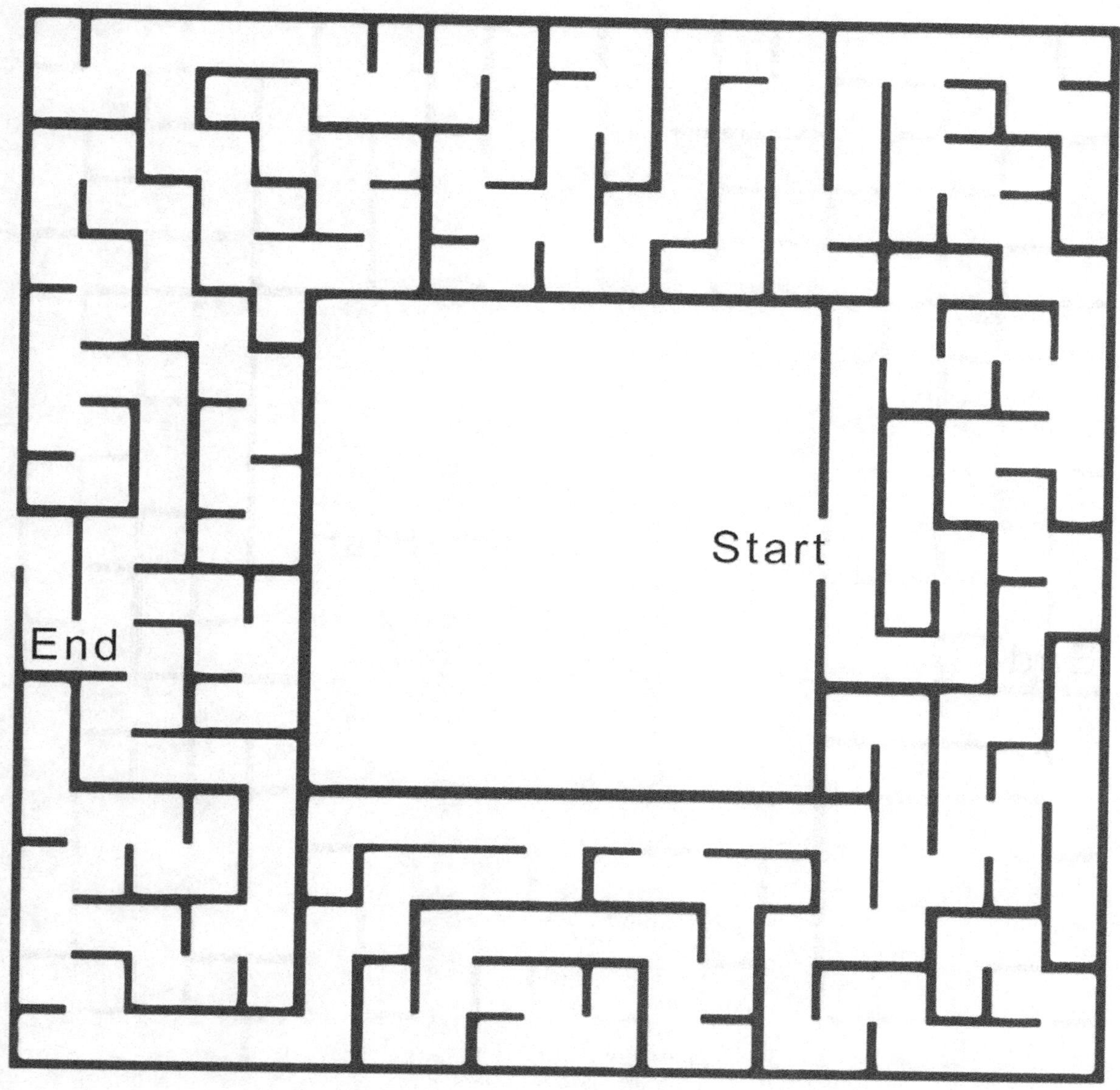

Start time: __________ End time: __________

Total time, maze 1: __________

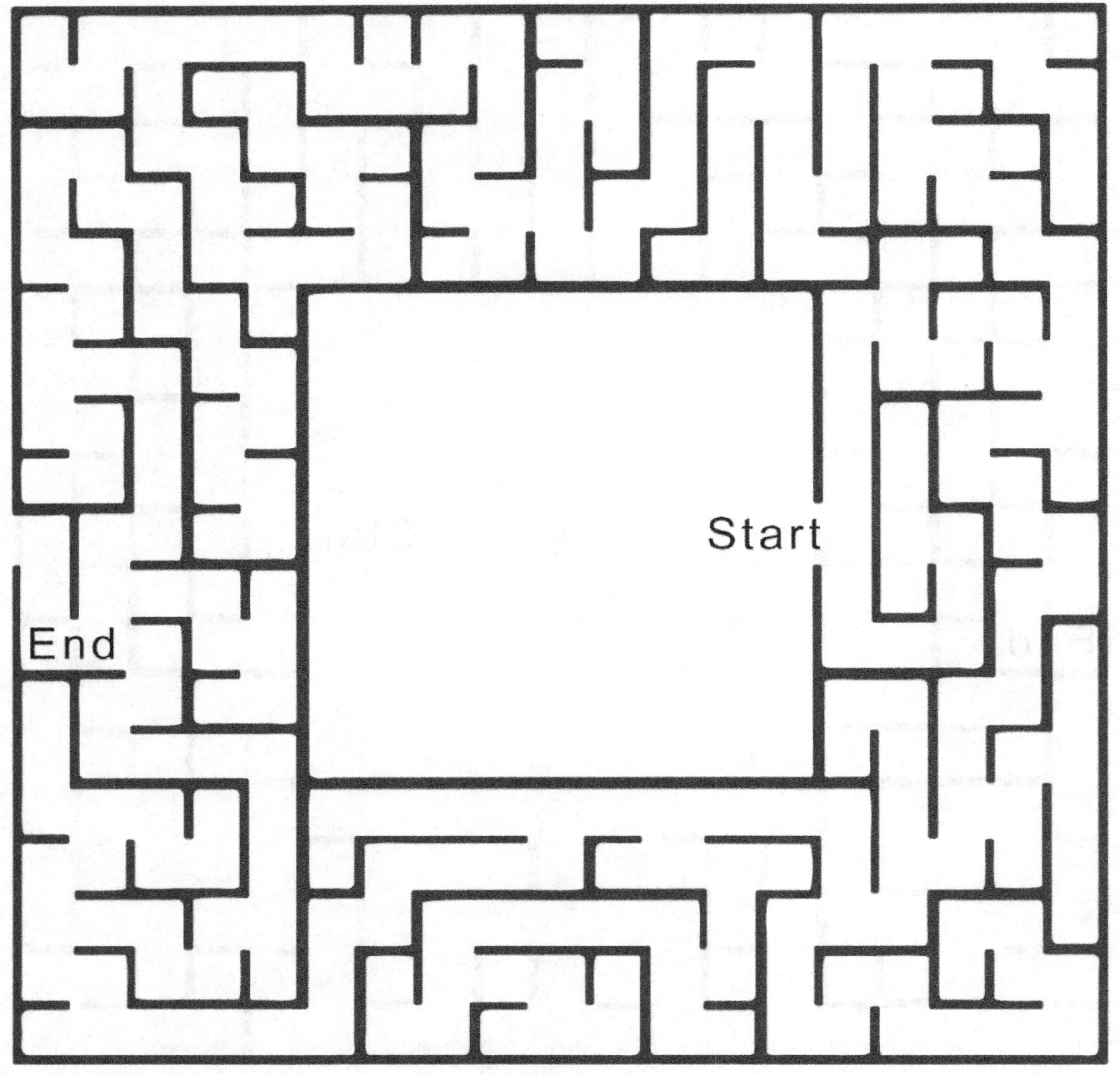

Start time: __________ End time: __________

Total time, maze 2: __________

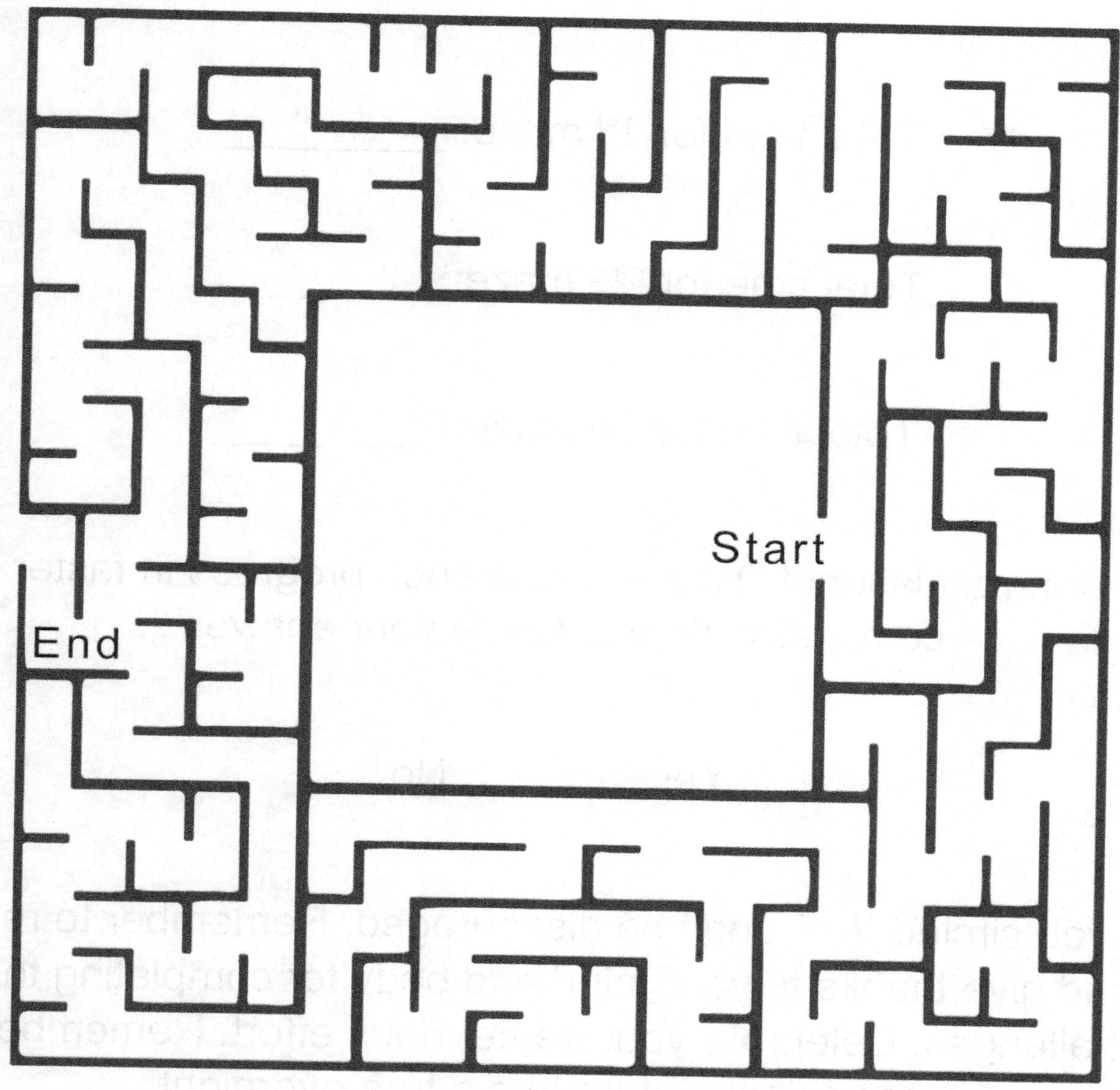

Start time: __________ End time: __________

Total time, maze 3: __________

Total time for 1st maze: __________

Total time for 2nd maze: __________

Total time for 3rd maze: __________

Congratulations! Did you experience progress in faster completion times? Circle your answer.

Yes No

If you circled "No" don't be discouraged. Remember to rest and give thanks to your mind and body for completing the challenges. Celebrate your tremendous effort. Remember, a seed doesn't turn into a tree overnight.

Stop beating yourself up. You are a work in progress - which means you get there a little at a time, not all at once.

—*Unknown*

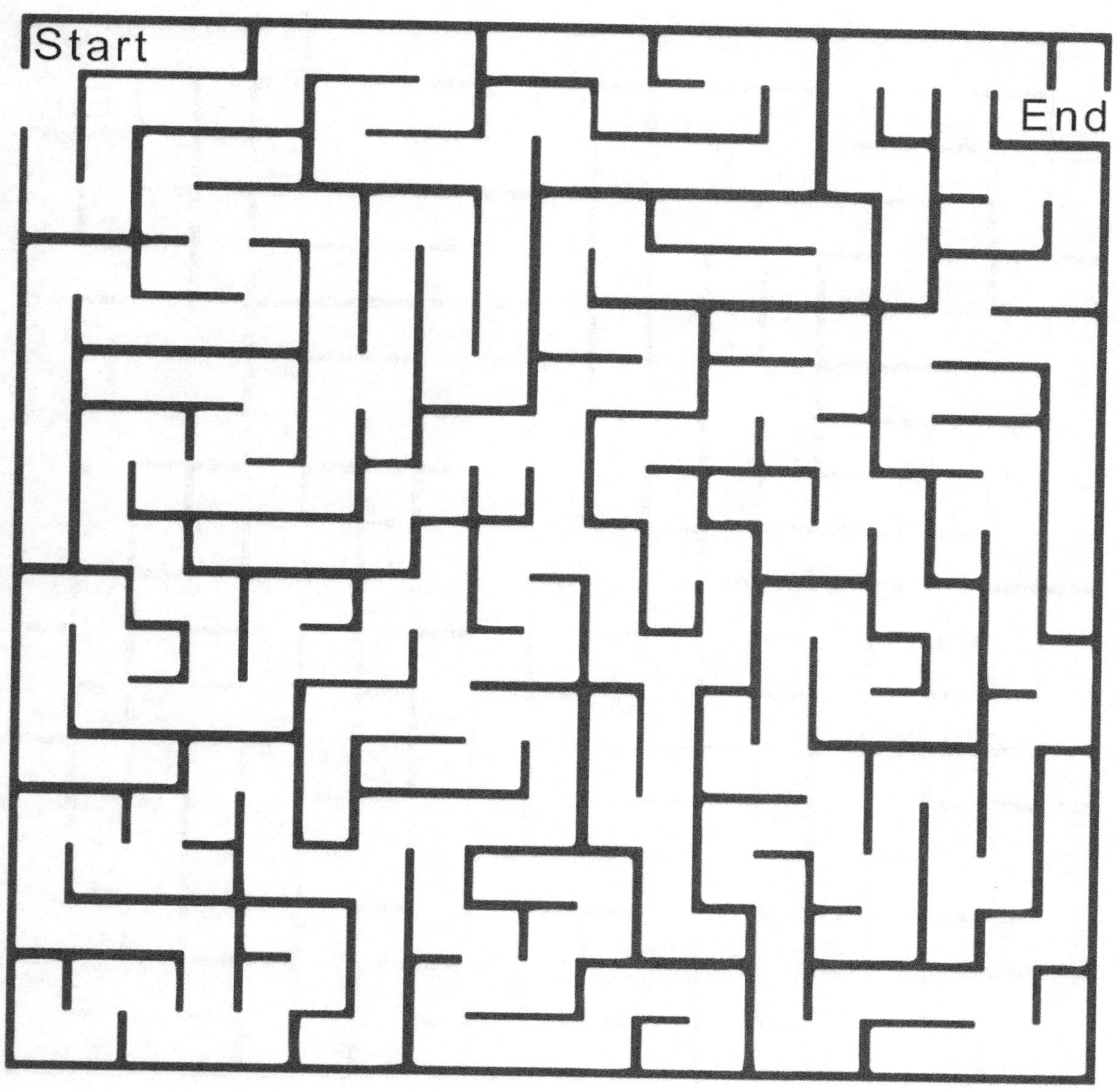

Start time: __________ End time: __________

Total time, maze 1: __________

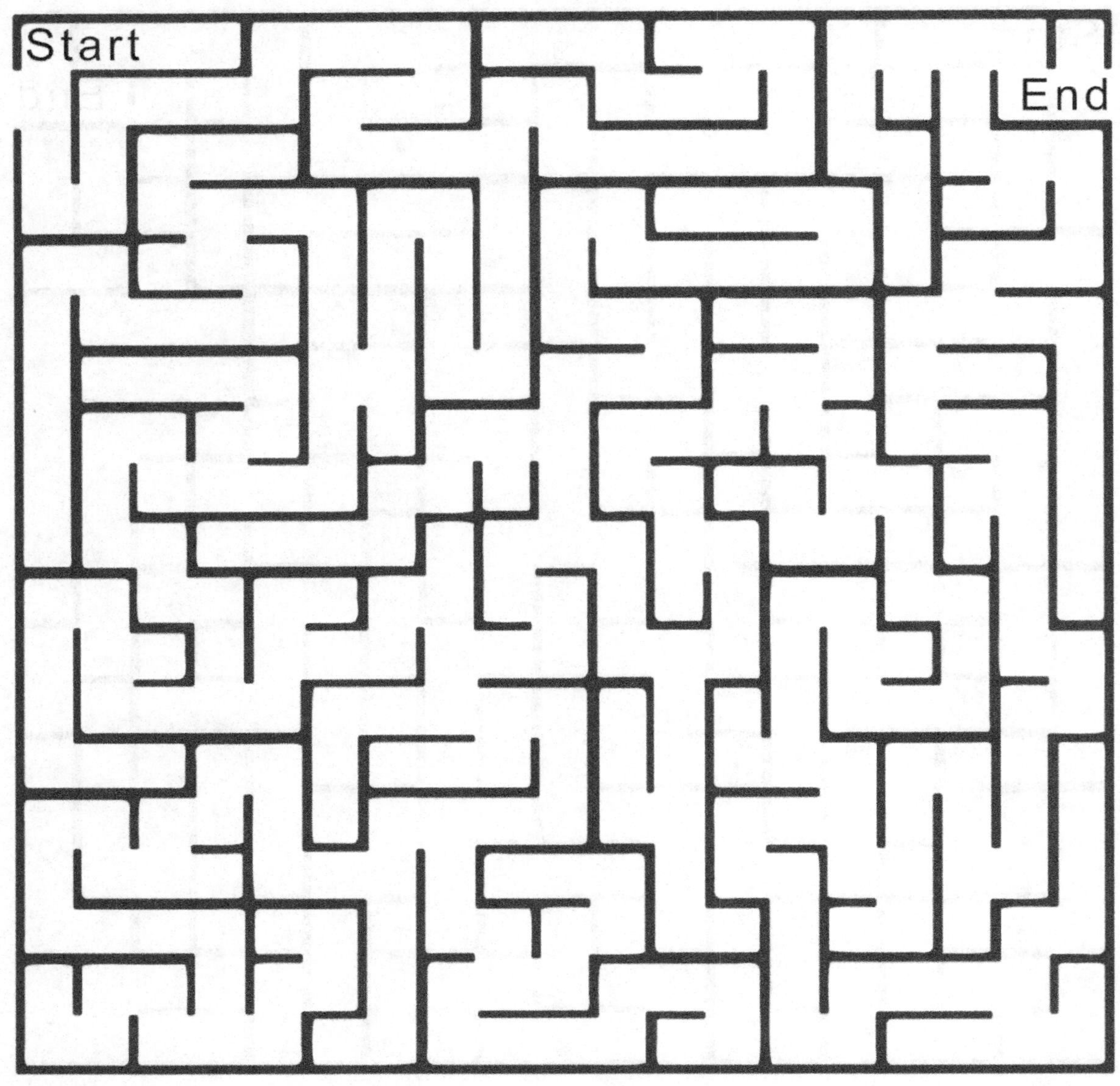

Start time: __________ End time: __________

Total time, maze 2: __________

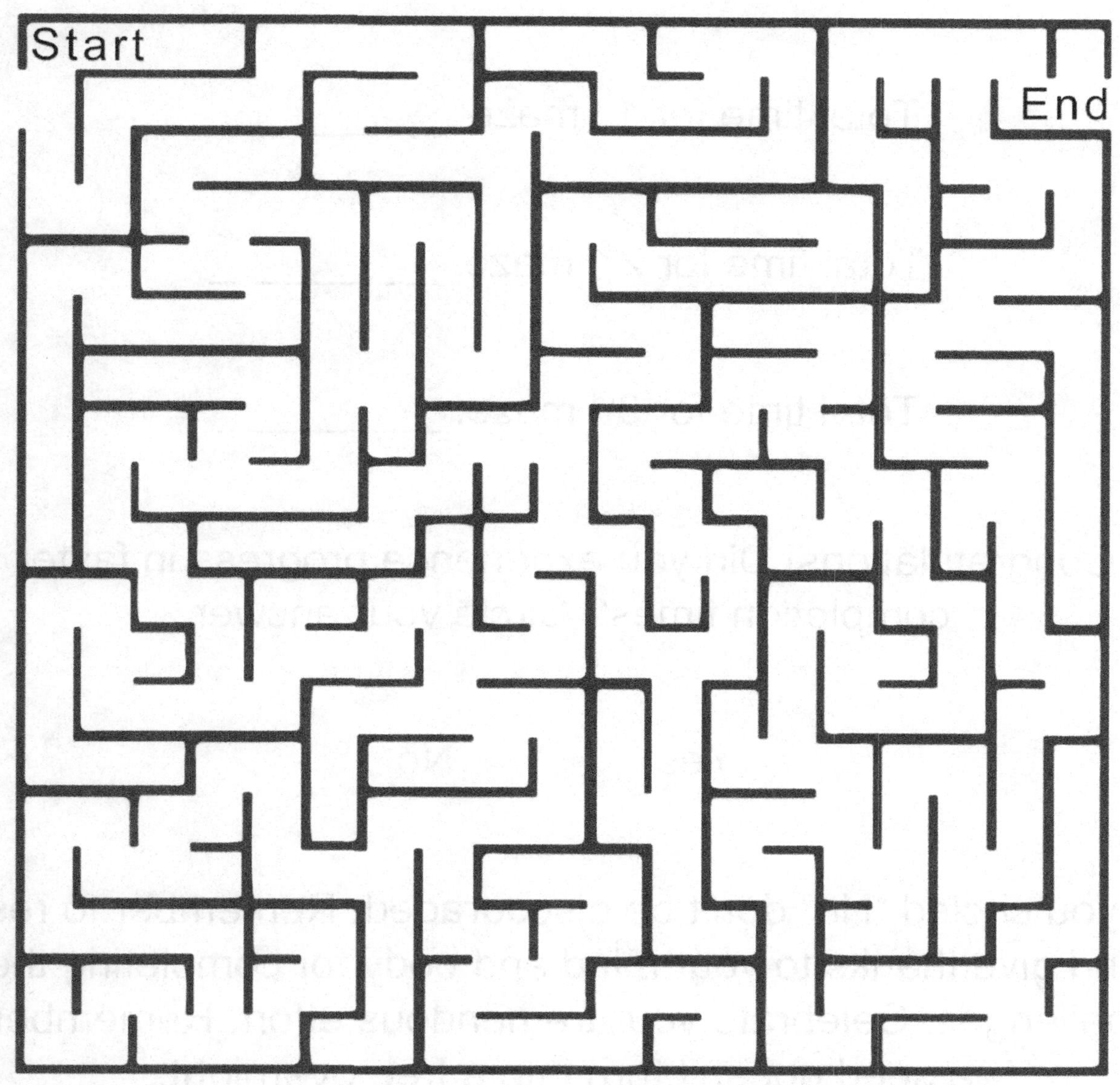

Start time: __________ End time: __________

Total time, maze 3: __________

Total time for 1st maze: __________

Total time for 2nd maze: __________

Total time for 3rd maze: __________

Congratulations! Did you experience progress in faster completion times? Circle your answer.

Yes No

If you circled "No" don't be discouraged. Remember to rest and give thanks to your mind and body for completing the challenges. Celebrate your tremendous effort. Remember, a seed doesn't turn into a tree overnight.

Yesterday I was clever so I wanted to change the world. Today I am wise, so I am changing myself.

—*Rumi*

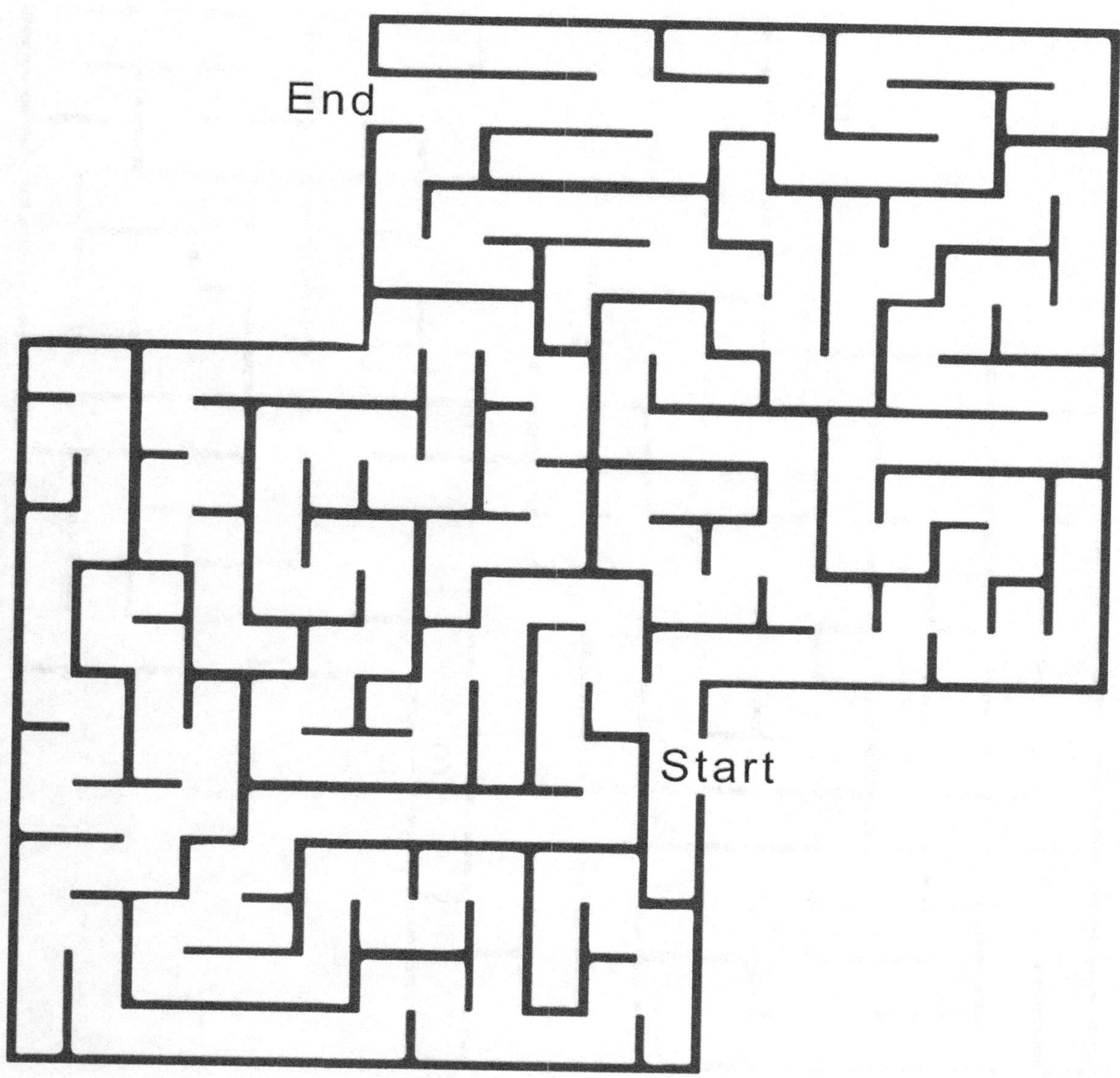

Start time: __________ End time: __________

Total time, maze 1: __________

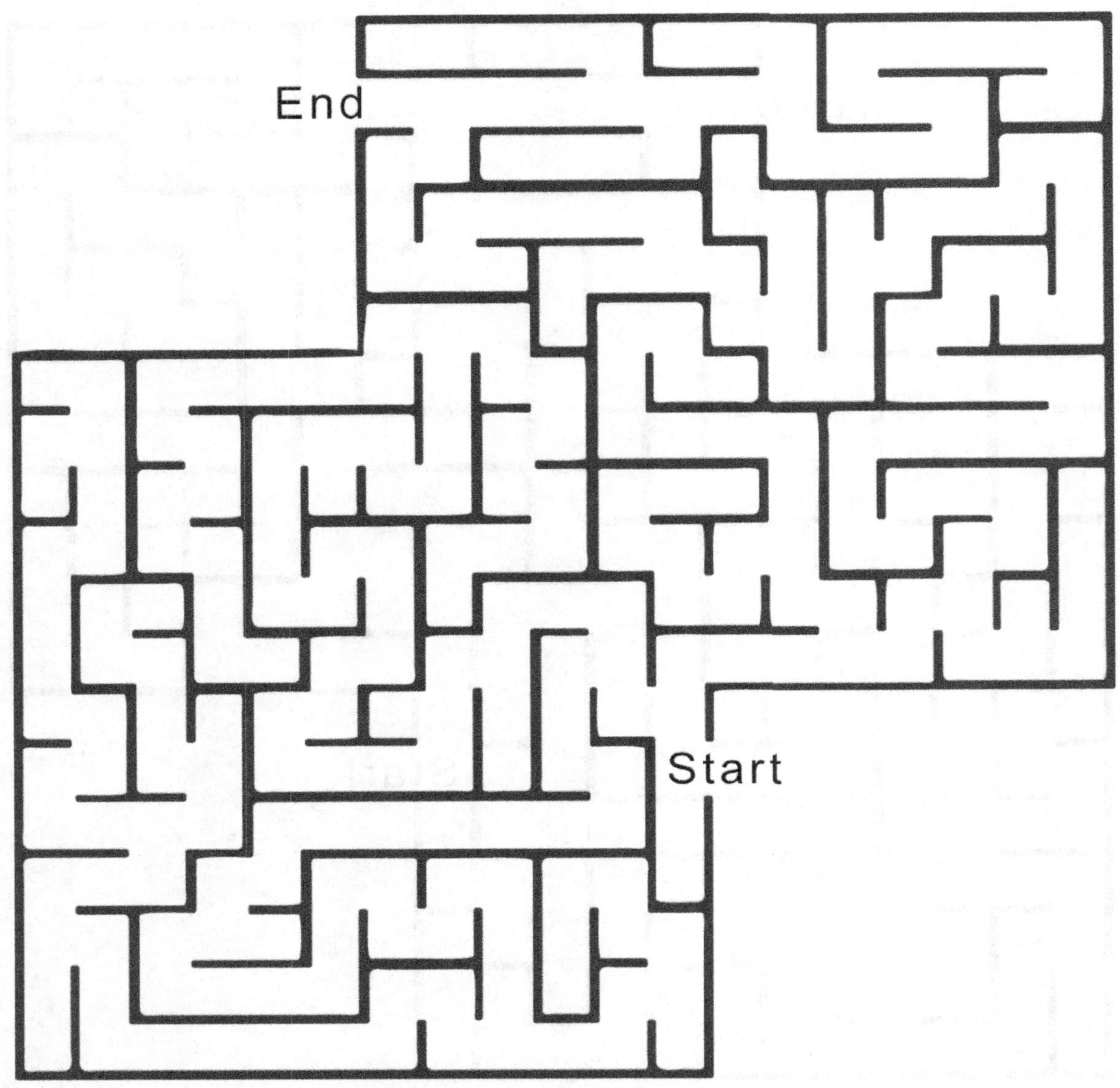

Start time: __________ End time: __________

Total time, maze 2: __________

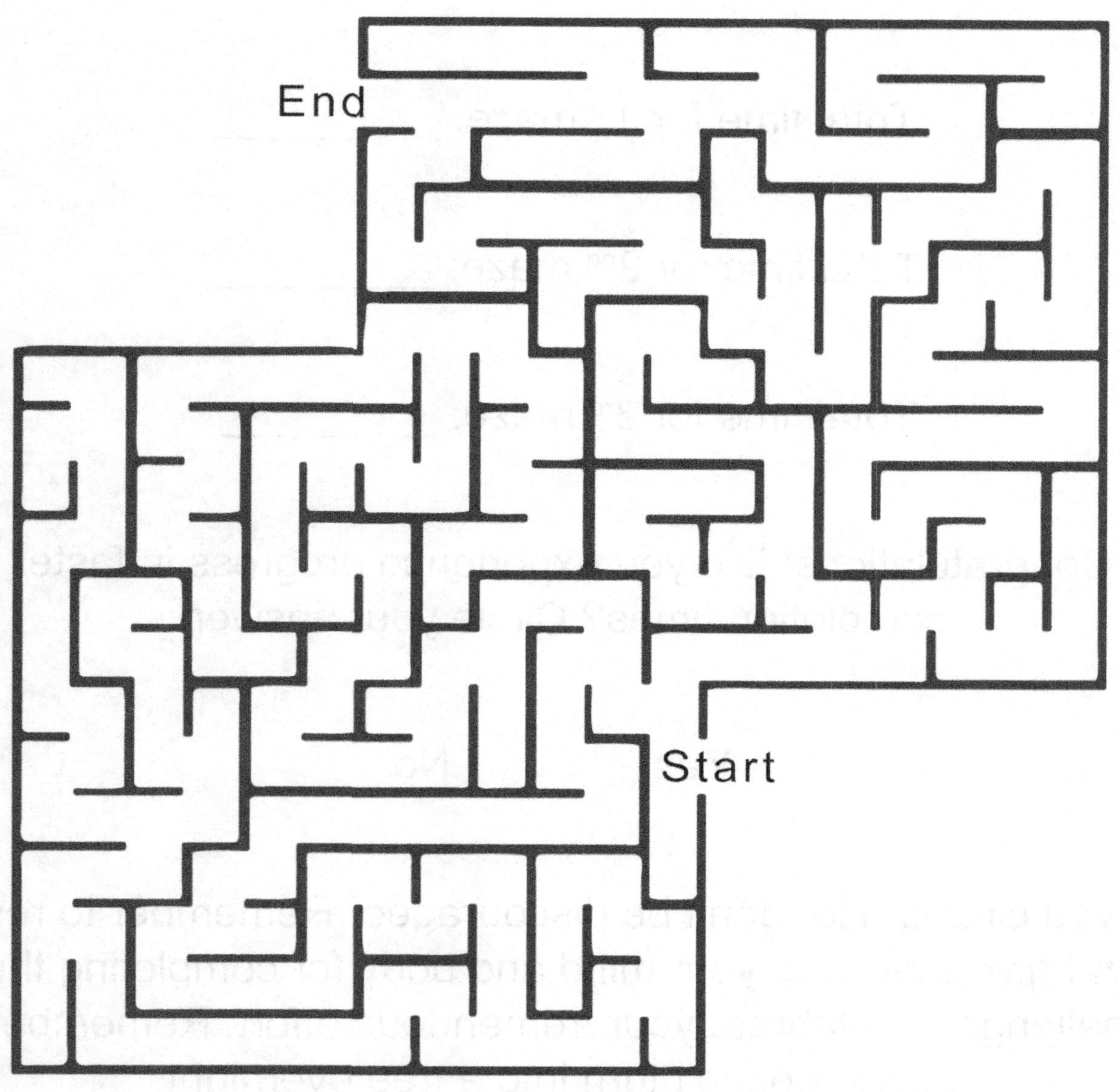

Start time: __________ End time: __________

Total time, maze 3: __________

Total time for 1st maze: __________

Total time for 2nd maze: __________

Total time for 3rd maze: __________

Congratulations! Did you experience progress in faster completion times? Circle your answer.

Yes No

If you circled "No" don't be discouraged. Remember to rest and give thanks to your mind and body for completing the challenges. Celebrate your tremendous effort. Remember, a seed doesn't turn into a tree overnight.

If you really want to do something, you'll find a way. If you don't, you'll find an excuse.

—Jim Rohn

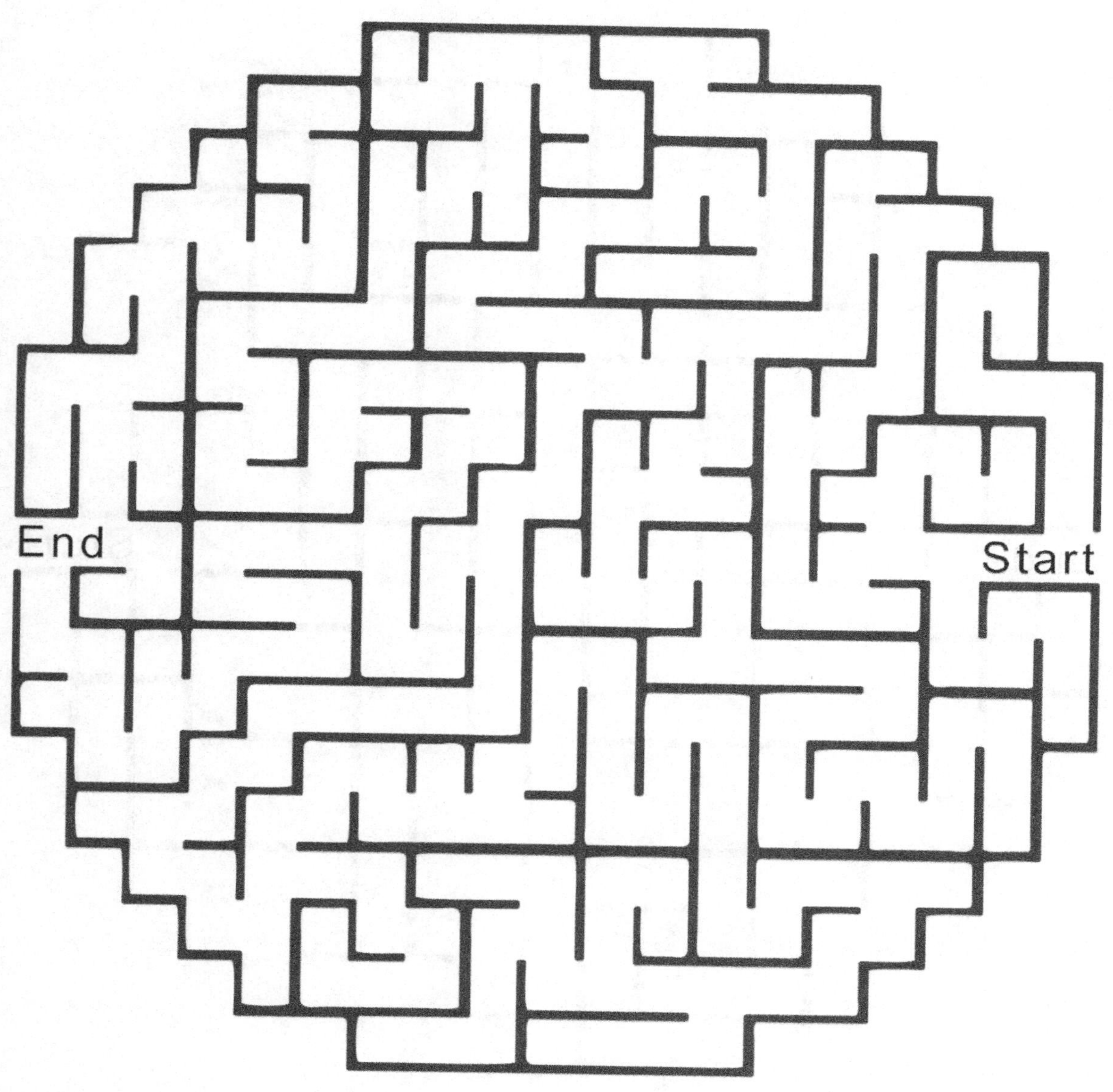

Start time: __________ End time: __________

Total time, maze 1: __________

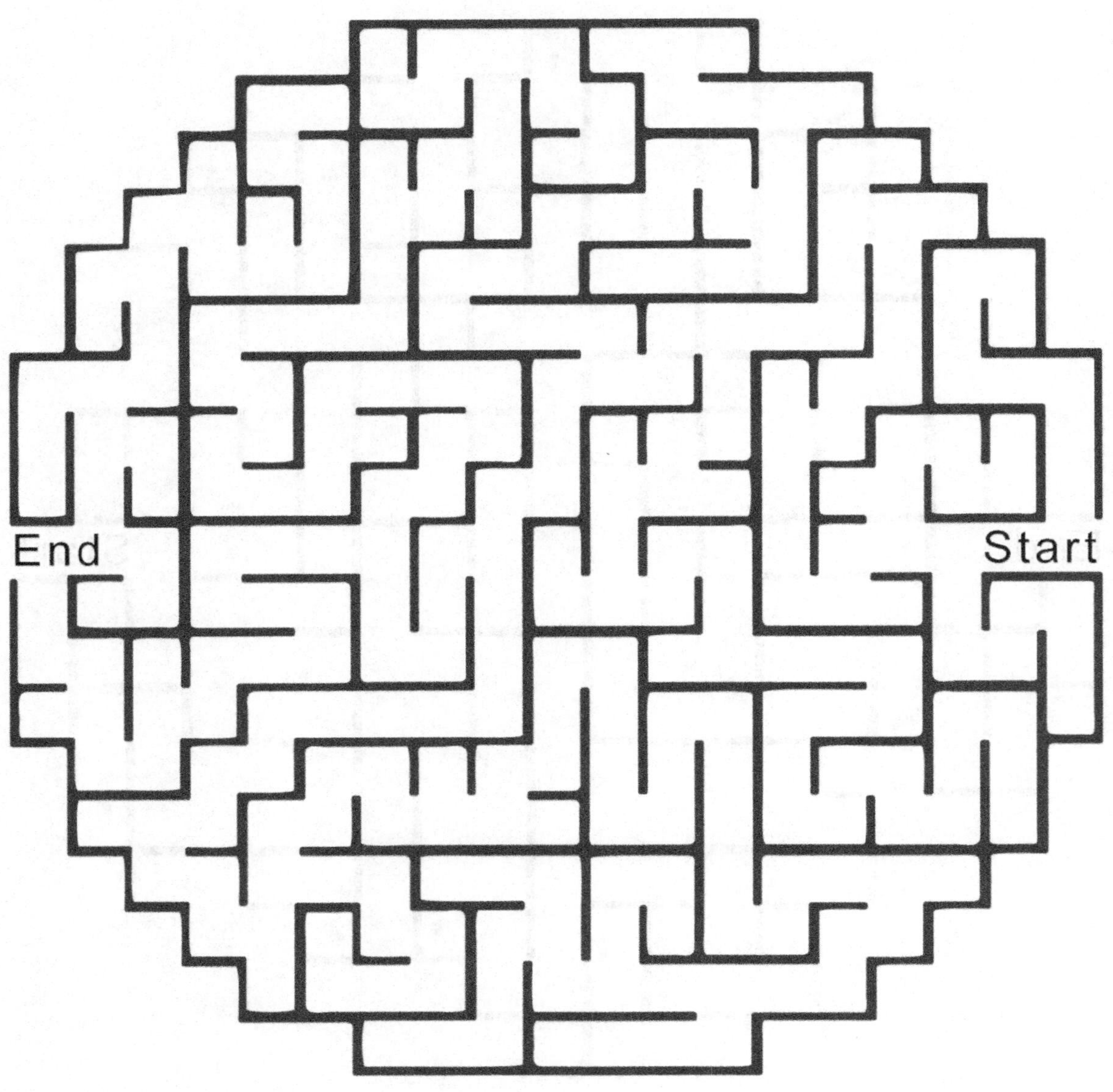

Start time: __________ End time: __________

Total time, maze 2: __________

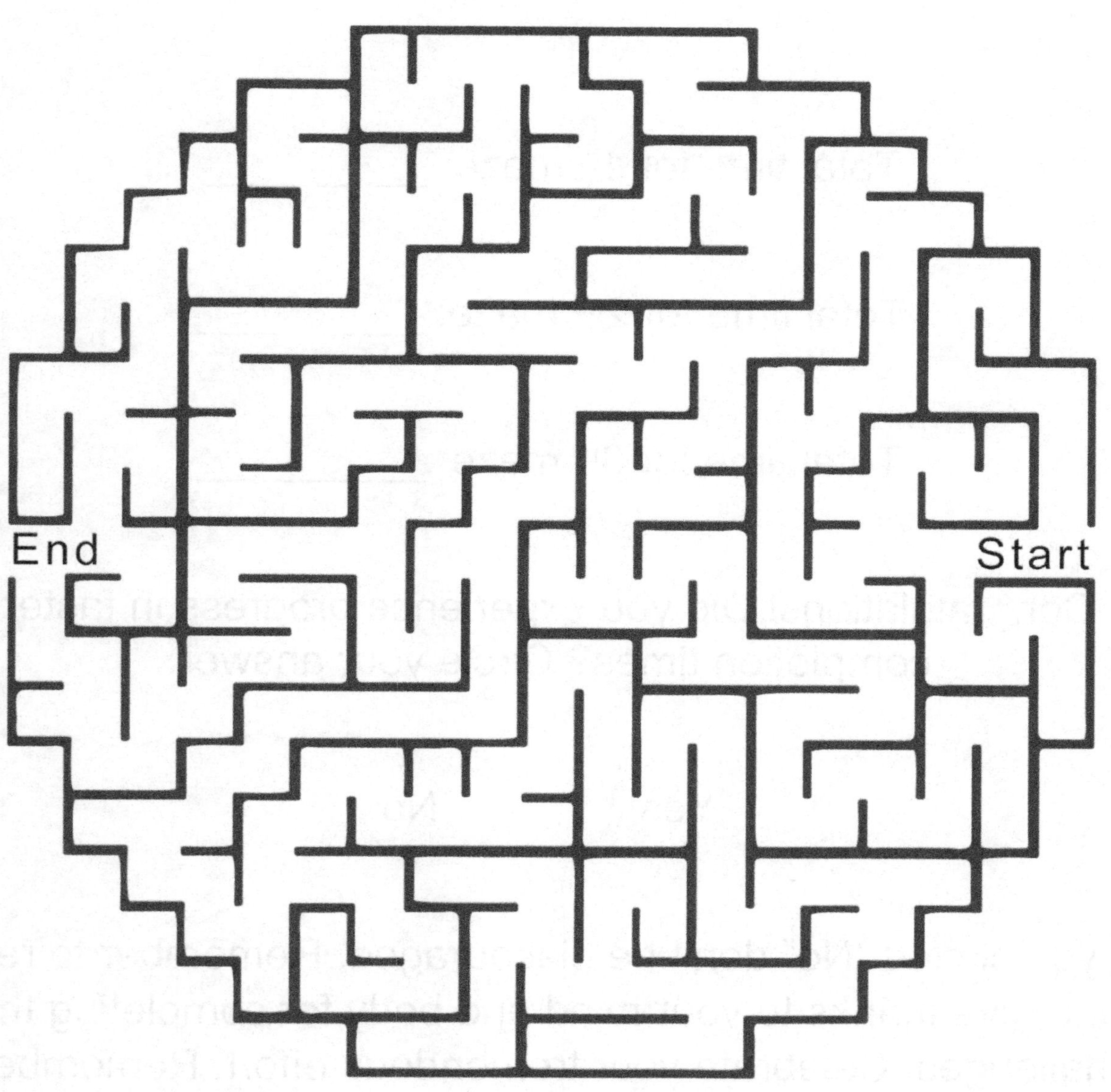

Start time: __________ End time: __________

Total time, maze 3: __________

Total time for 1st maze: __________

Total time for 2nd maze: __________

Total time for 3rd maze: __________

Congratulations! Did you experience progress in faster completion times? Circle your answer.

Yes No

If you circled "No" don't be discouraged. Remember to rest and give thanks to your mind and body for completing the challenges. Celebrate your tremendous effort. Remember, a seed doesn't turn into a tree overnight.

F.E.A.R: has two meanings: 1). Forget Everything And Run or 2). Face Everything And Rise; the choice is yours!

—Zig Ziglar

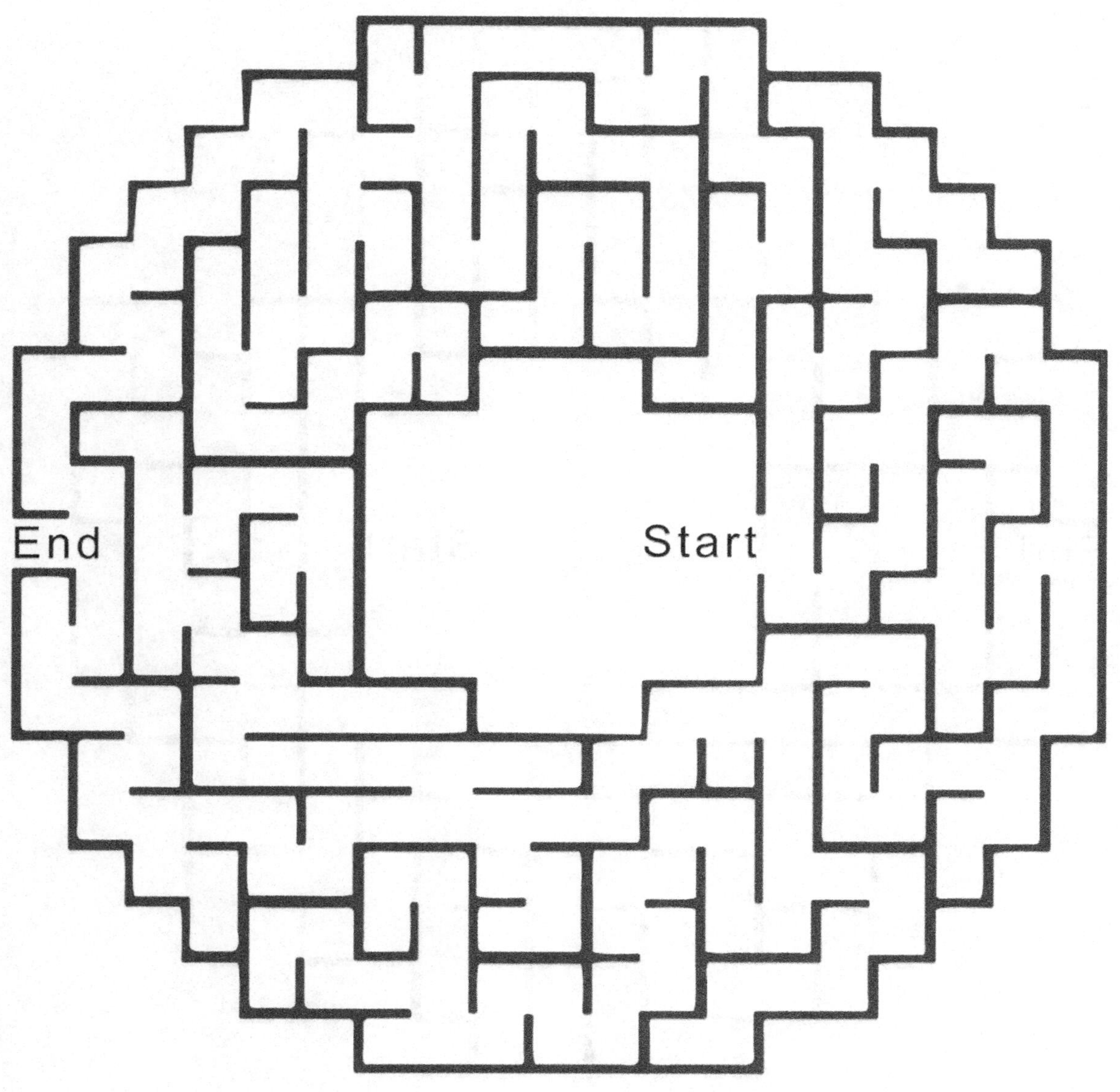

Start time: __________ End time: __________

Total time, maze 1: __________

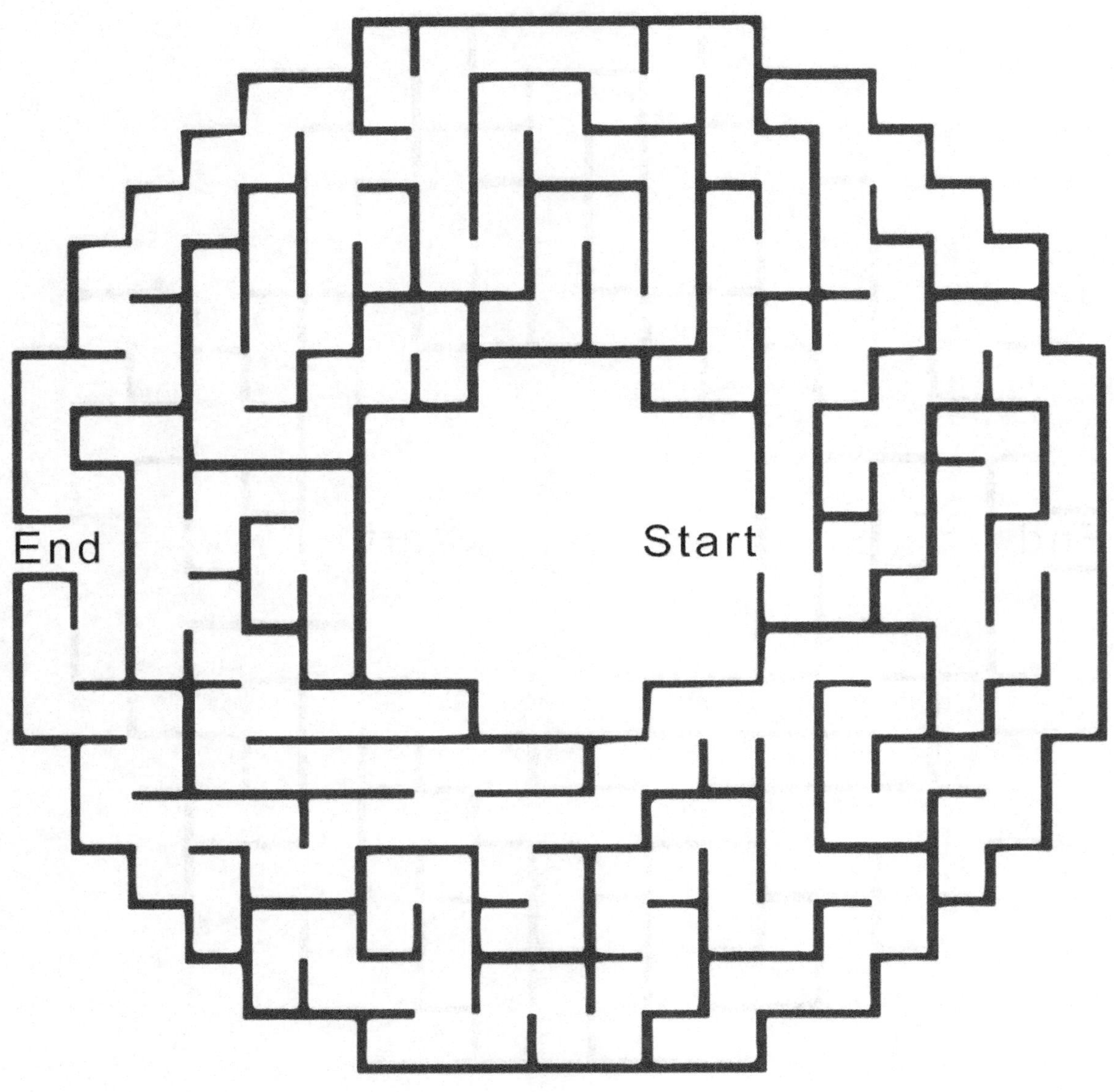

Start time: __________ End time: __________

Total time, maze 2: __________

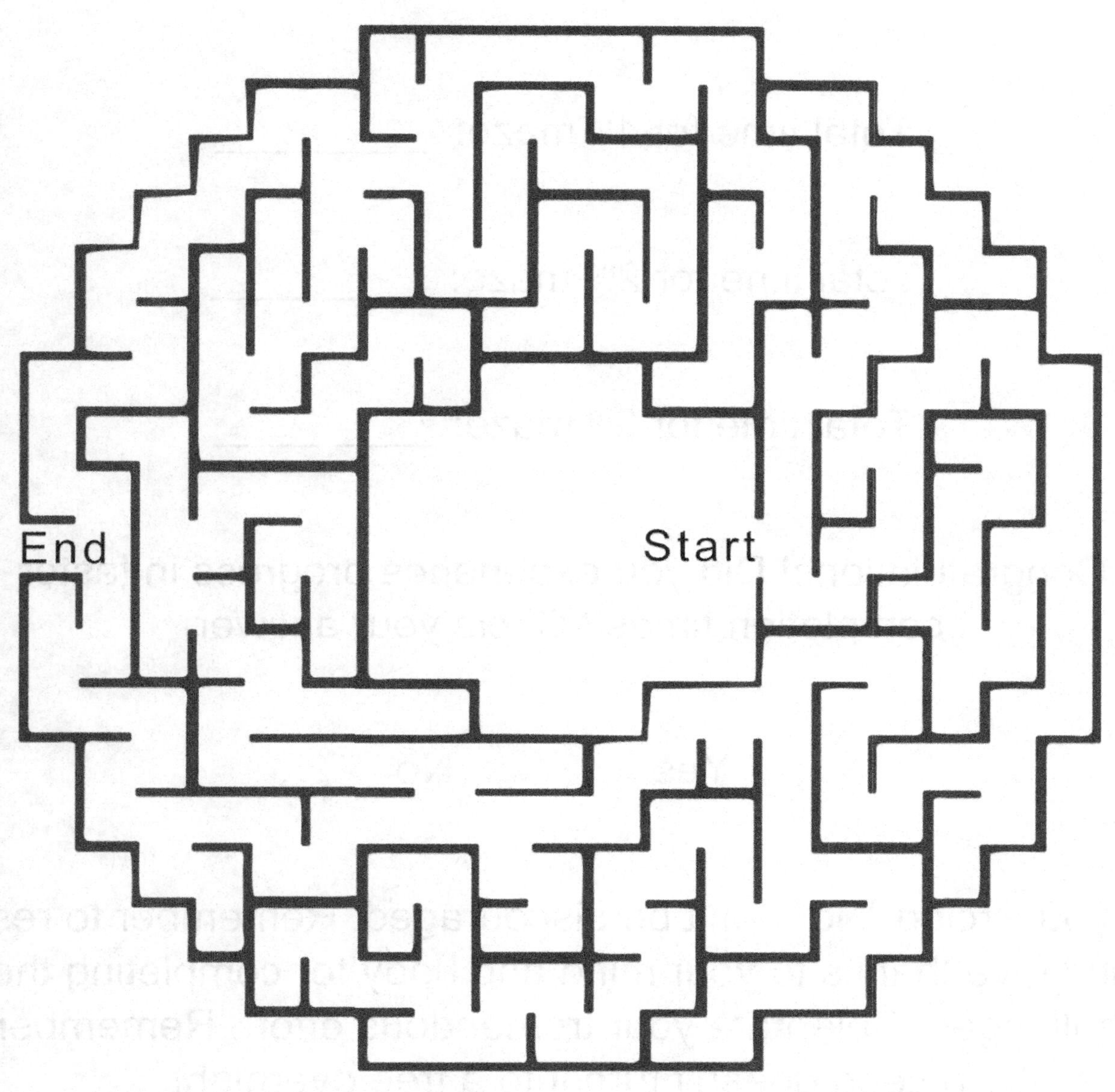

Start time: __________ End time: __________

Total time, maze 3: __________

Total time for 1st maze: __________

Total time for 2nd maze: __________

Total time for 3rd maze: __________

Congratulations! Did you experience progress in faster completion times? Circle your answer.

Yes No

If you circled "No" don't be discouraged. Remember to rest and give thanks to your mind and body for completing the challenges. Celebrate your tremendous effort. Remember, a seed doesn't turn into a tree overnight.

Life is like a camera… Focus on what's important, Capture the good times, Develop from the negatives, and if things don't work out, take another shot.

—*Unknown*

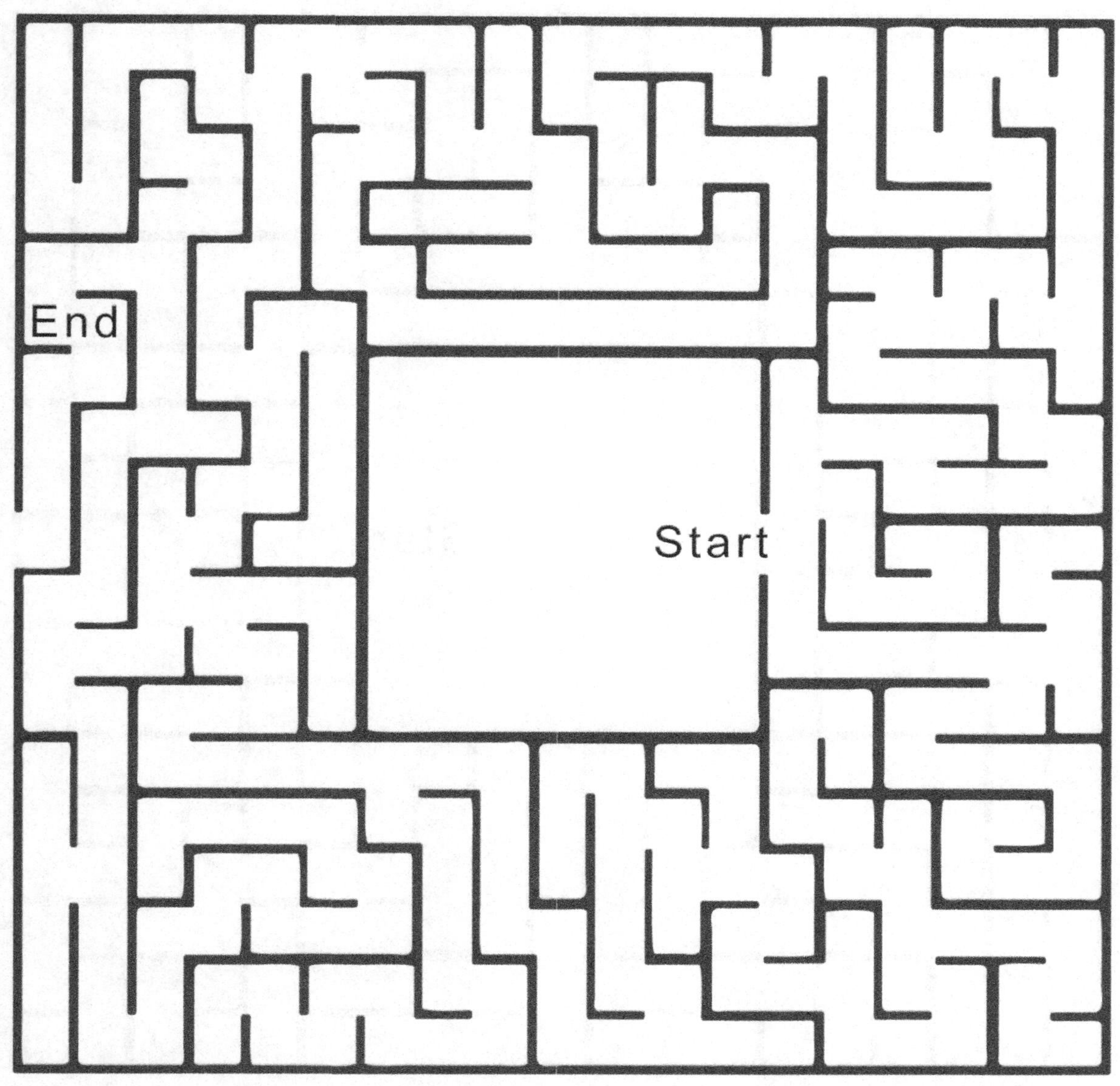

Start time: __________ End time: __________

Total time, maze 1: __________

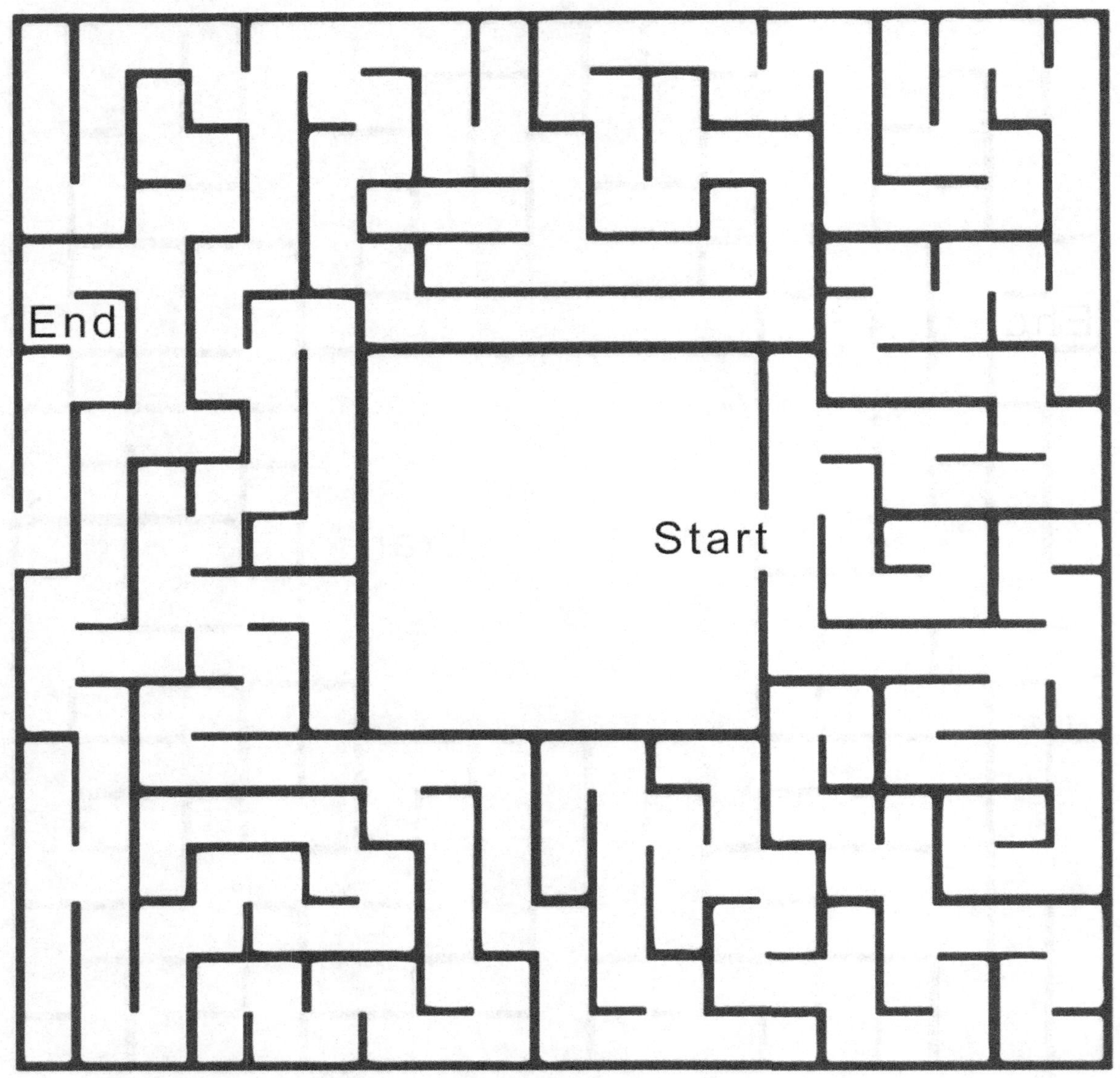

Start time: __________ End time: __________

Total time, maze 2: __________

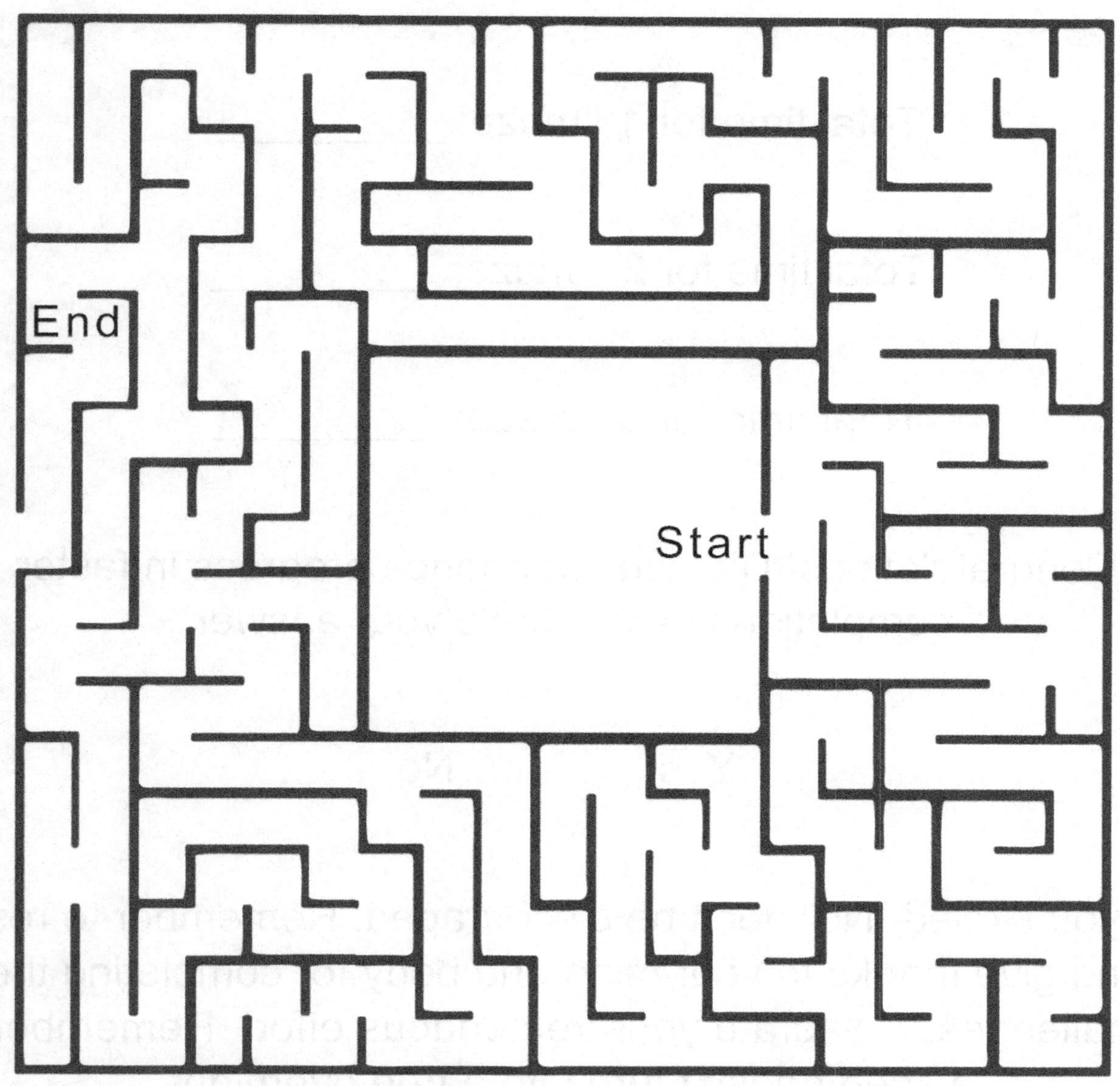

Start time: __________ End time: __________

Total time, maze 3: __________

Total time for 1st maze: __________

Total time for 2nd maze: __________

Total time for 3rd maze: __________

Congratulations! Did you experience progress in faster completion times? Circle your answer.

Yes No

If you circled "No" don't be discouraged. Remember to rest and give thanks to your mind and body for completing the challenges. Celebrate your tremendous effort. Remember, a seed doesn't turn into a tree overnight.

Keep watering, keep planting, keep cultivating, and one day your garden will bloom.

Nourishing myself is a joyful experience,
and I am worth the time spent on my healing.

—Louise Hay

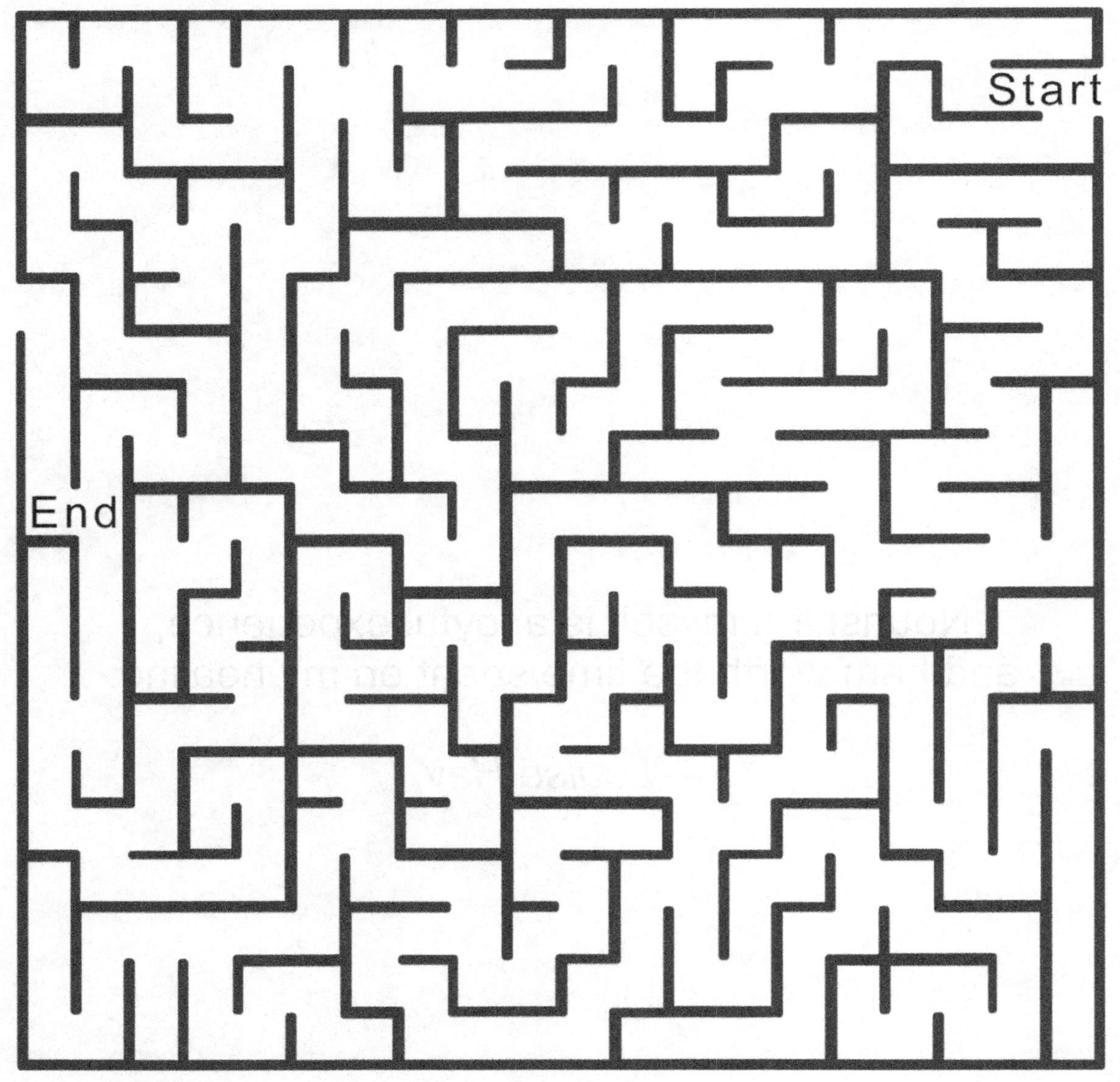

Start time: __________ End time: __________

Total time, maze 1: __________

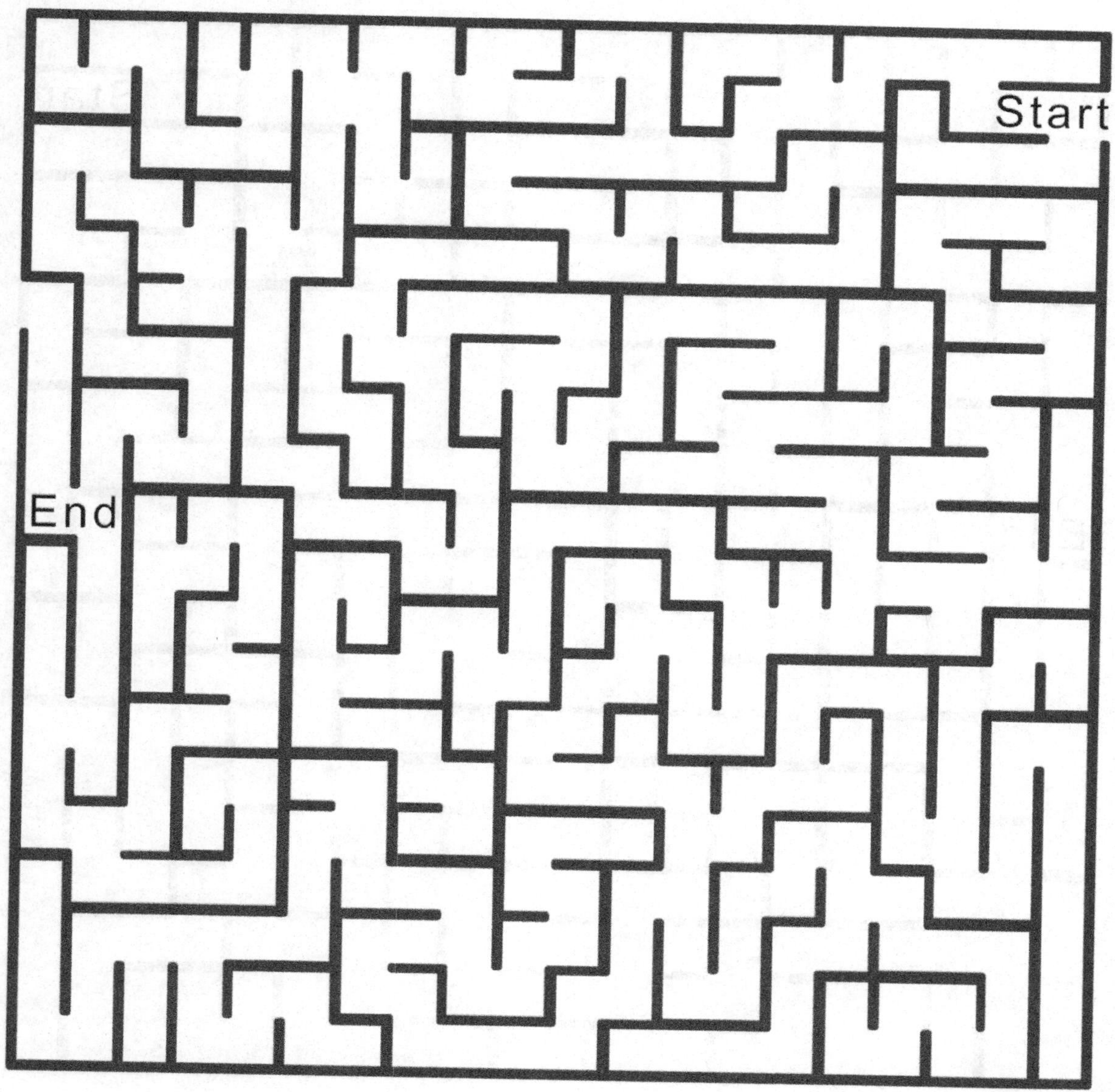

Start time: __________ End time: __________

Total time, maze 2: __________

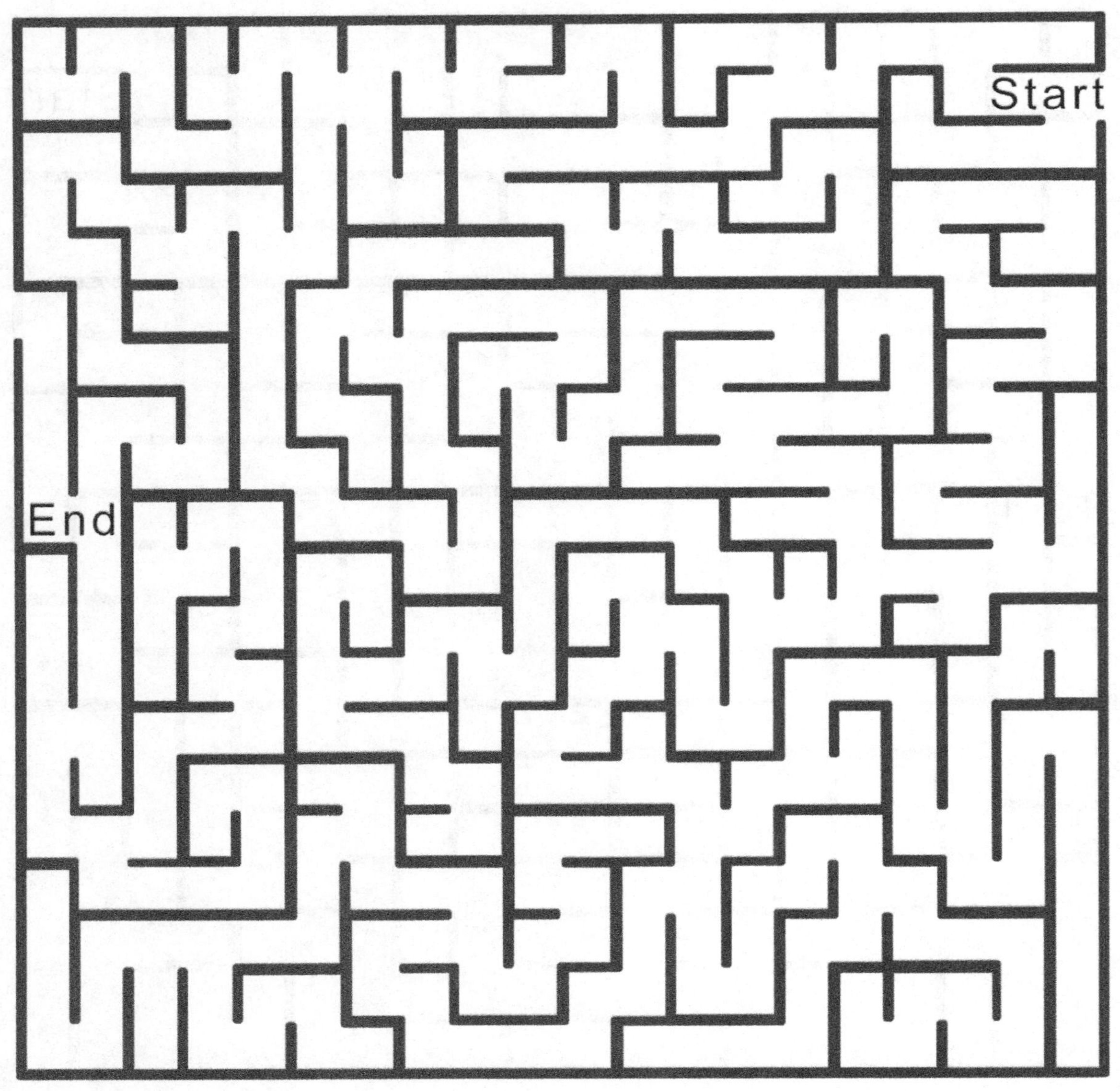

Start time: __________ End time: __________

Total time, maze 3: __________

Total time for 1st maze: __________

Total time for 2nd maze: __________

Total time for 3rd maze: __________

Congratulations! Did you experience progress in faster completion times? Circle your answer.

Yes No

If you circled “No” don’t be discouraged. Remember to rest and give thanks to your mind and body for completing the challenges. Celebrate your tremendous effort. Remember, a seed doesn’t turn into a tree overnight.

One of the things I learned the hard way was that it doesn't pay to get discouraged. Keeping busy and making optimism a way of life can restore your faith in yourself.

—Lucille Ball

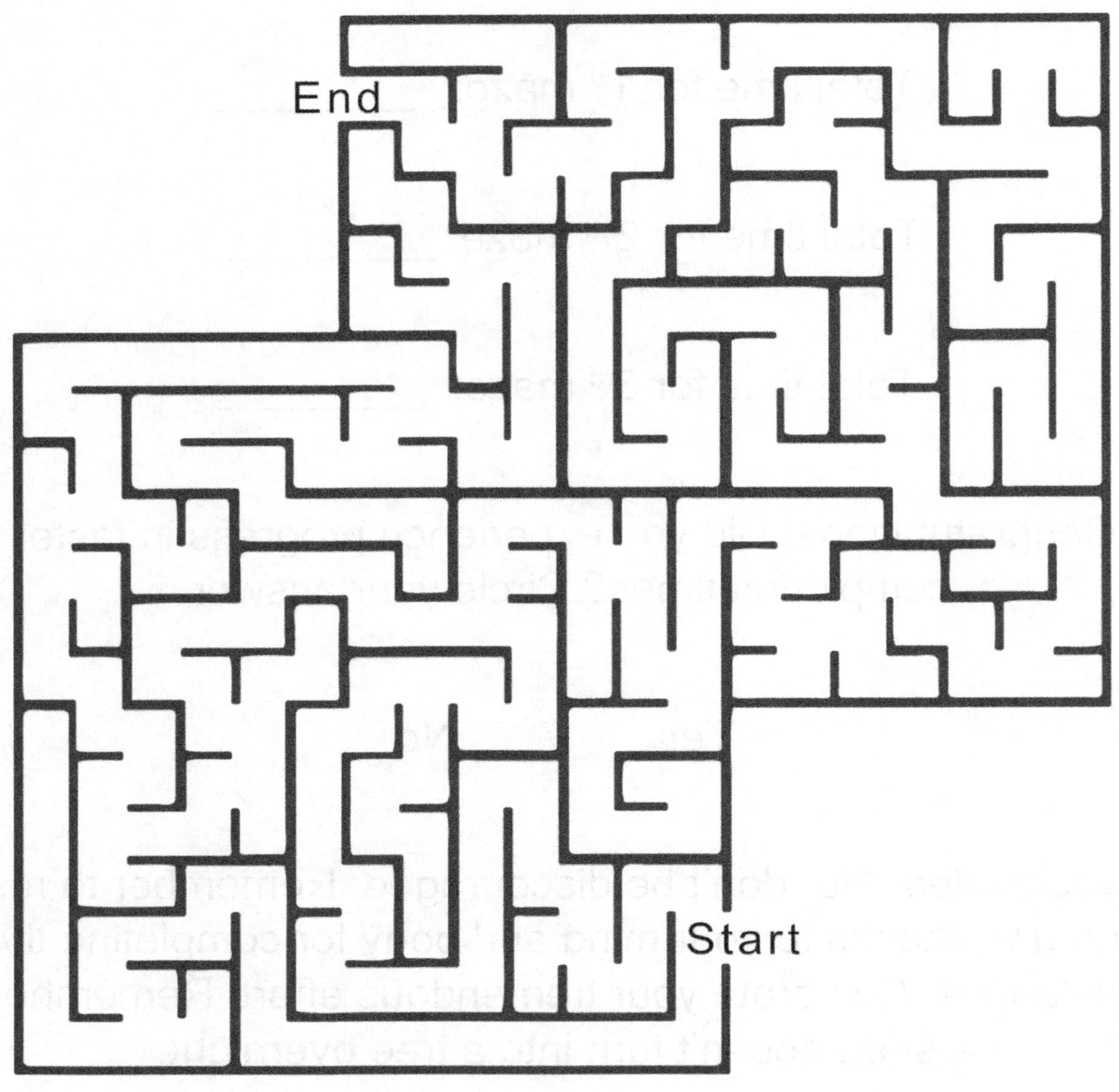

Start time: __________ End time: __________

Total time, maze 1: __________

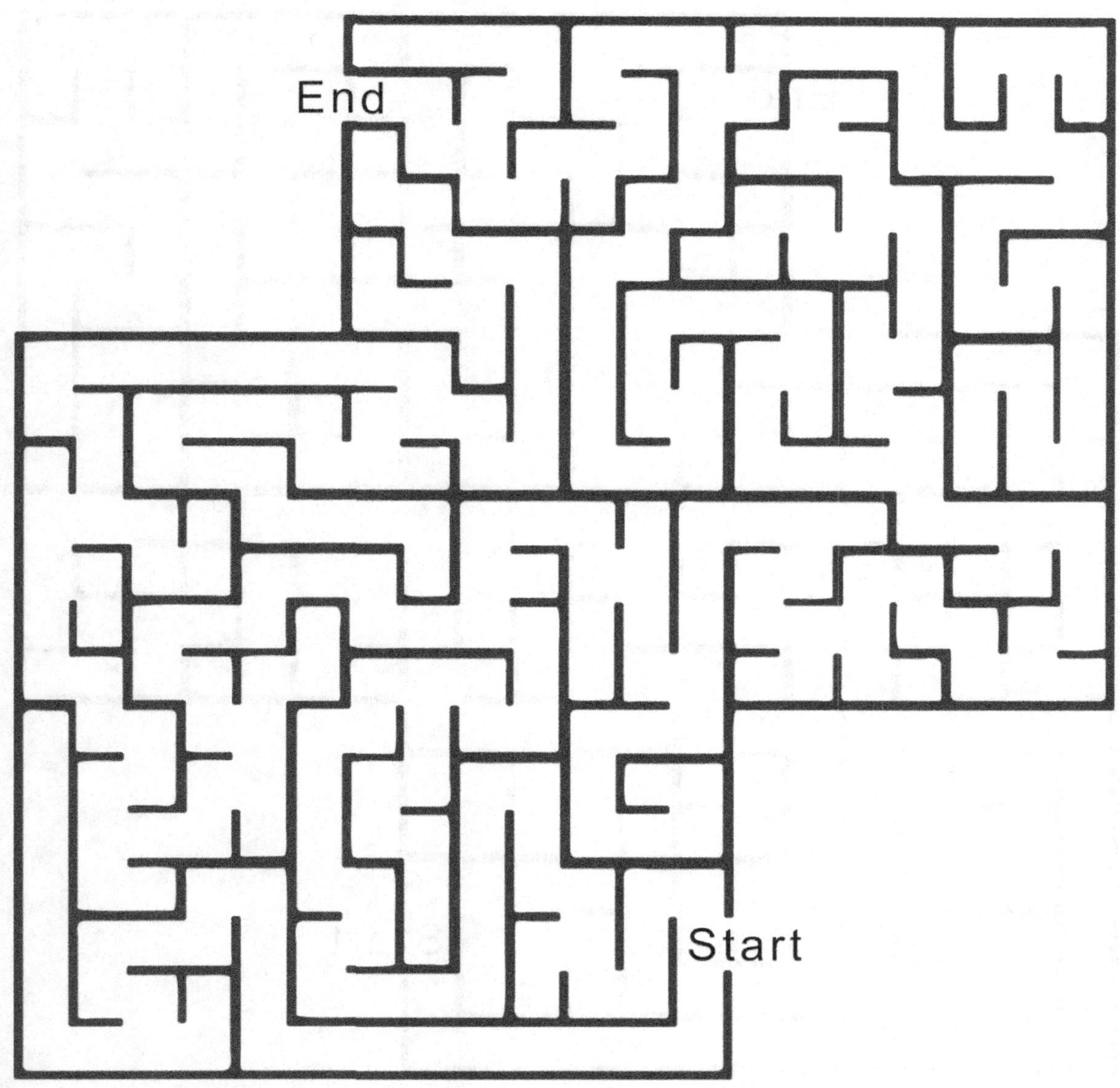

Start time: __________ End time: __________

Total time, maze 2: __________

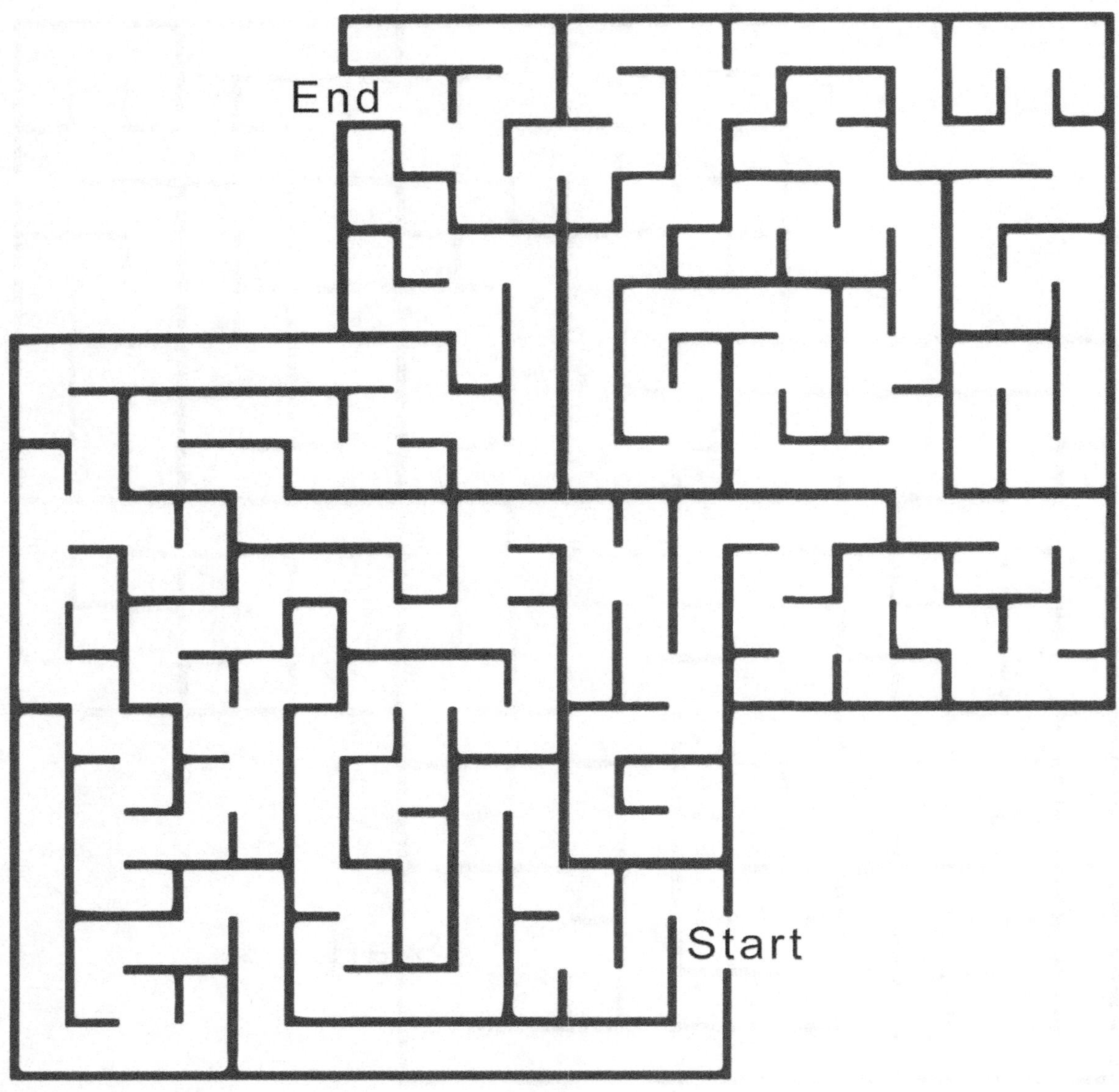

Start time: __________ End time: __________

Total time, maze 3: __________

Total time for 1st maze: __________

Total time for 2nd maze: __________

Total time for 3rd maze: __________

Congratulations! Did you experience progress in faster completion times? Circle your answer.

Yes No

If you circled "No" don't be discouraged. Remember to rest and give thanks to your mind and body for completing the challenges. Celebrate your tremendous effort. Remember, a seed doesn't turn into a tree overnight.

Edison failed 10,000 times before he made the electric light. Do not be discouraged if you fail a few times.

—Napoleon Hill

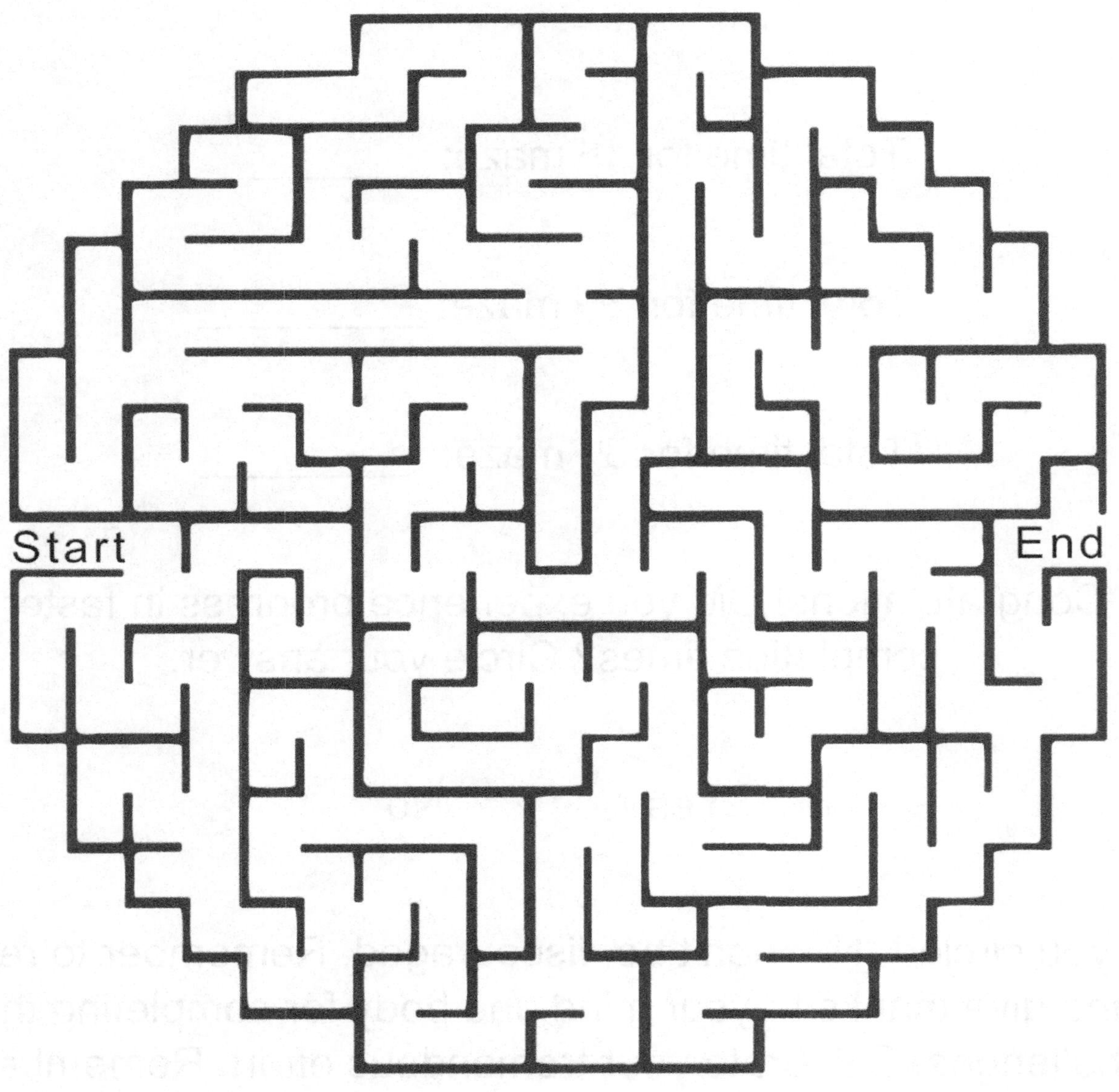

Start time: __________ End time: __________

Total time, maze 1: __________

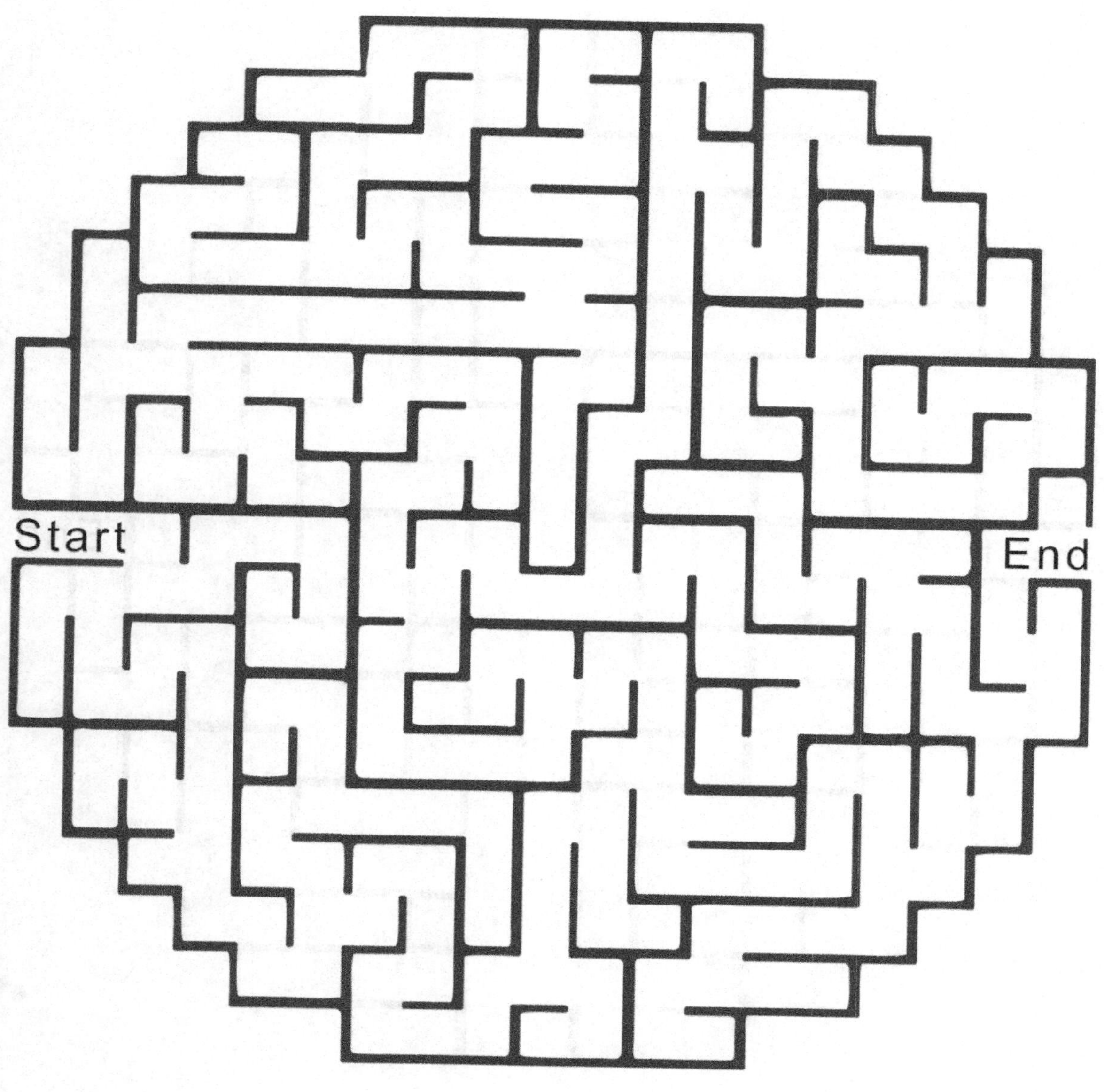

Start time: __________ End time: __________

Total time, maze 2: __________

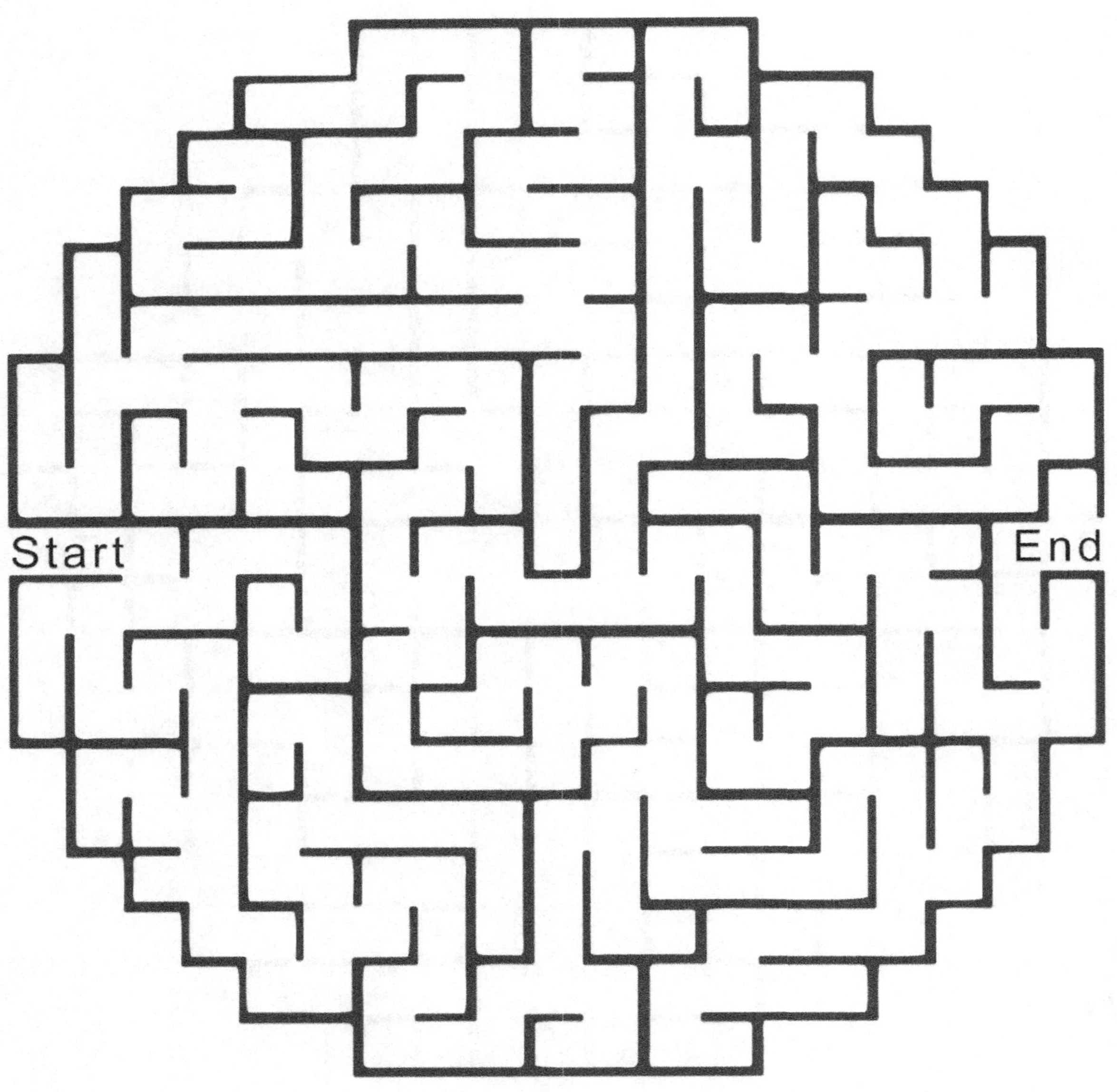

Start time: __________ End time: __________

Total time, maze 3: __________

Total time for 1st maze: __________

Total time for 2nd maze: __________

Total time for 3rd maze: __________

Congratulations! Did you experience progress in faster completion times? Circle your answer.

Yes No

If you circled "No" don't be discouraged. Remember to rest and give thanks to your mind and body for completing the challenges. Celebrate your tremendous effort. Remember, a seed doesn't turn into a tree overnight.

A man can get discouraged many times but he is not a failure until he begins to blame somebody else and stops trying.

—*John Burroughs*

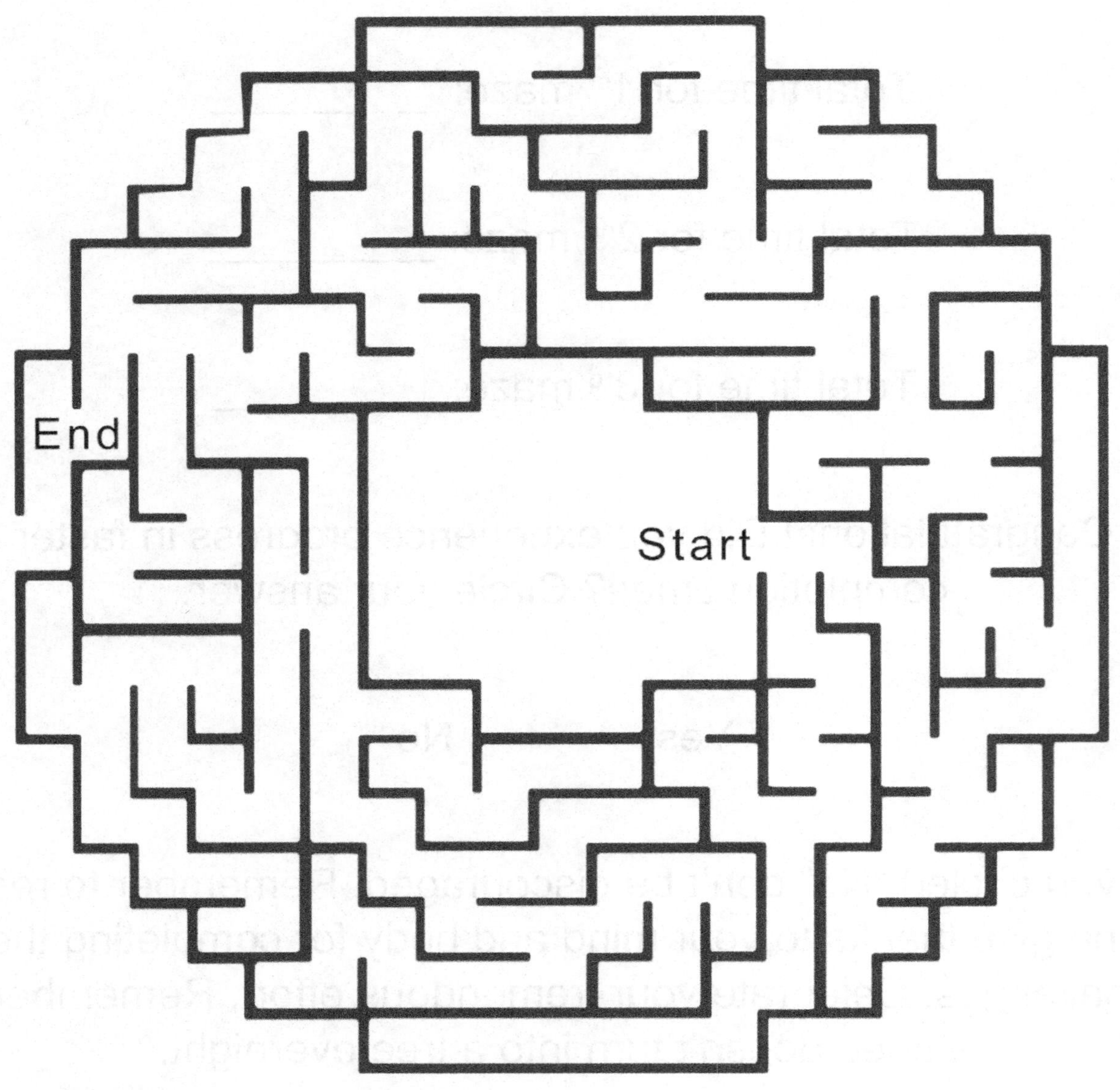

Start time: __________ End time: __________

Total time, maze 1: __________

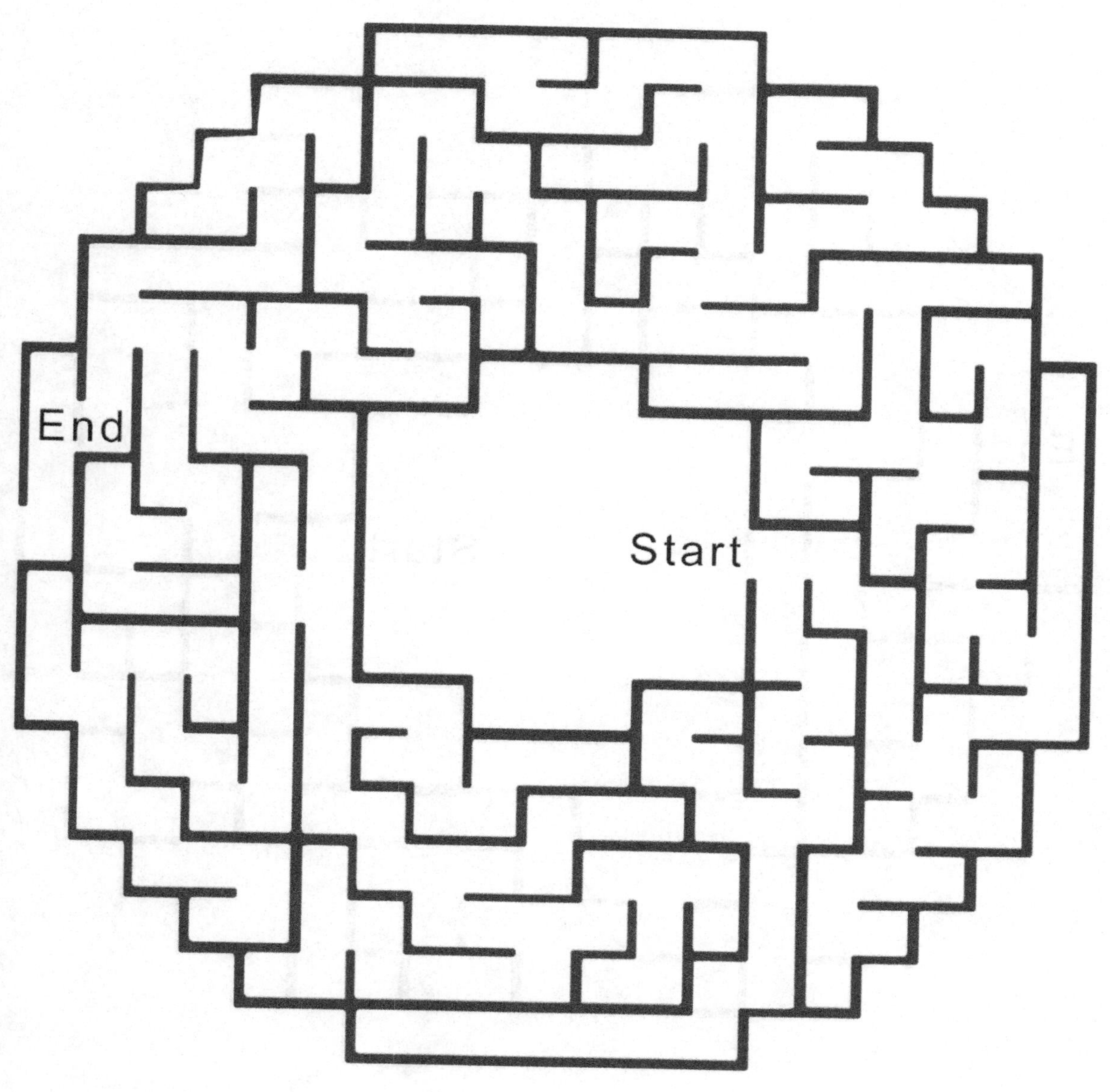

Start time: __________ End time: __________

Total time, maze 2: __________

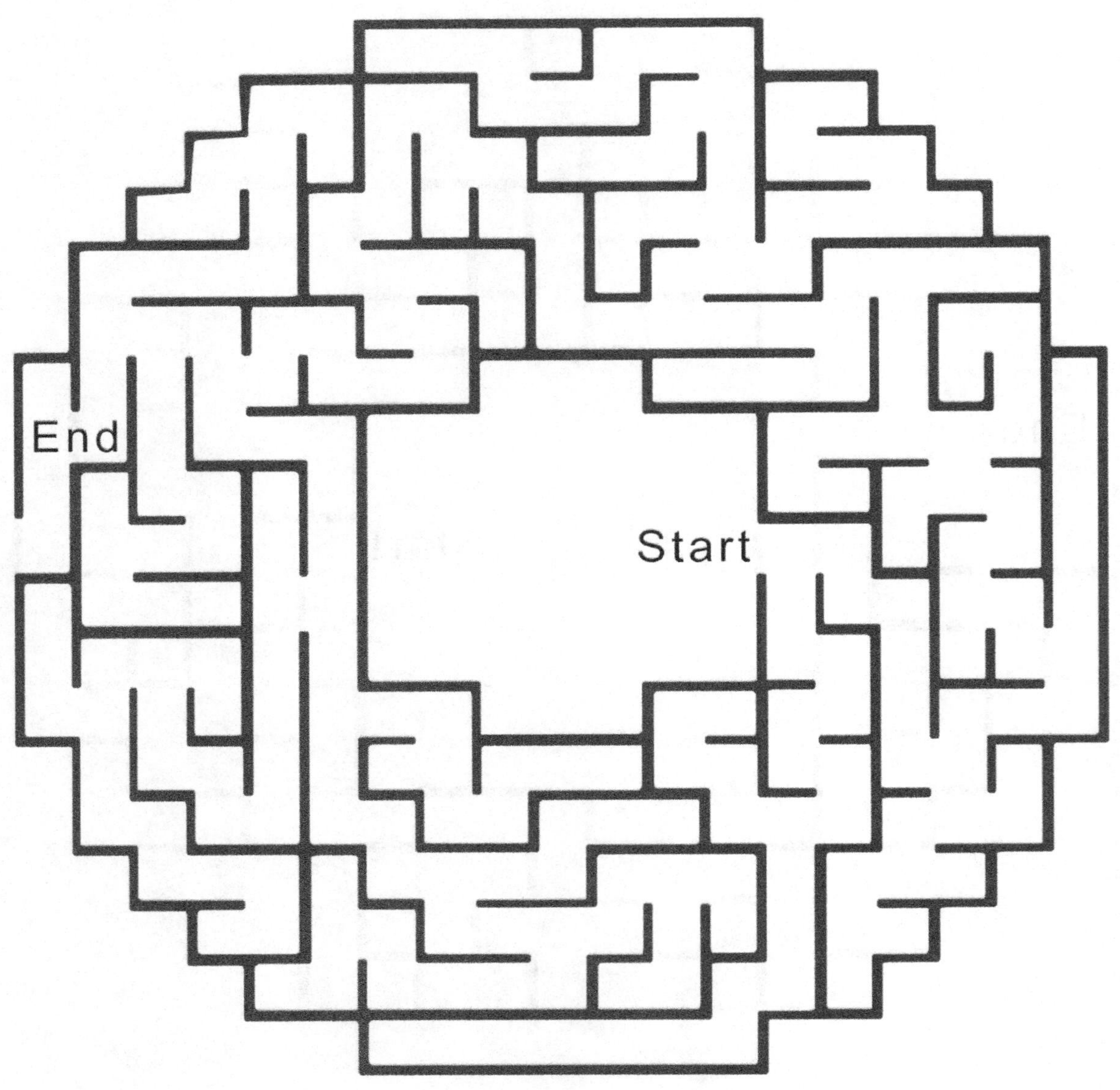

Start time: __________ End time: __________

Total time, maze 3: __________

Total time for 1st maze: __________

Total time for 2nd maze: __________

Total time for 3rd maze: __________

Congratulations! Did you experience progress in faster completion times? Circle your answer.

Yes No

If you circled "No" don't be discouraged. Remember to rest and give thanks to your mind and body for completing the challenges. Celebrate your tremendous effort. Remember, a seed doesn't turn into a tree overnight.

Continuous, unflagging effort, persistence and determination will win. Let not the man be discouraged who has these.

—*James Whitcomb Riley*

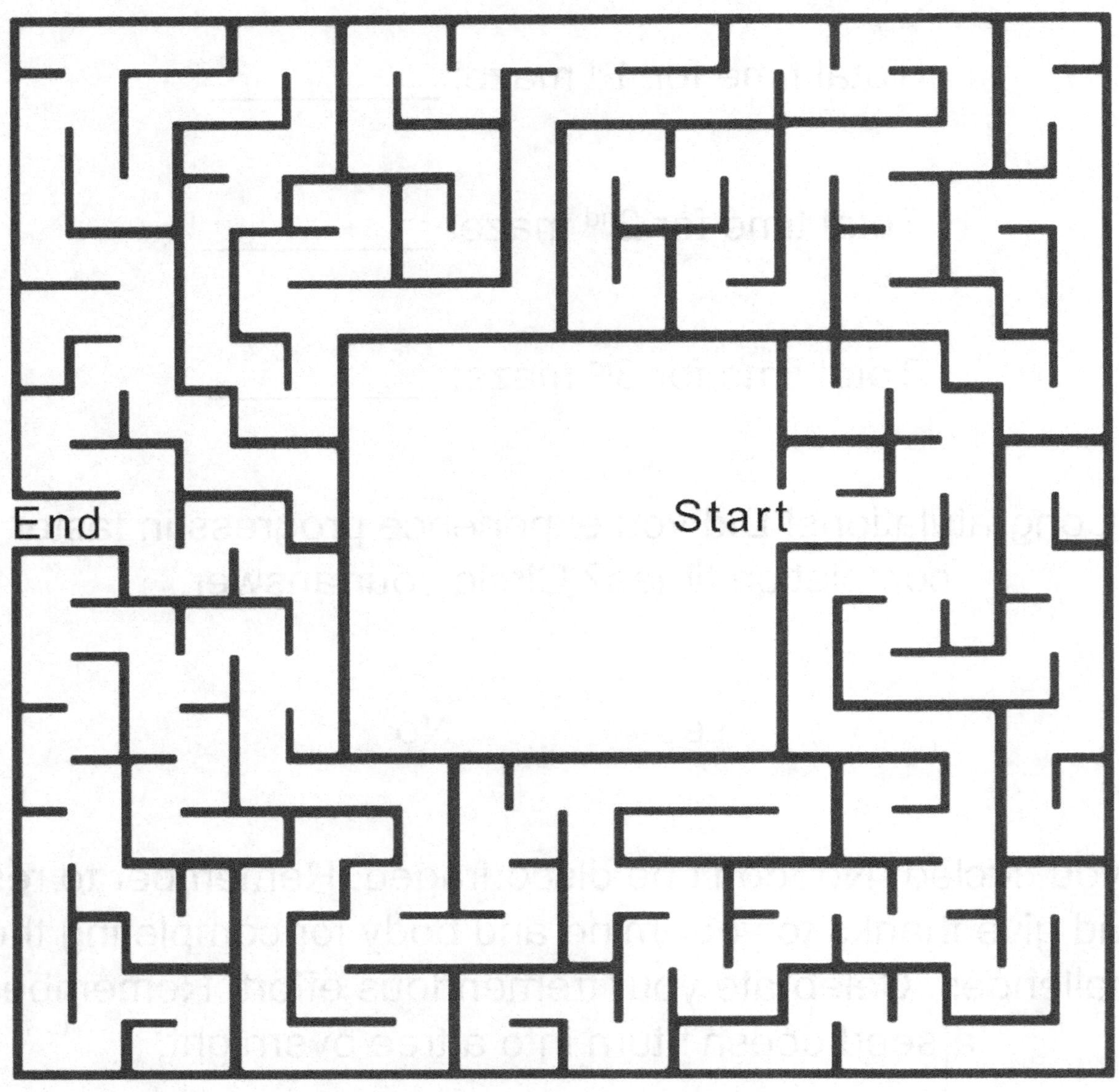

Start time: __________ End time: __________

Total time, maze 1: __________

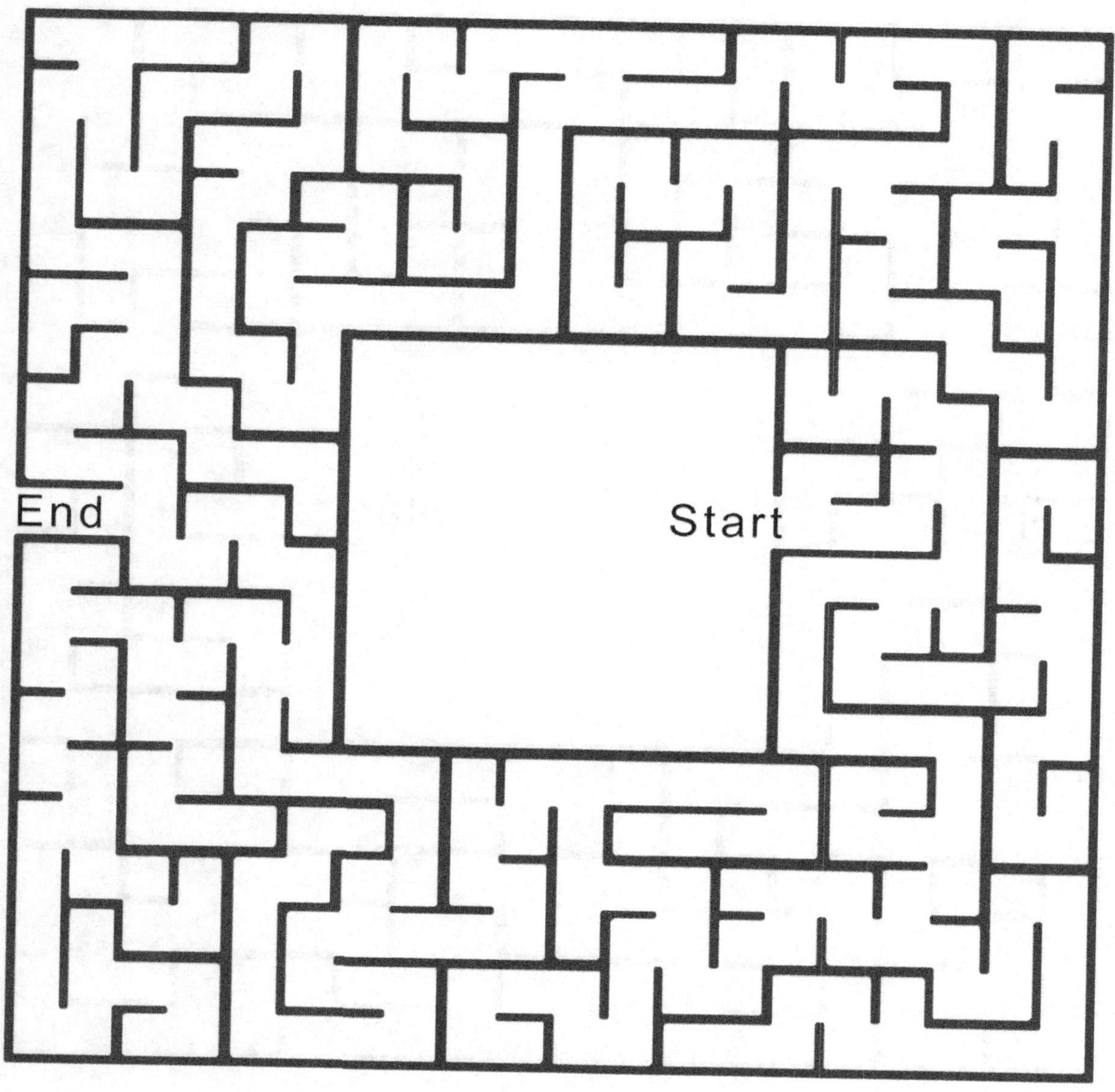

Start time: __________ End time: __________

Total time, maze 2: __________

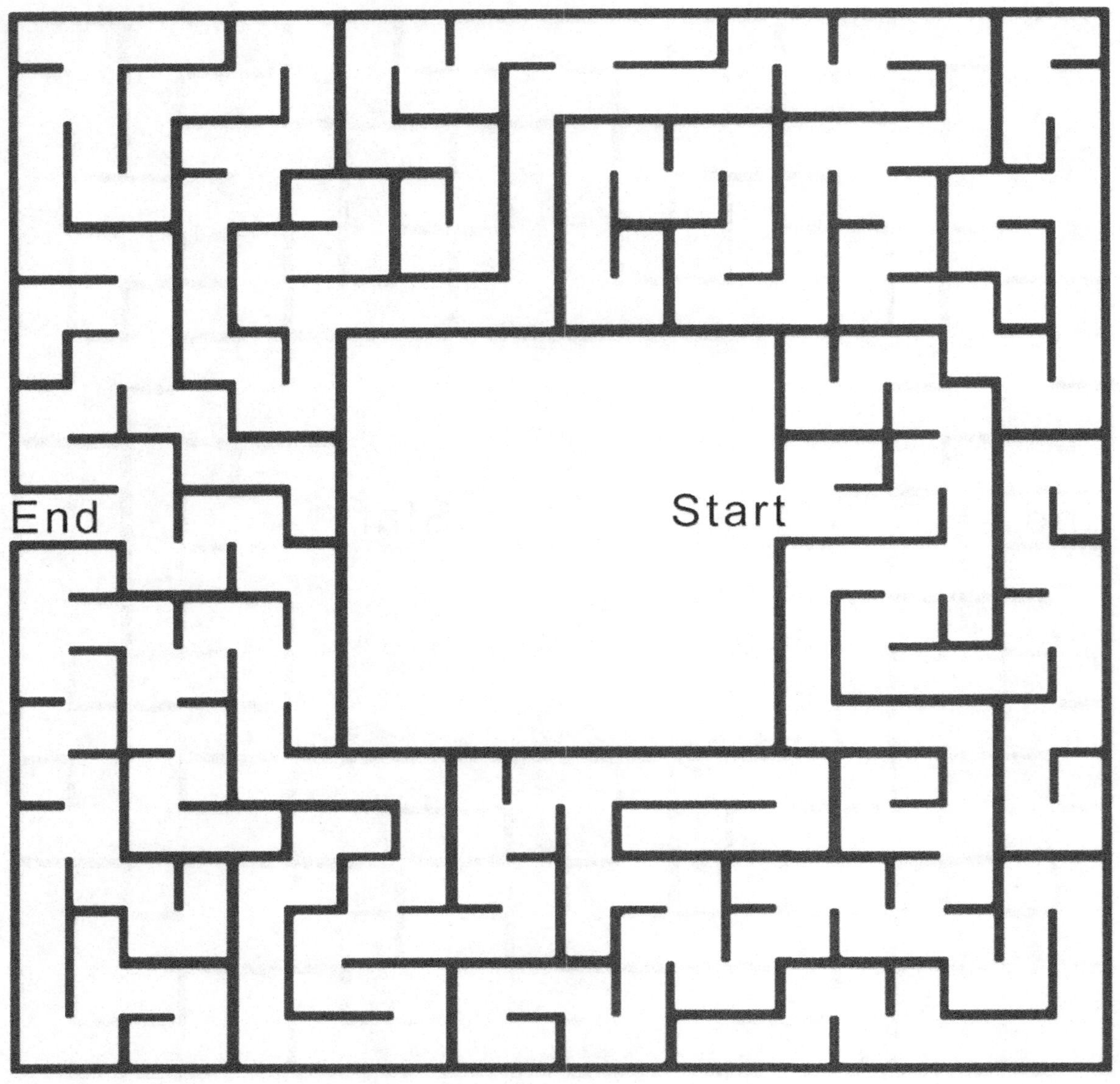

Start time: __________ End time: __________

Total time, maze 3: __________

Total time for 1st maze: __________

Total time for 2nd maze: __________

Total time for 3rd maze: __________

Congratulations! Did you experience progress in faster completion times? Circle your answer.

Yes No

If you circled "No" don't be discouraged. Remember to rest and give thanks to your mind and body for completing the challenges. Celebrate your tremendous effort. Remember, a seed doesn't turn into a tree overnight.

What is important is to believe in something so strongly that you're never discouraged.

—*Salma Hayek*

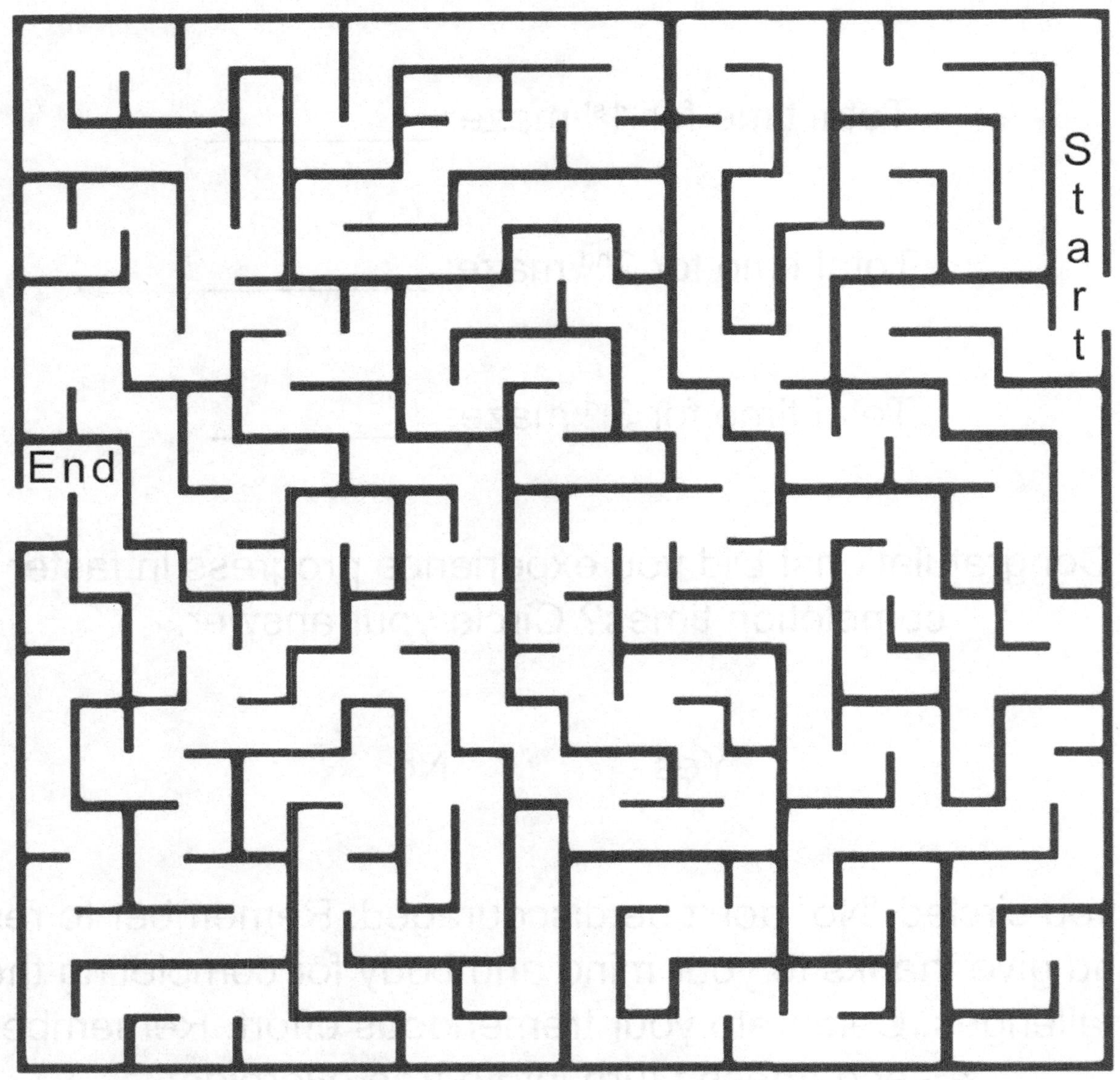

Start time: __________ End time: __________

Total time, maze 1: __________

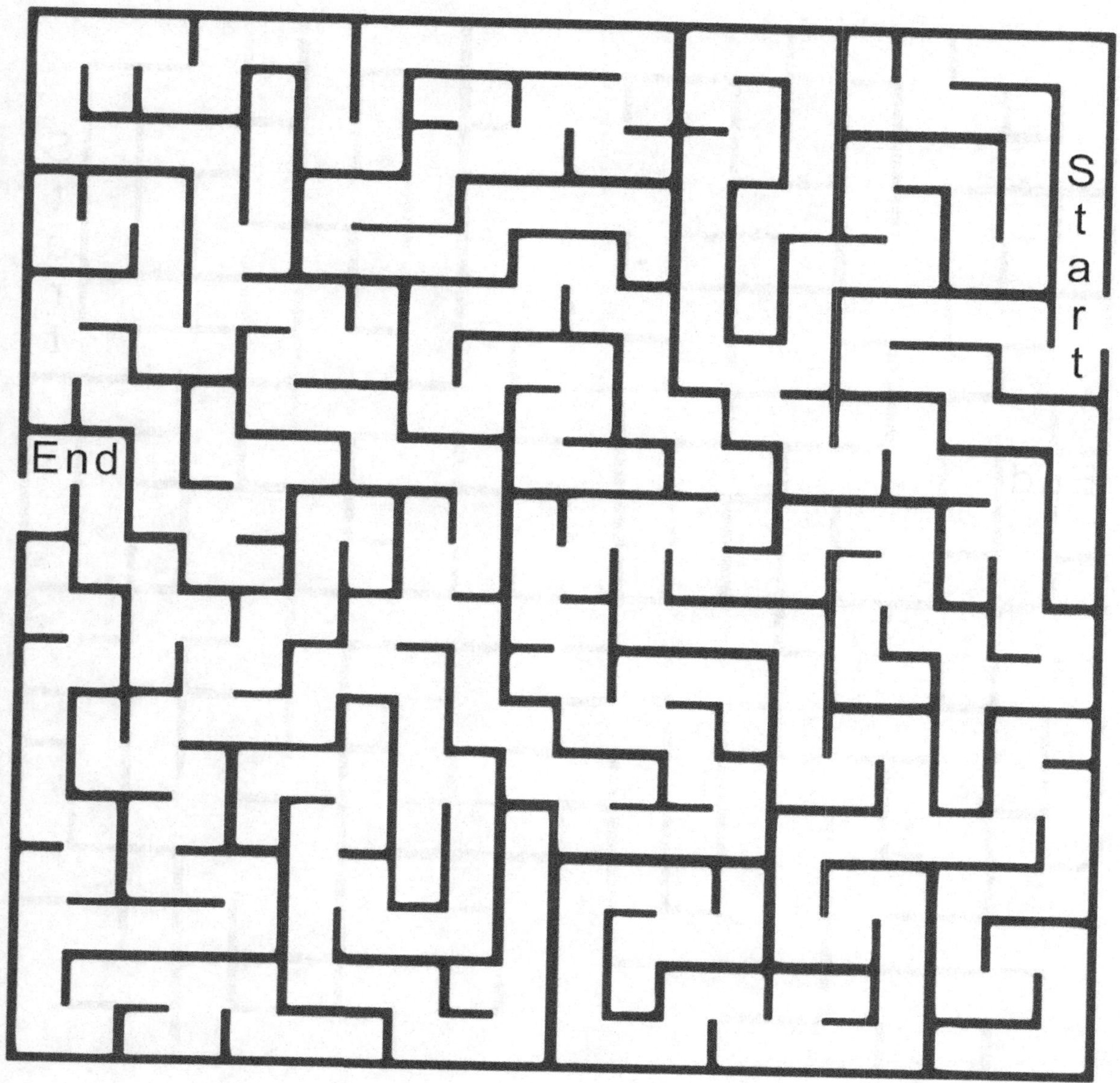

Start time: __________ End time: __________

Total time, maze 2: __________

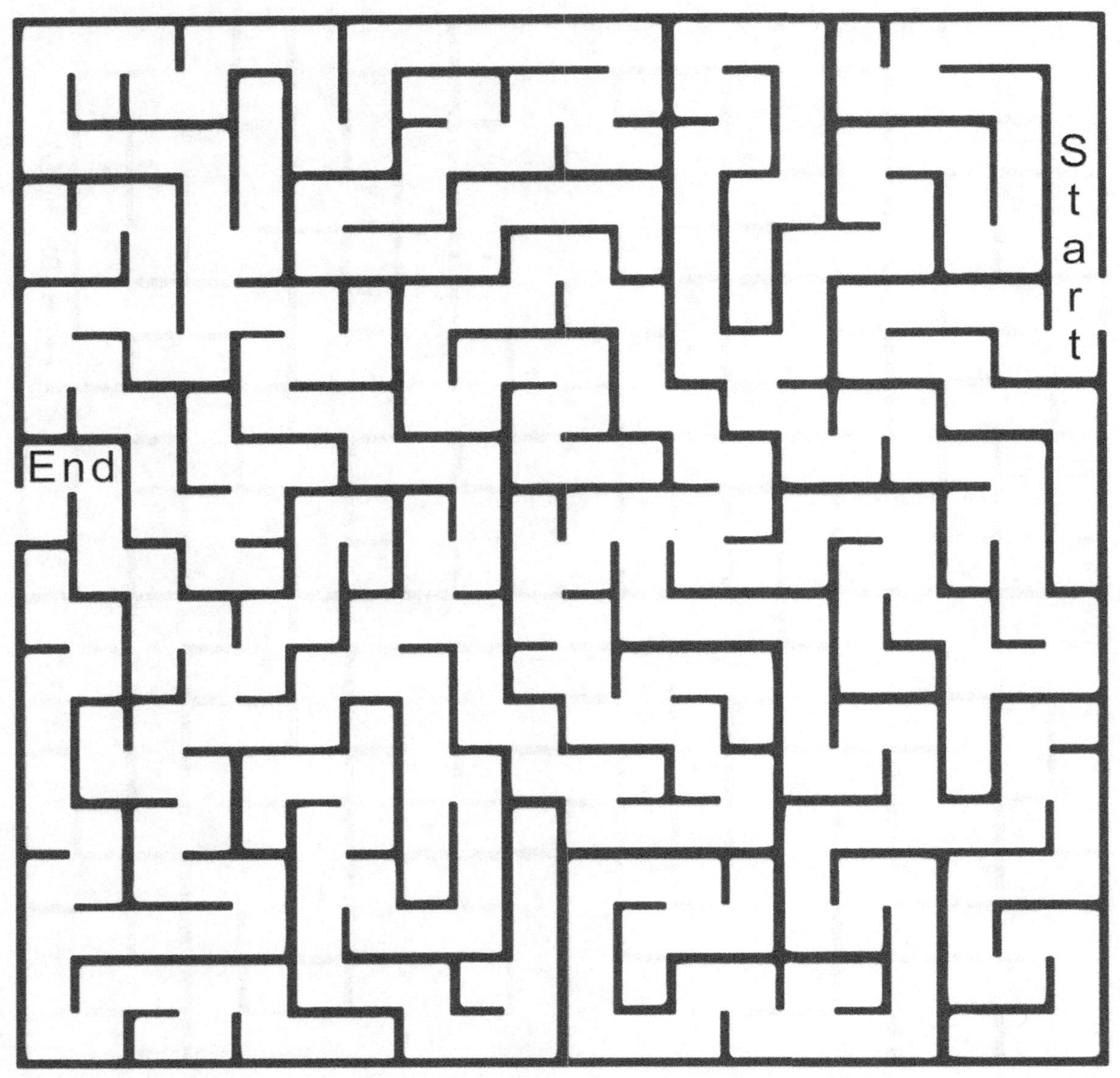

Start time: ___________ End time: ___________

Total time, maze 3: ___________

Total time for 1st maze: __________

Total time for 2nd maze: __________

Total time for 3rd maze: __________

Congratulations! Did you experience progress in faster completion times? Circle your answer.

Yes No

If you circled "No" don't be discouraged. Remember to rest and give thanks to your mind and body for completing the challenges. Celebrate your tremendous effort. Remember, a seed doesn't turn into a tree overnight.

Stop beating yourself up. You are a work in progress - which means you get there a little at a time, not all at once.

—Unknown

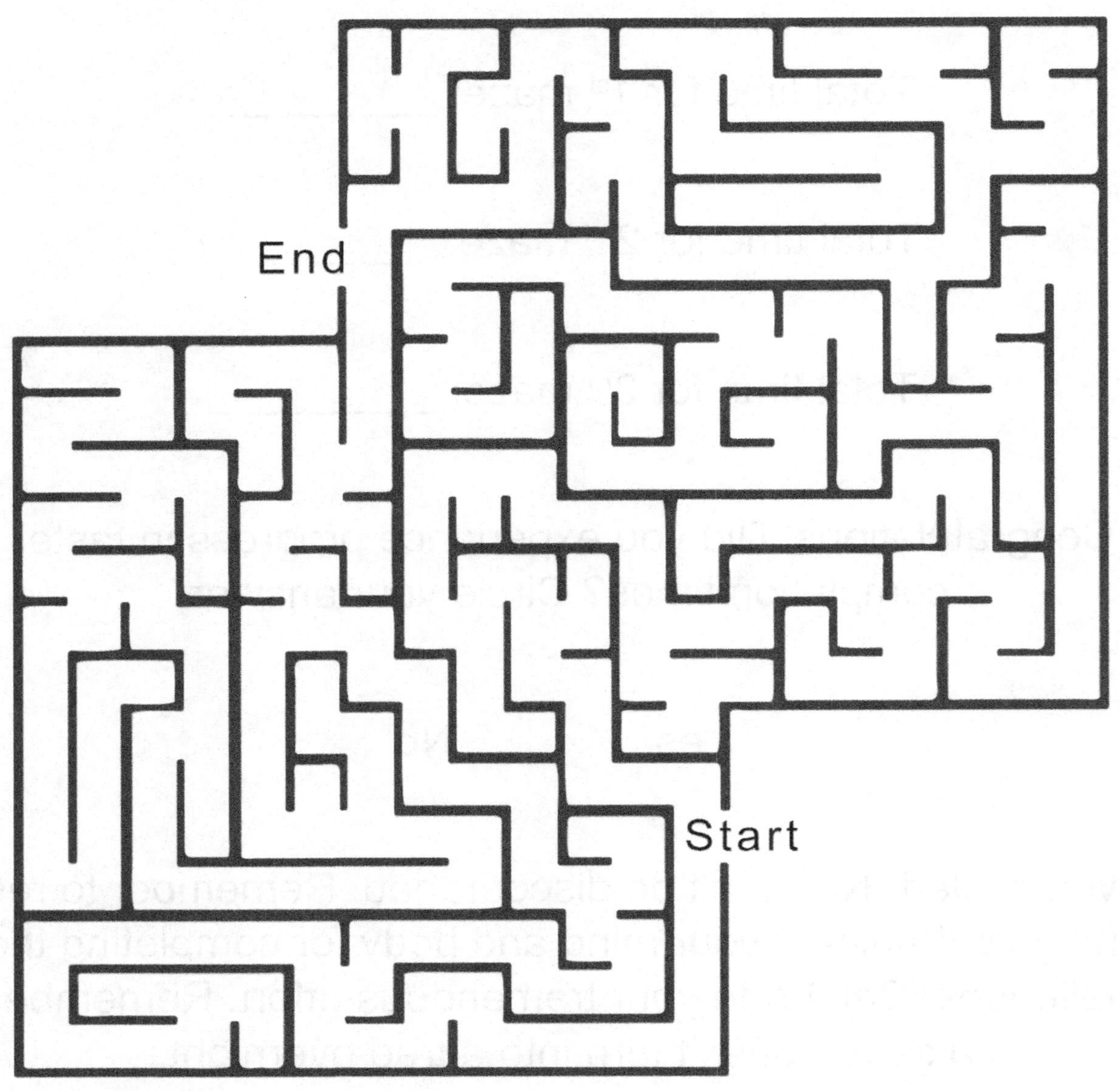

Start time: __________ End time: __________

Total time, maze 1: __________

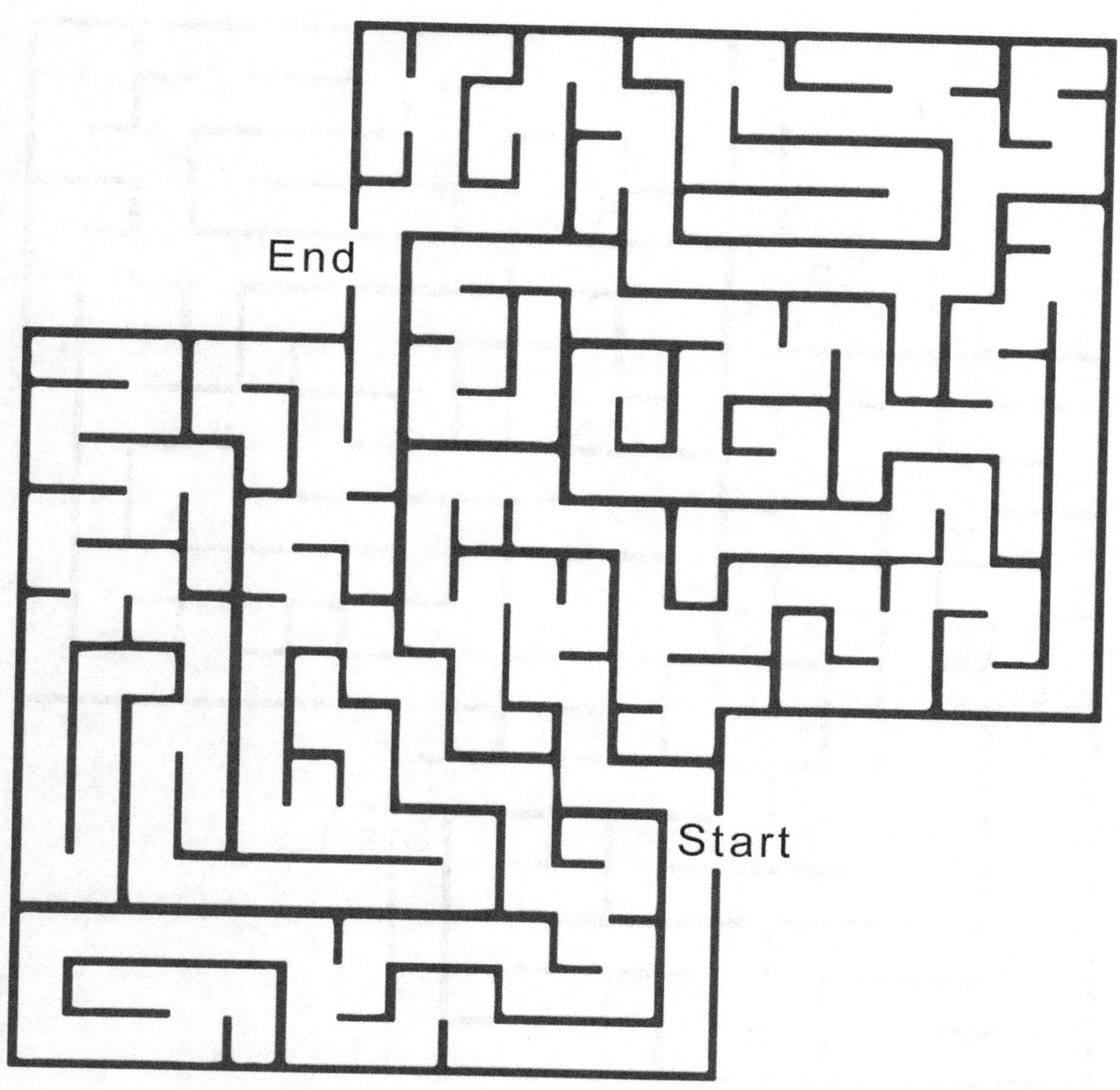

Start time: __________ End time: __________

Total time, maze 2: __________

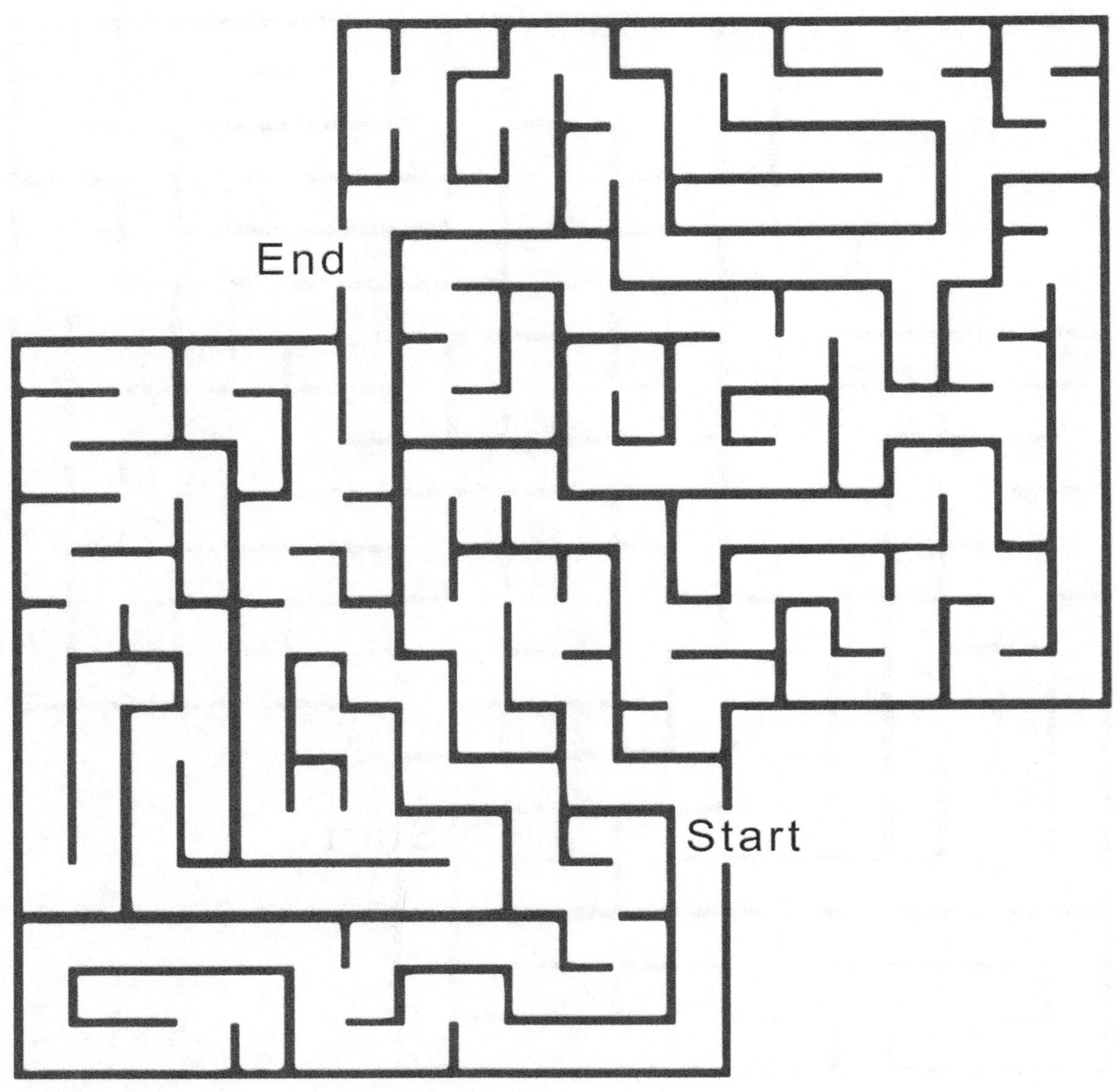

Start time: __________ End time: __________

Total time, maze 3: __________

Total time for 1st maze: __________

Total time for 2nd maze: __________

Total time for 3rd maze: __________

Congratulations! Did you experience progress in faster completion times? Circle your answer.

Yes No

If you circled "No" don't be discouraged. Remember to rest and give thanks to your mind and body for completing the challenges. Celebrate your tremendous effort. Remember, a seed doesn't turn into a tree overnight.

Yesterday I was clever so I wanted to change the world. Today I am wise, so I am changing myself.

—Rumi

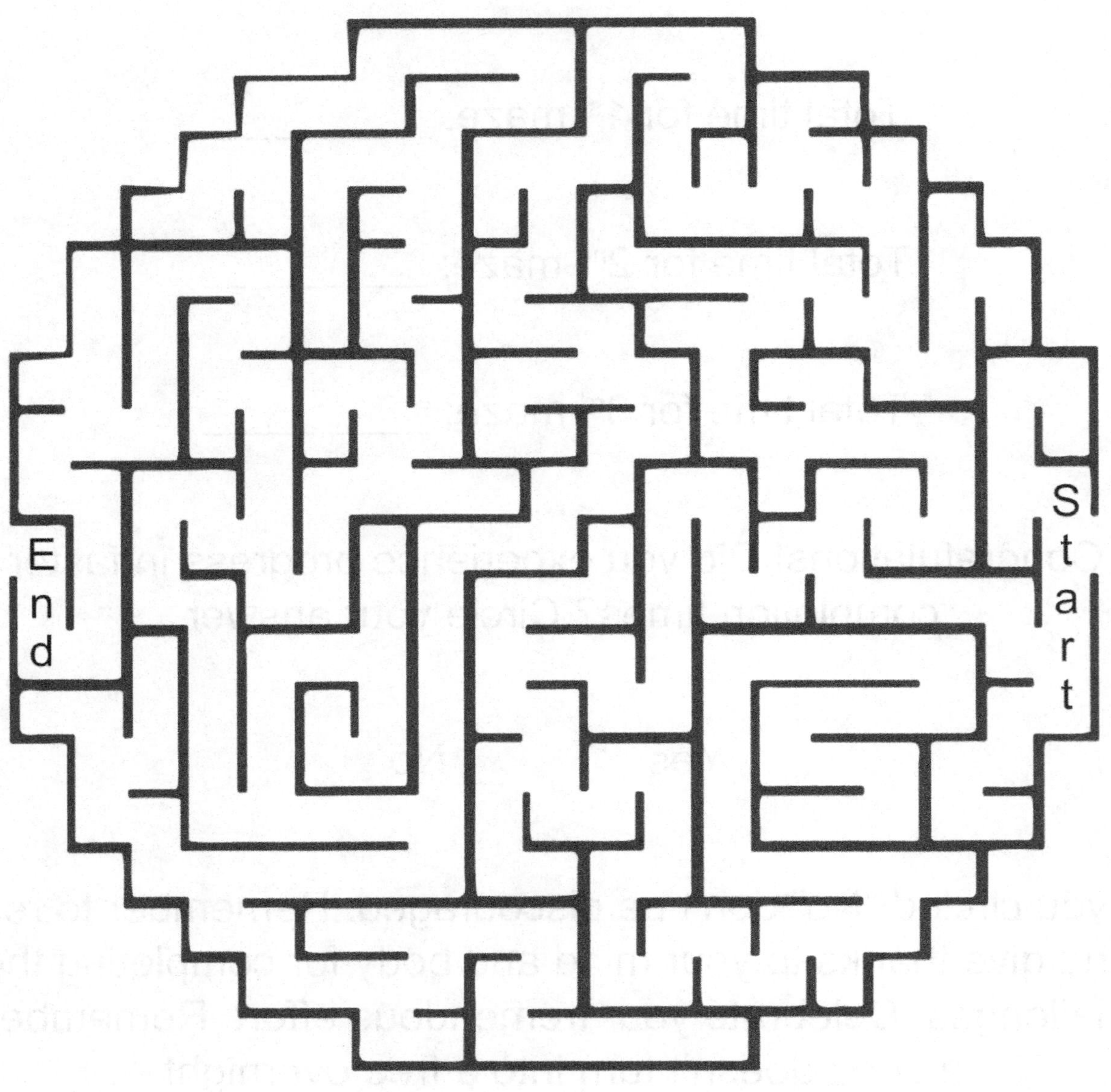

Start time: __________ End time: __________

Total time, maze 1: __________

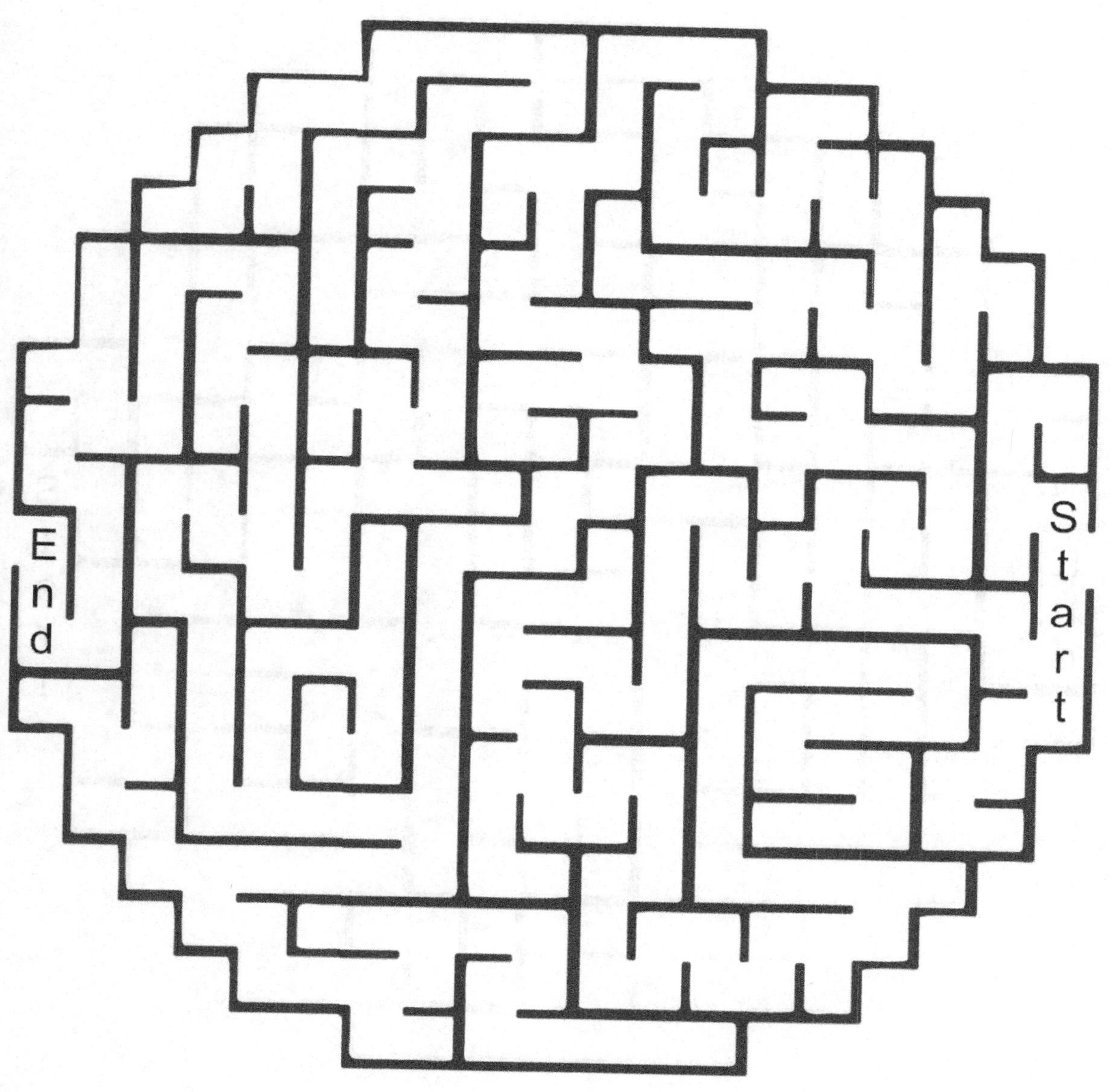

Start time: __________ End time: __________

Total time, maze 2: __________

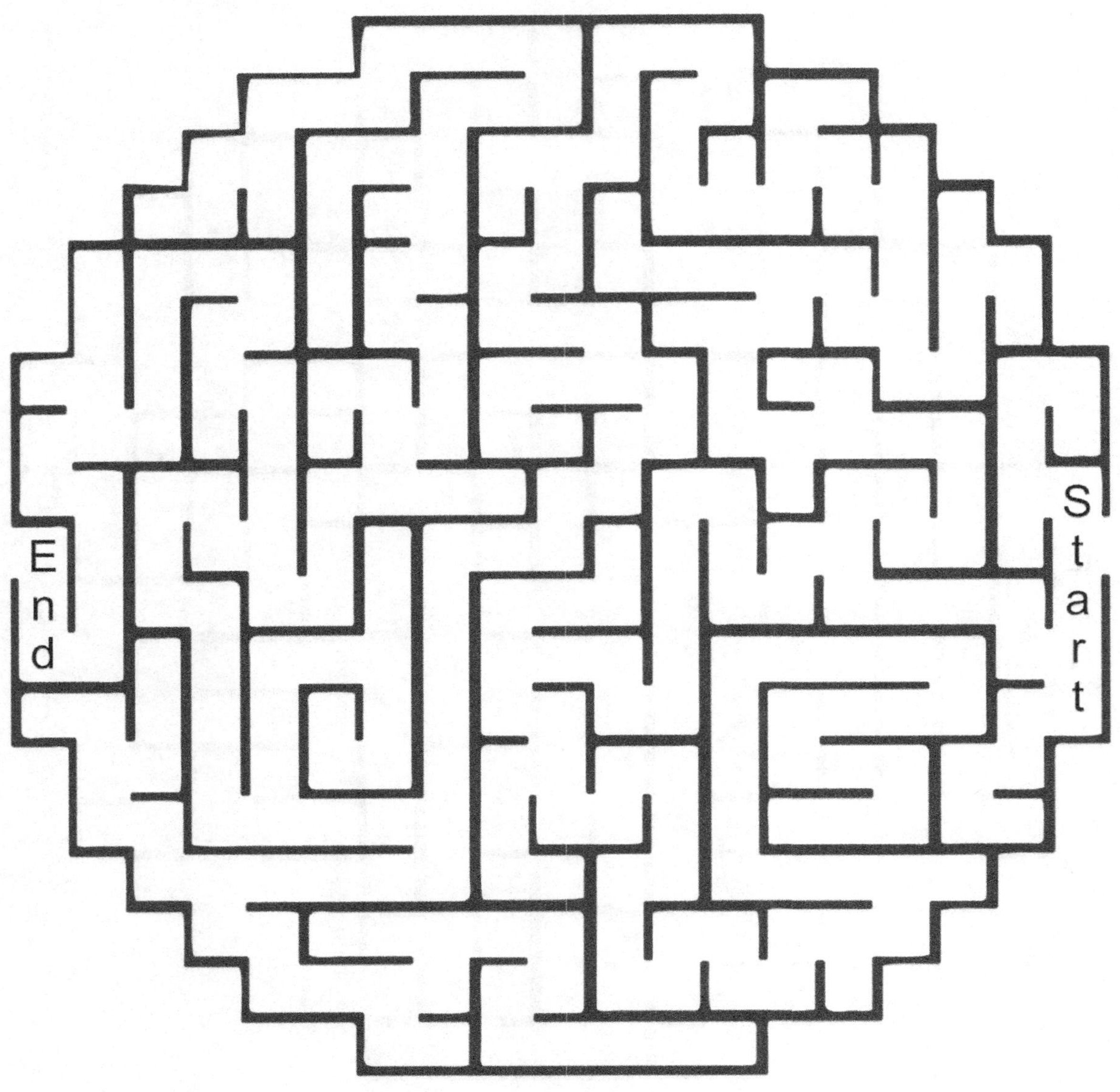

Start time: __________ End time: __________

Total time, maze 3: __________

Total time for 1st maze: __________

Total time for 2nd maze: __________

Total time for 3rd maze: __________

Congratulations! Did you experience progress in faster completion times? Circle your answer.

Yes No

If you circled "No" don't be discouraged. Remember to rest and give thanks to your mind and body for completing the challenges. Celebrate your tremendous effort. Remember, a seed doesn't turn into a tree overnight.

If you really want to do something, you'll find a way. If you don't, you'll find an excuse.

—*Jim Rohn*

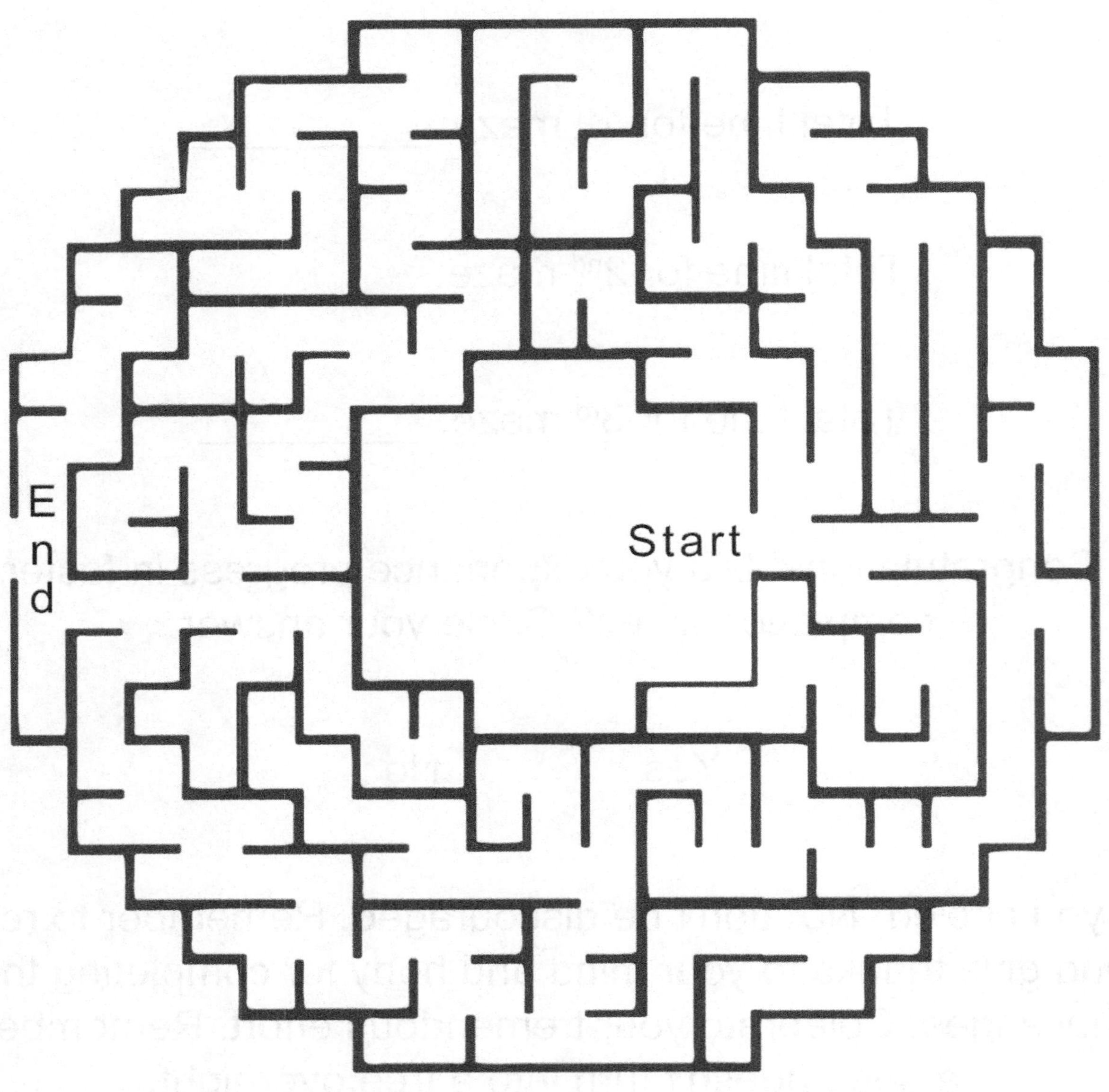

Start time: __________ End time: __________

Total time, maze 1: __________

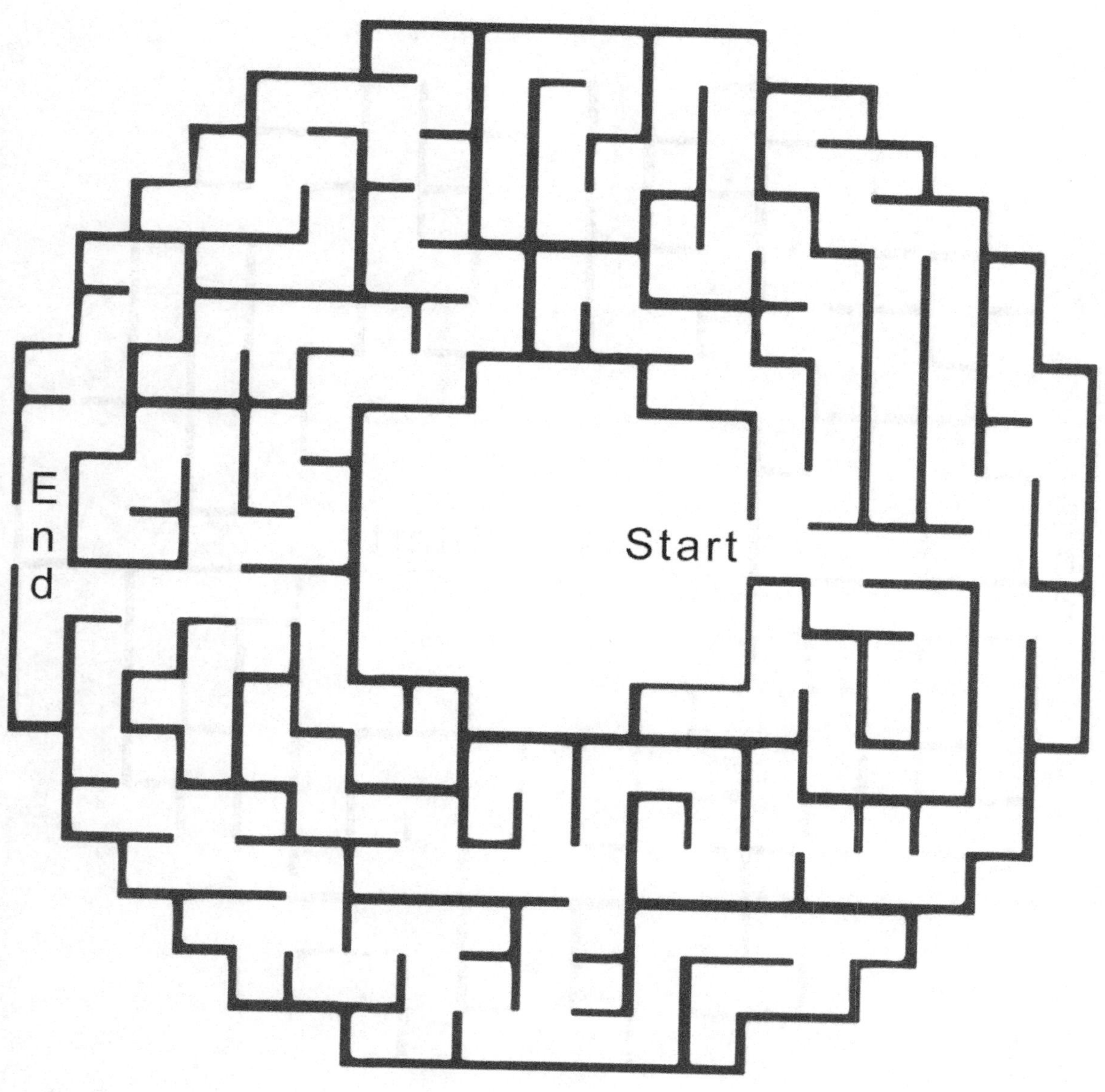

Start time: __________ End time: __________

Total time, maze 2: __________

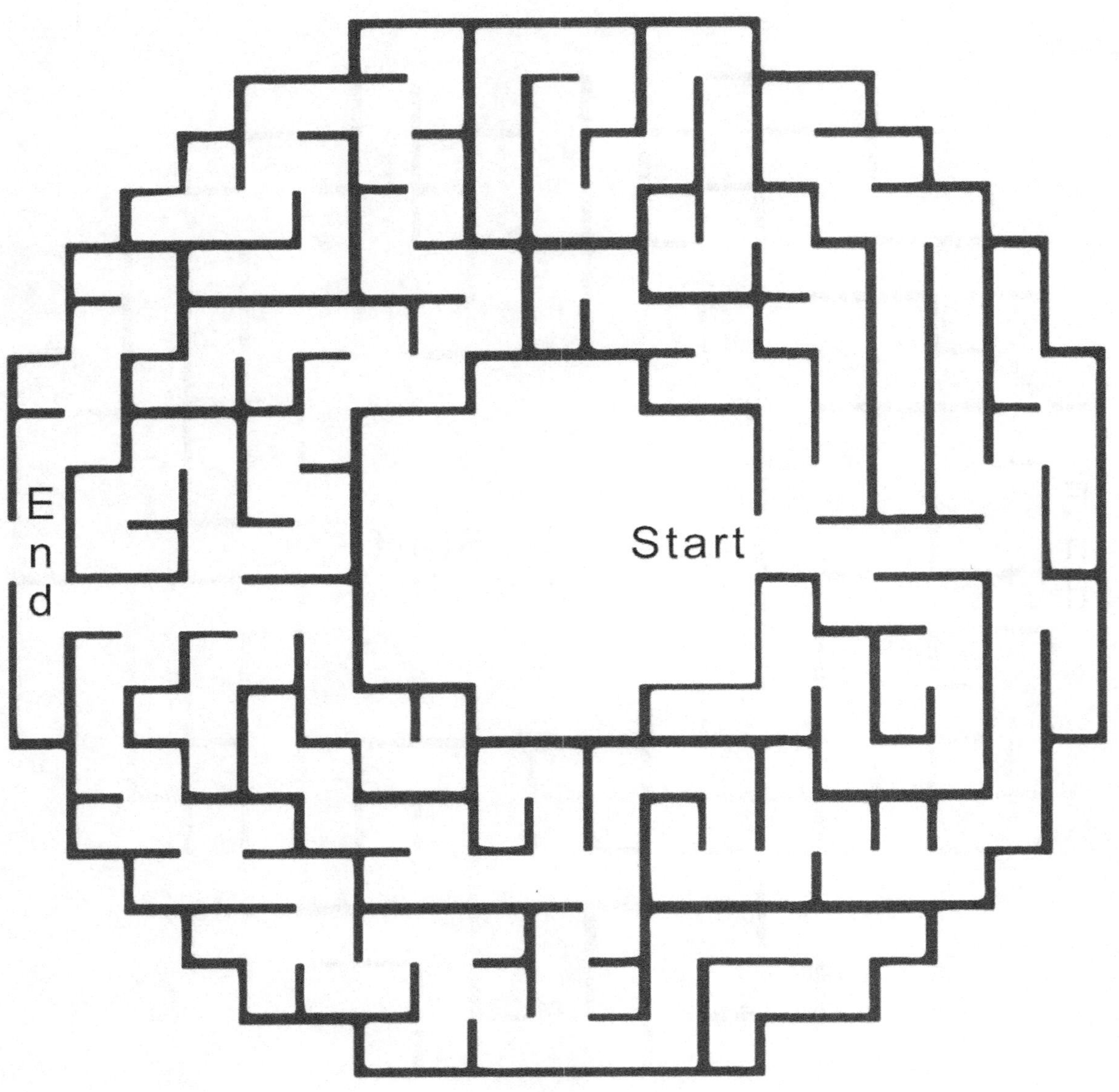

Start time: __________ End time: __________

Total time, maze 3: __________

Total time for 1st maze: __________

Total time for 2nd maze: __________

Total time for 3rd maze: __________

Congratulations! Did you experience progress in faster completion times? Circle your answer.

Yes No

If you circled "No" don't be discouraged. Remember to rest and give thanks to your mind and body for completing the challenges. Celebrate your tremendous effort. Remember, a seed doesn't turn into a tree overnight.

F.E.A.R: has two meanings: 1). Forget Everything And Run or 2). Face Everything And Rise; the choice is yours!

—Zig Ziglar

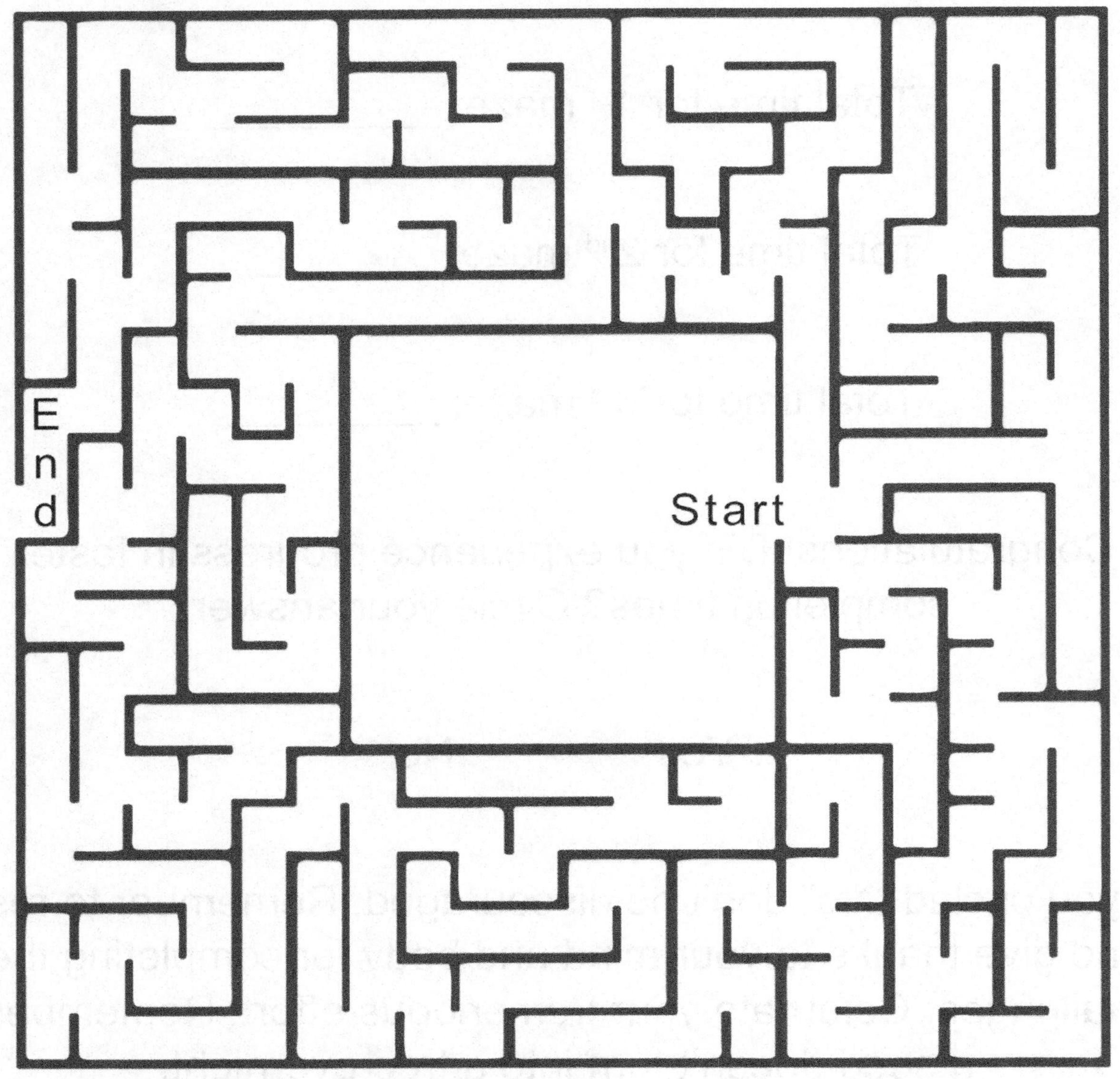

Start time: __________ End time: __________

Total time, maze 1: __________

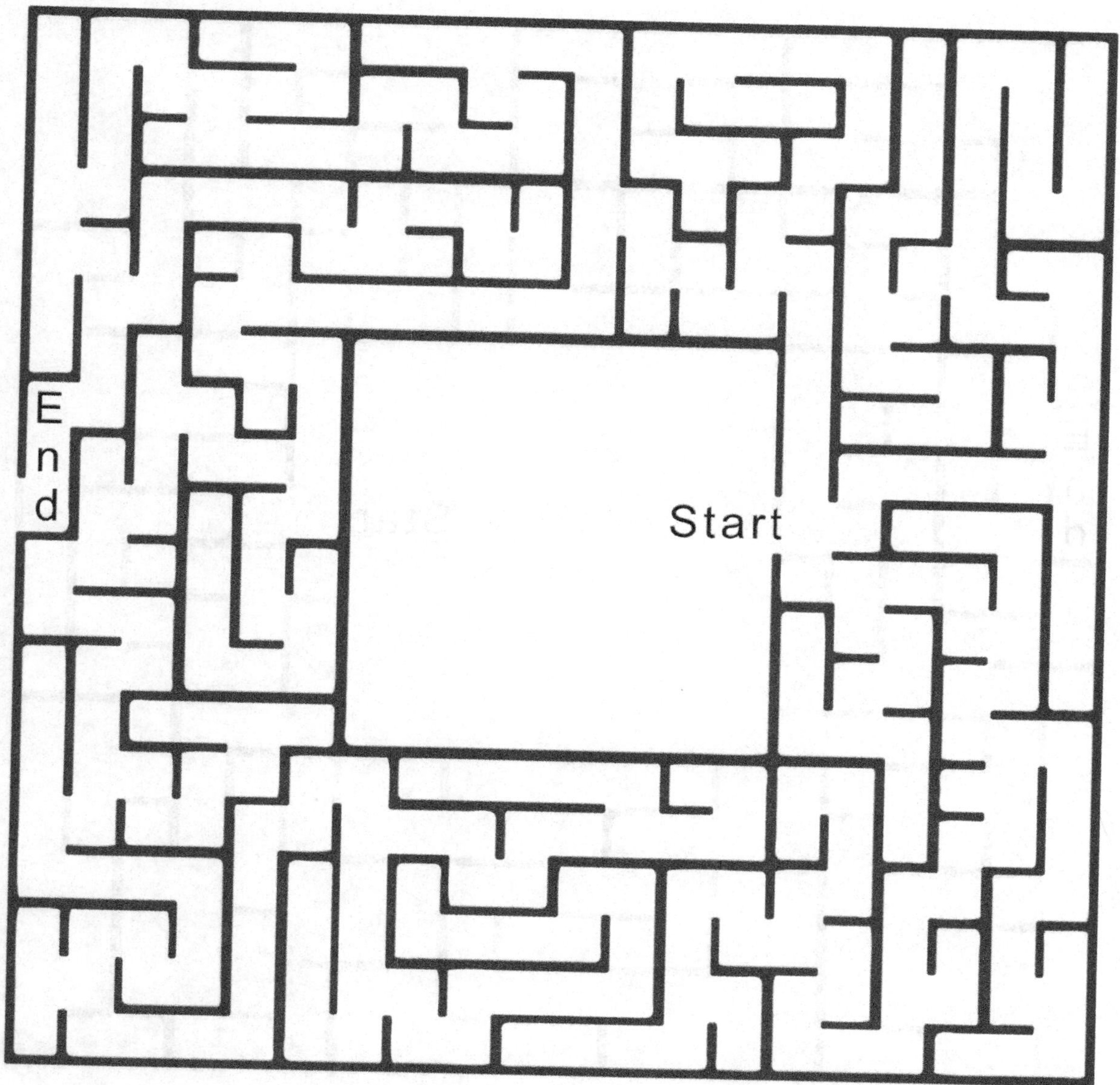

Start time: __________ End time: __________

Total time, maze 2: __________

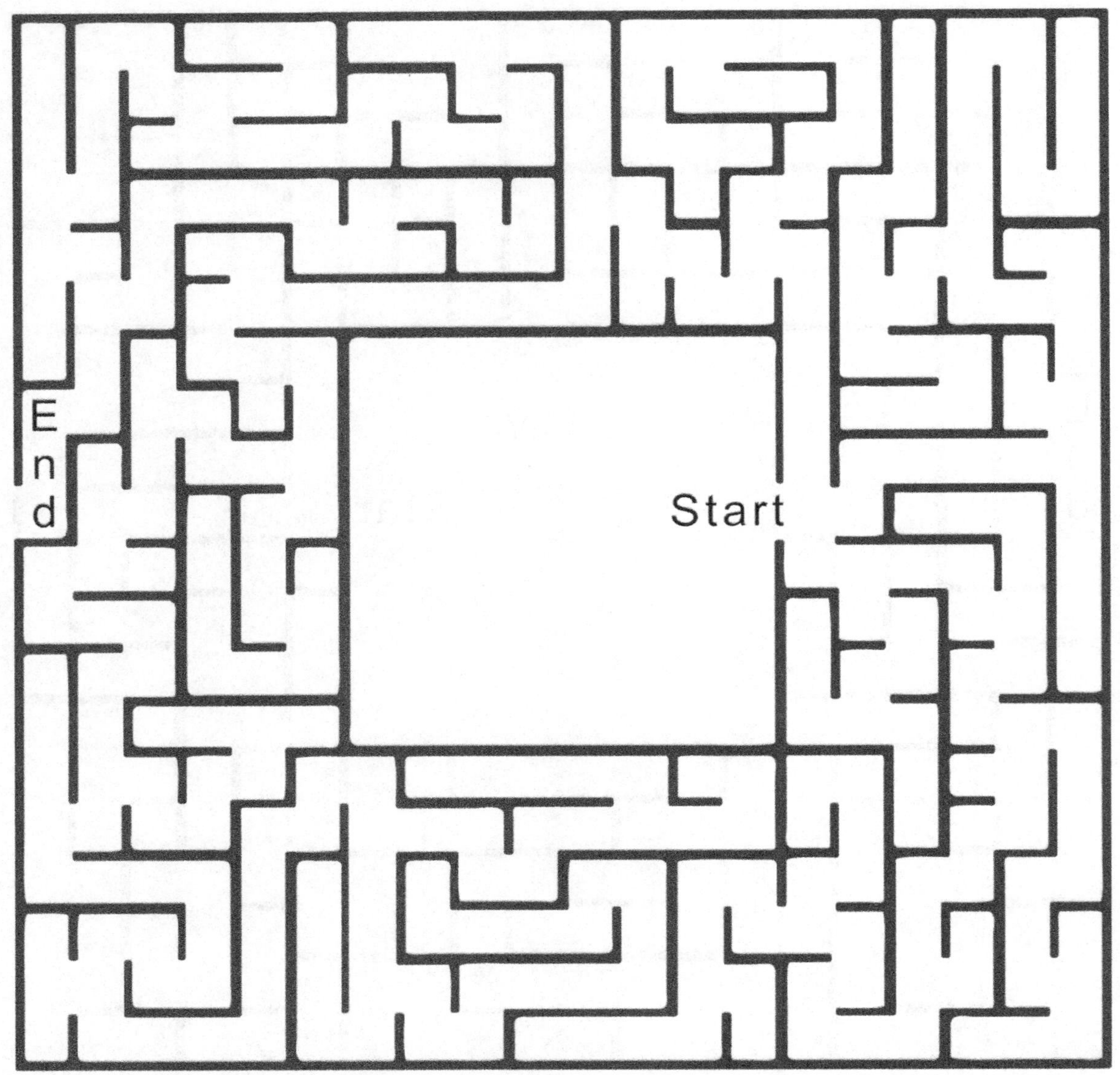

Start time: __________ End time: __________

Total time, maze 3: __________

Total time for 1st maze: __________

Total time for 2nd maze: __________

Total time for 3rd maze: __________

Congratulations! Did you experience progress in faster completion times? Circle your answer.

Yes No

If you circled "No" don't be discouraged. Remember to rest and give thanks to your mind and body for completing the challenges. Celebrate your tremendous effort. Remember, a seed doesn't turn into a tree overnight.

Life is like a camera… Focus on what's important, Capture the good times, Develop from the negatives, and if things don't work out, take another shot.

—*Unknown*

Only those who risk going too far
can possibly find out how far one can go.

—*T.S. Eliot*

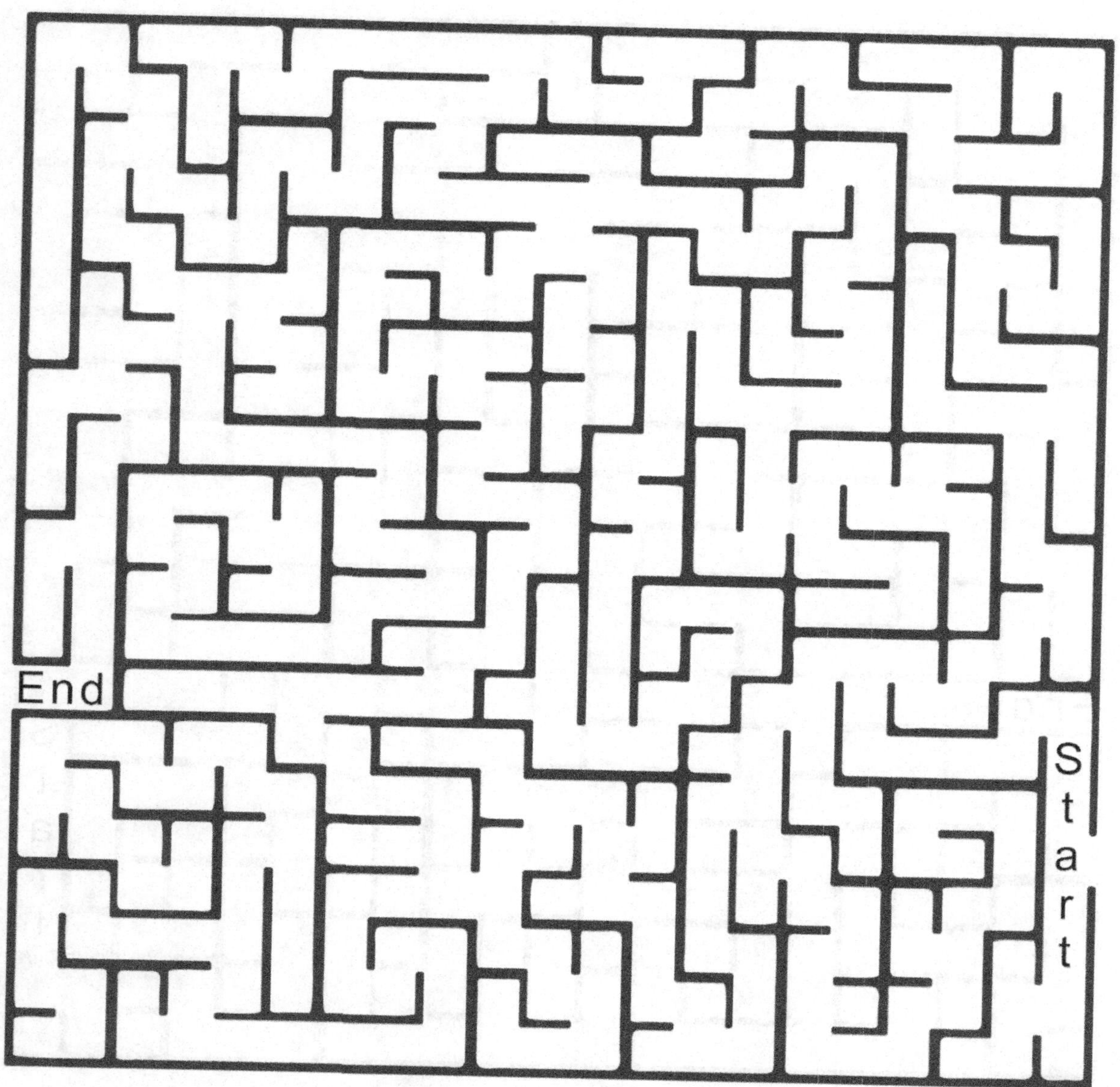

Start time: __________ End time: __________

Total time, maze 1: __________

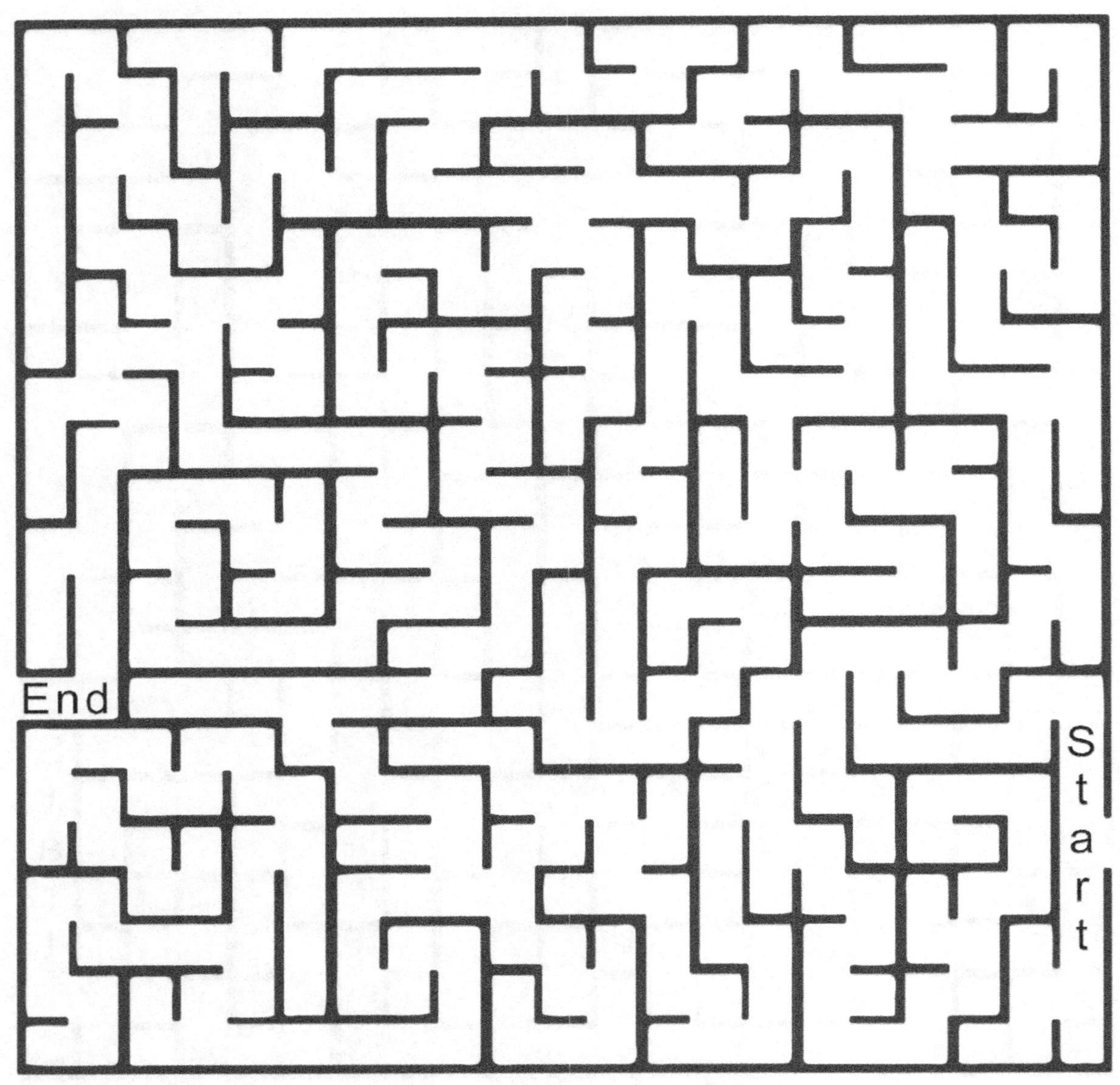

Start time: ___________ End time: ___________

Total time, maze 2: ___________

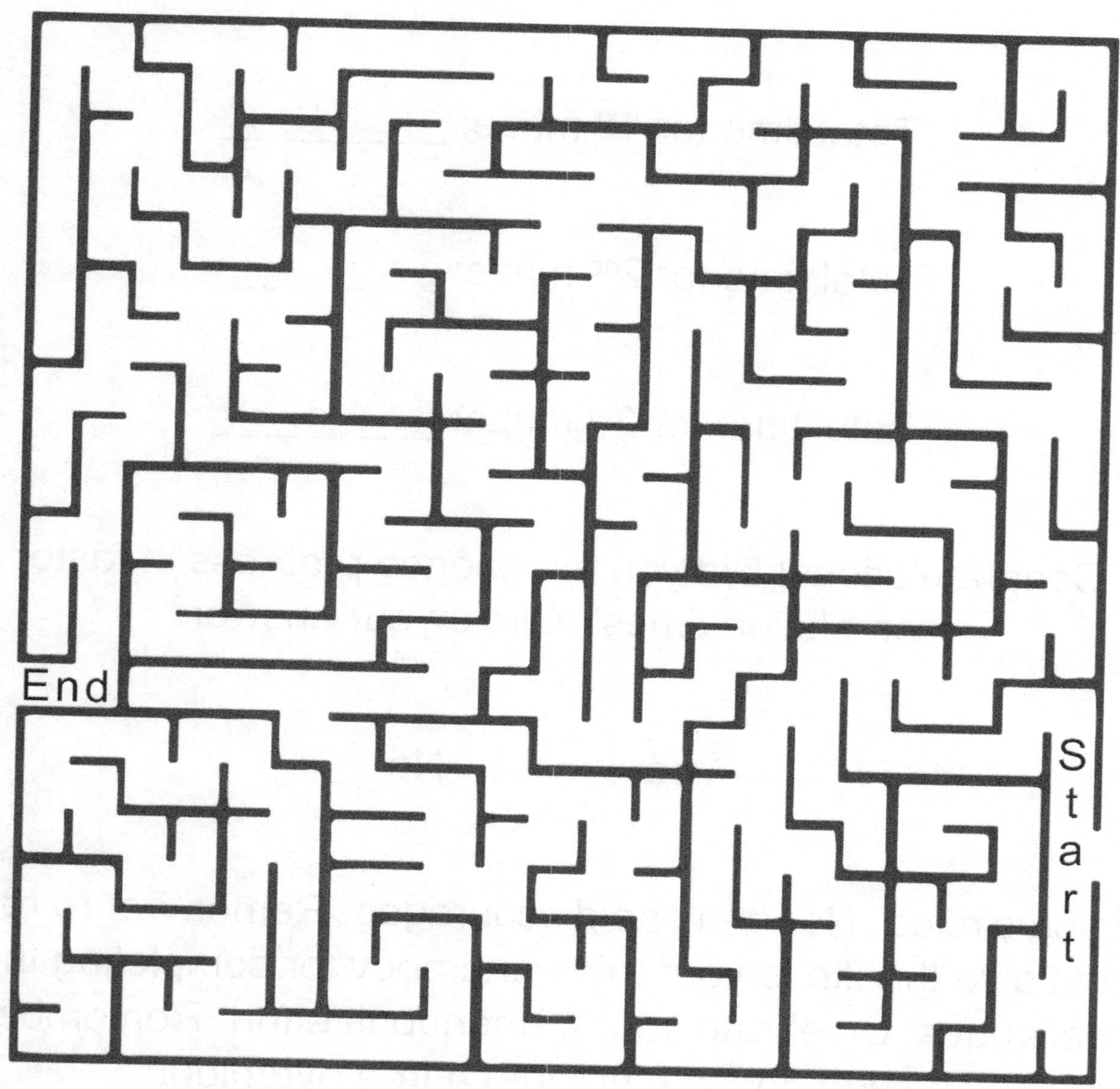

Start time: __________ End time: __________

Total time, maze 3: __________

Total time for 1st maze: __________

Total time for 2nd maze: __________

Total time for 3rd maze: __________

Congratulations! Did you experience progress in faster completion times? Circle your answer.

Yes No

If you circled "No" don't be discouraged. Remember to rest and give thanks to your mind and body for completing the challenges. Celebrate your tremendous effort. Remember, a seed doesn't turn into a tree overnight.

Keep watering, keep planting, keep cultivating, and one day your garden will bloom.

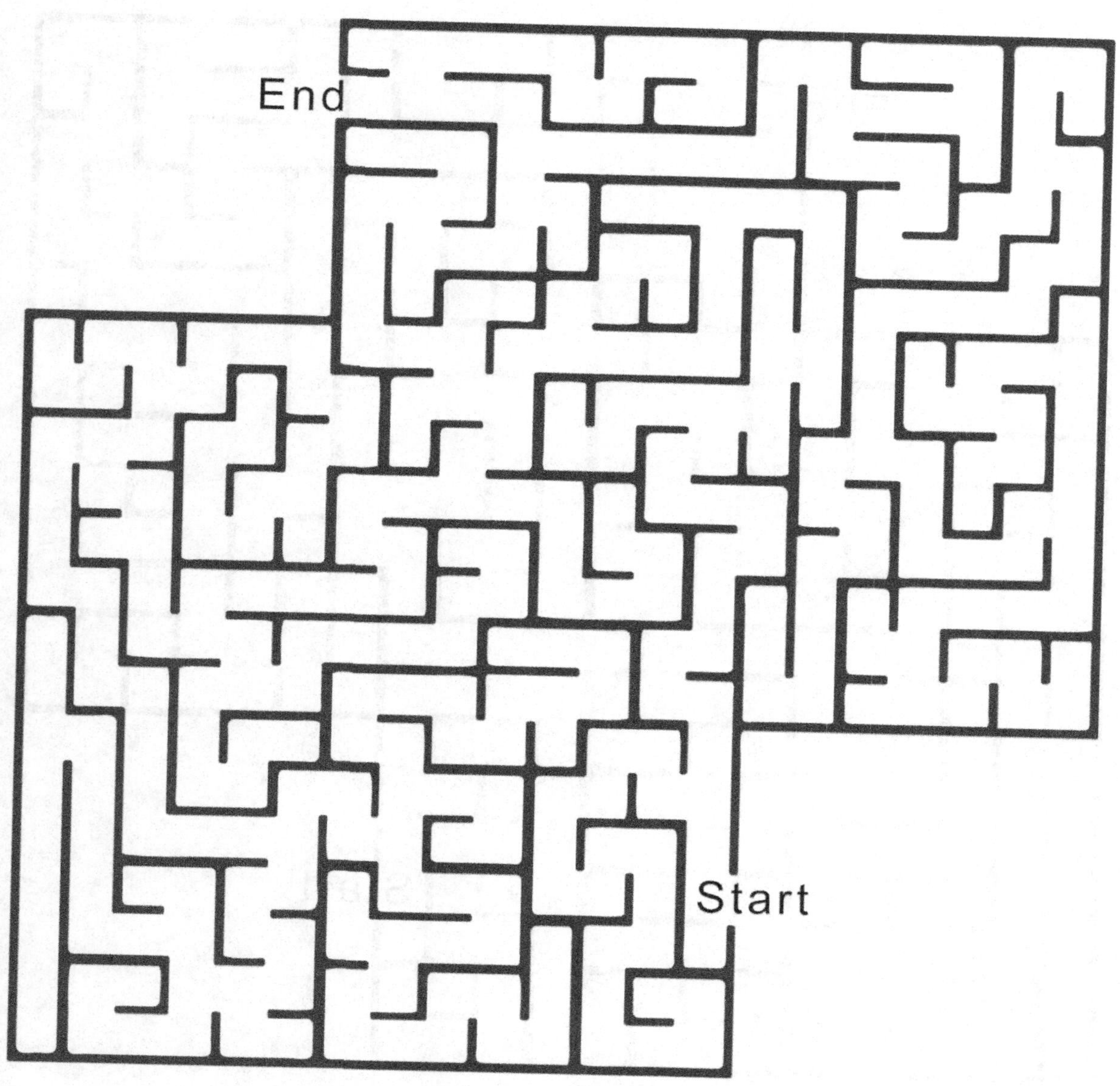

Start time: ___________ End time: ___________

Total time, maze 1: ___________

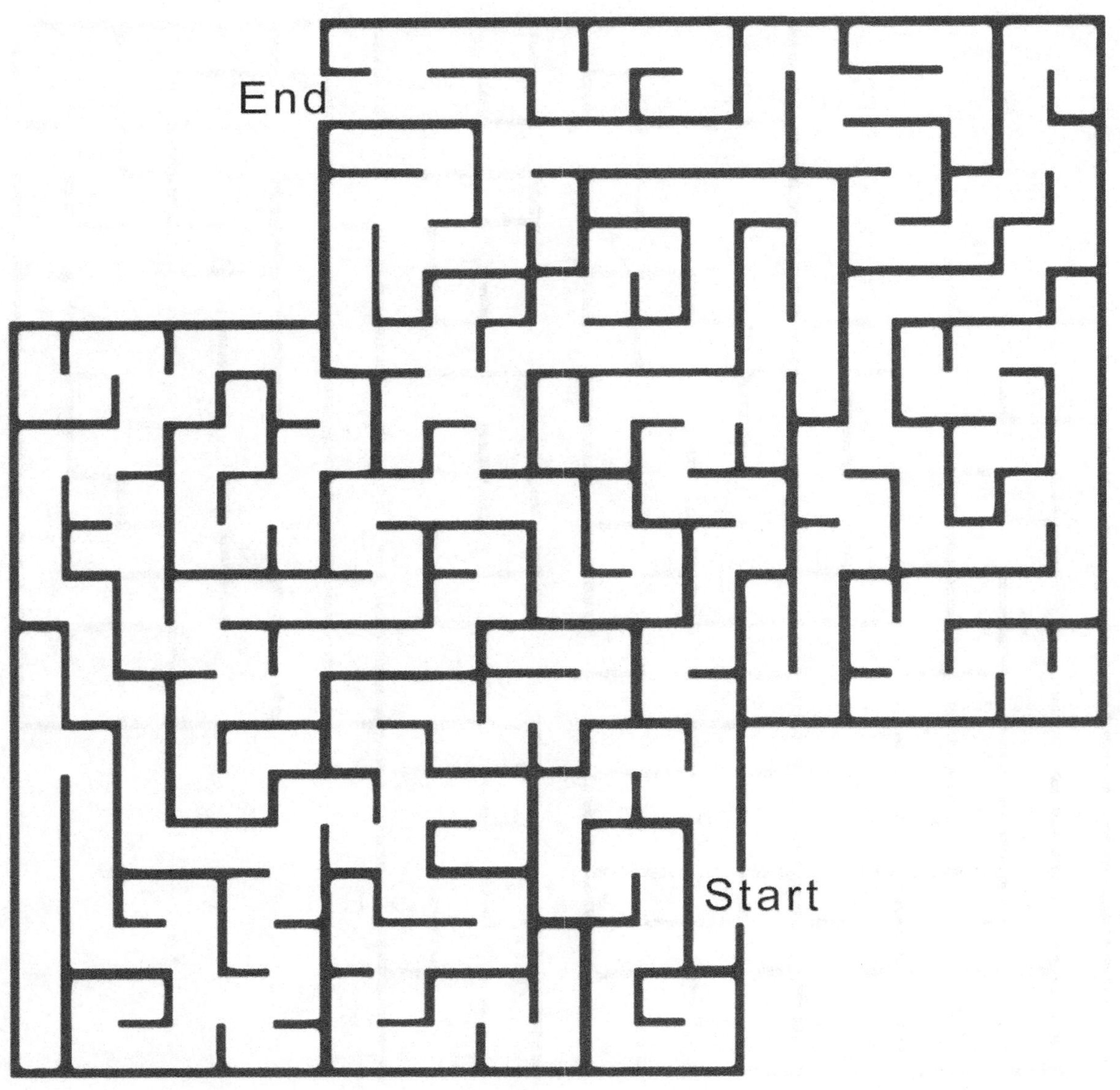

Start time: __________ End time: __________

Total time, maze 2: __________

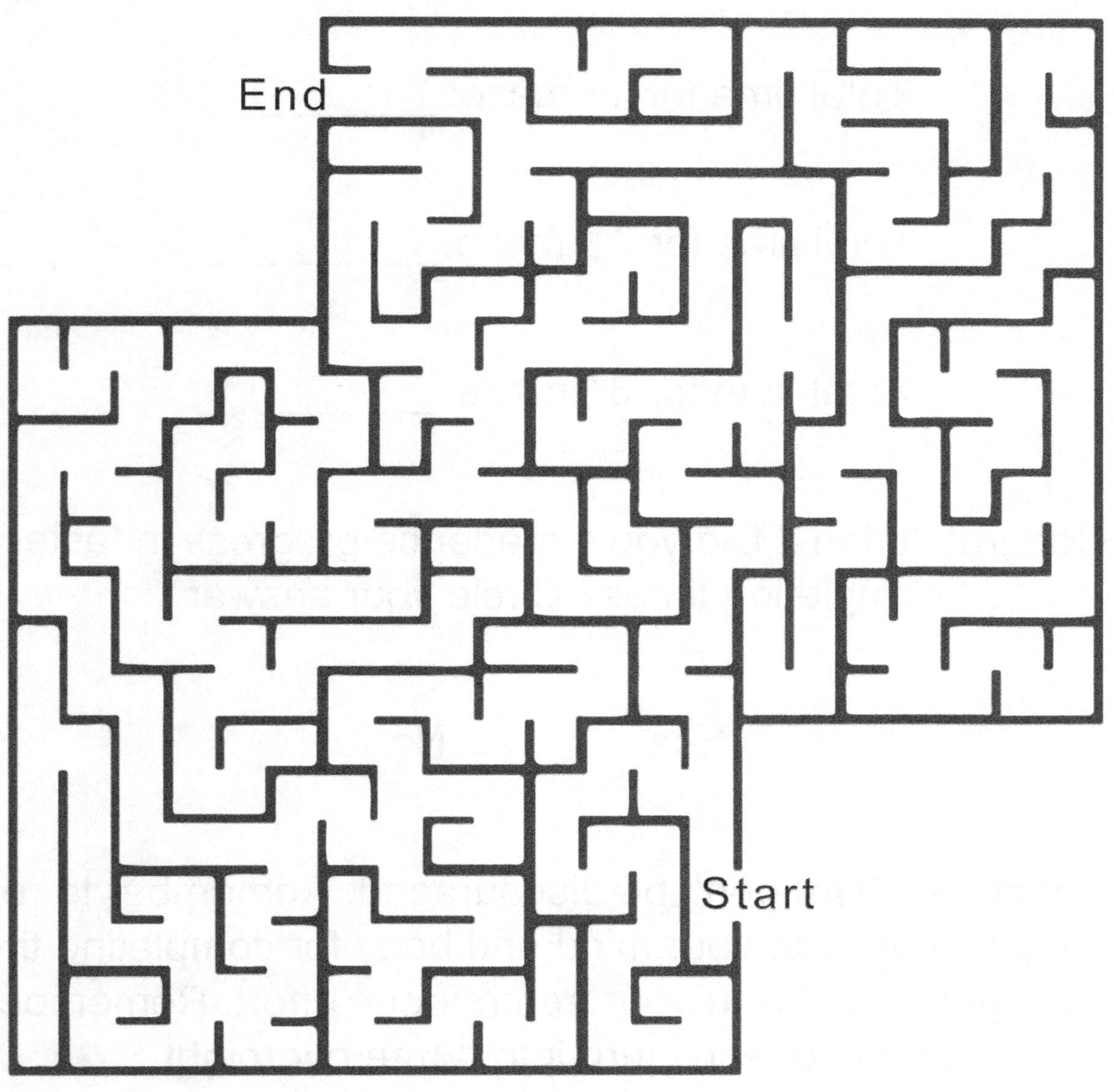

Start time: __________ End time: __________

Total time, maze 3: __________

Total time for 1st maze: __________

Total time for 2nd maze: __________

Total time for 3rd maze: __________

Congratulations! Did you experience progress in faster completion times? Circle your answer.

Yes No

If you circled "No" don't be discouraged. Remember to rest and give thanks to your mind and body for completing the challenges. Celebrate your tremendous effort. Remember, a seed doesn't turn into a tree overnight.

One of the things I learned the hard way was that it doesn't pay to get discouraged. Keeping busy and making optimism a way of life can restore your faith in yourself.

—Lucille Ball

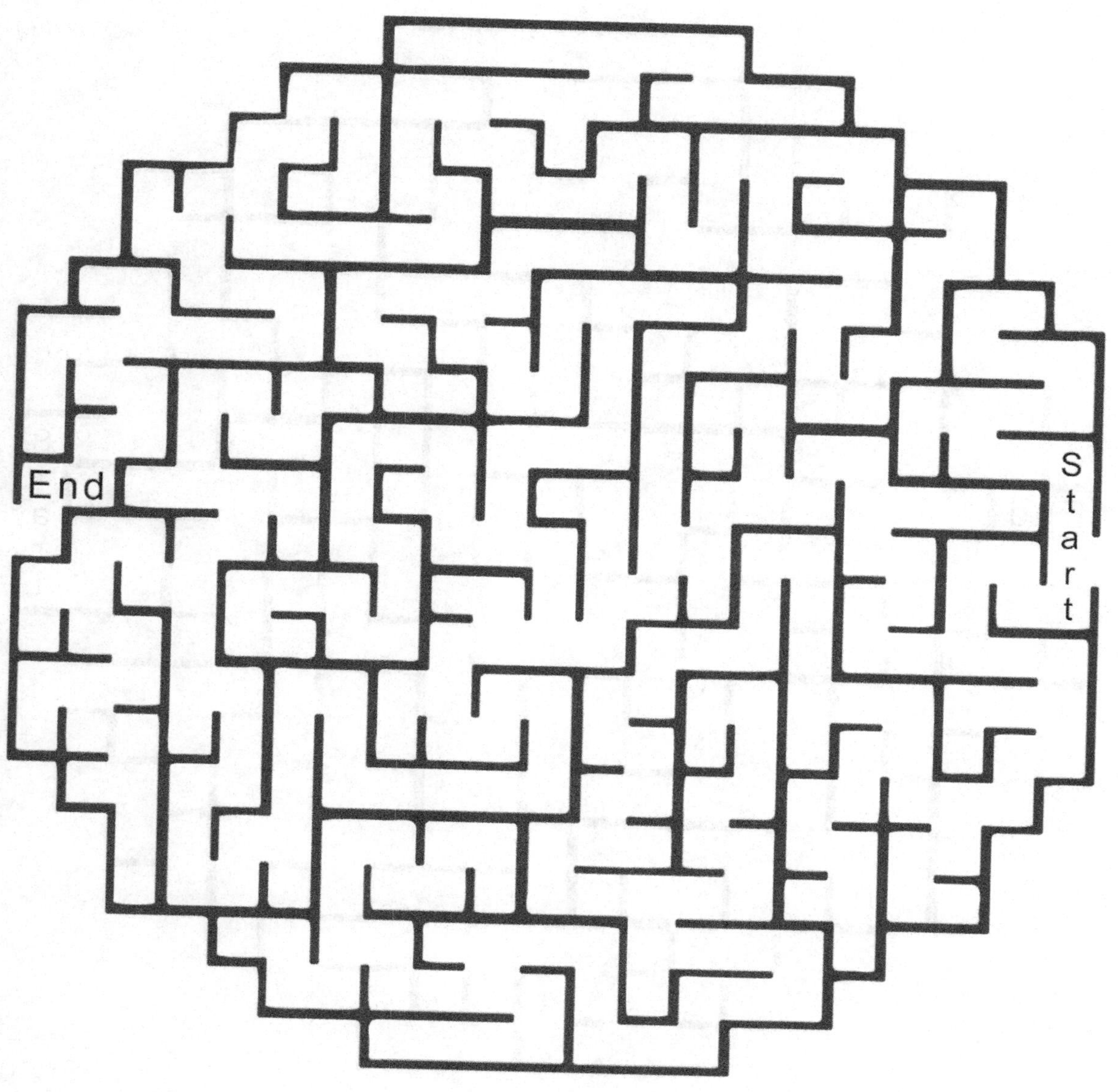

Start time: ___________ End time: ___________

Total time, maze 1: ___________

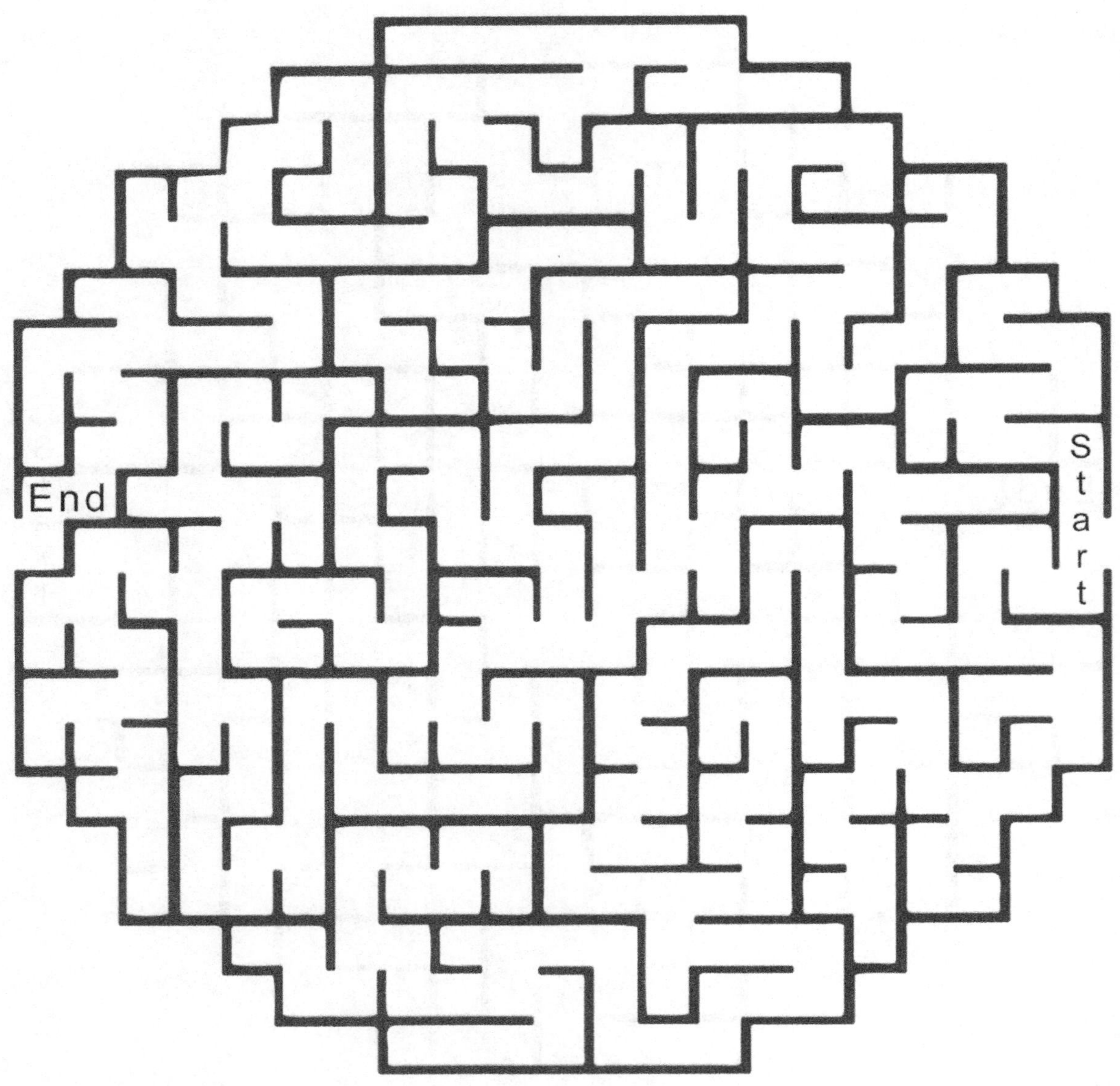

Start time: __________ End time: __________

Total time, maze 2: __________

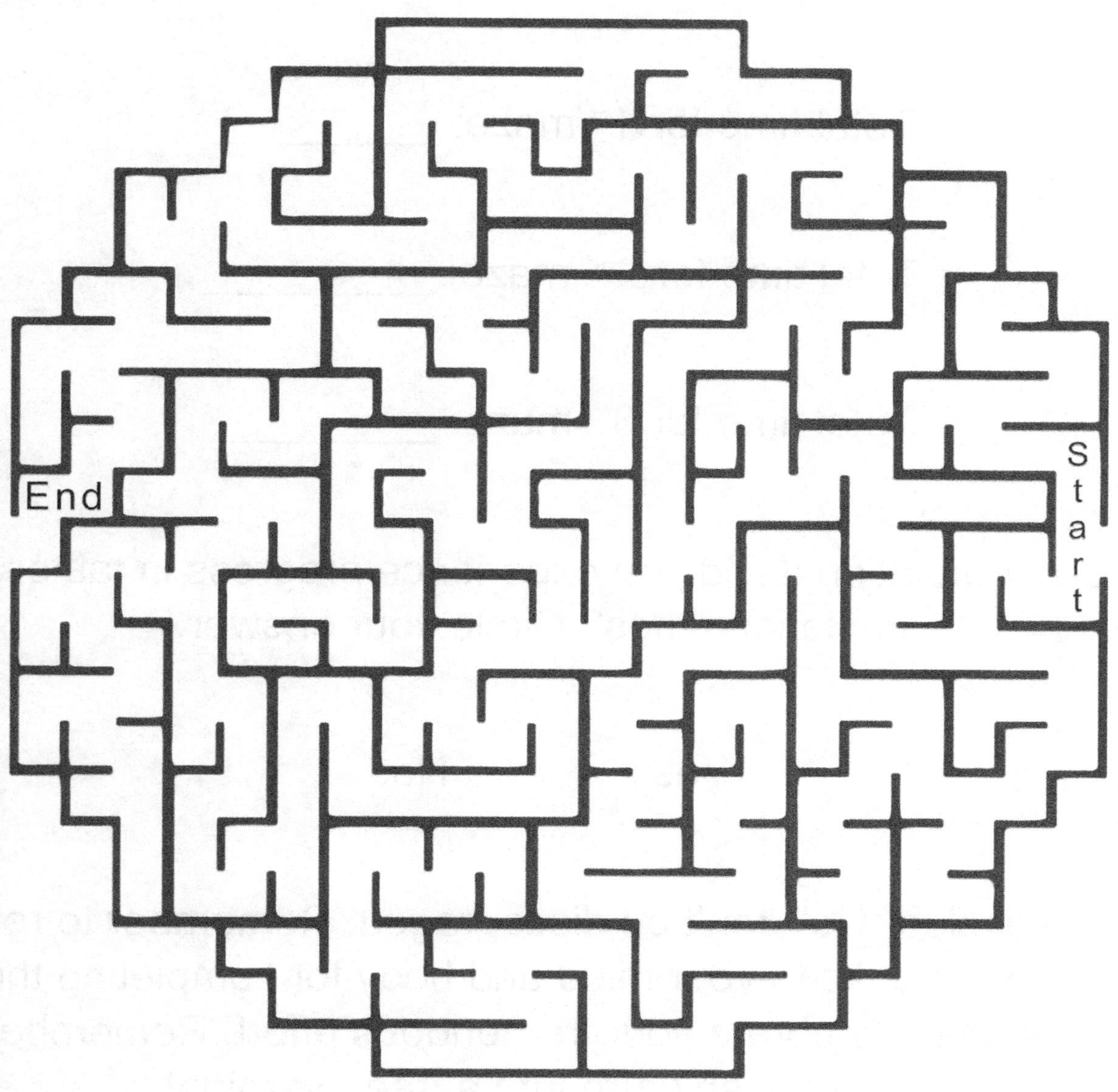

Start time: __________ End time: __________

Total time, maze 3: __________

Total time for 1st maze: __________

Total time for 2nd maze: __________

Total time for 3rd maze: __________

Congratulations! Did you experience progress in faster completion times? Circle your answer.

Yes No

If you circled "No" don't be discouraged. Remember to rest and give thanks to your mind and body for completing the challenges. Celebrate your tremendous effort. Remember, a seed doesn't turn into a tree overnight.

Edison failed 10,000 times before he made the electric light. Do not be discouraged if you fail a few times.

—*Napoleon Hill*

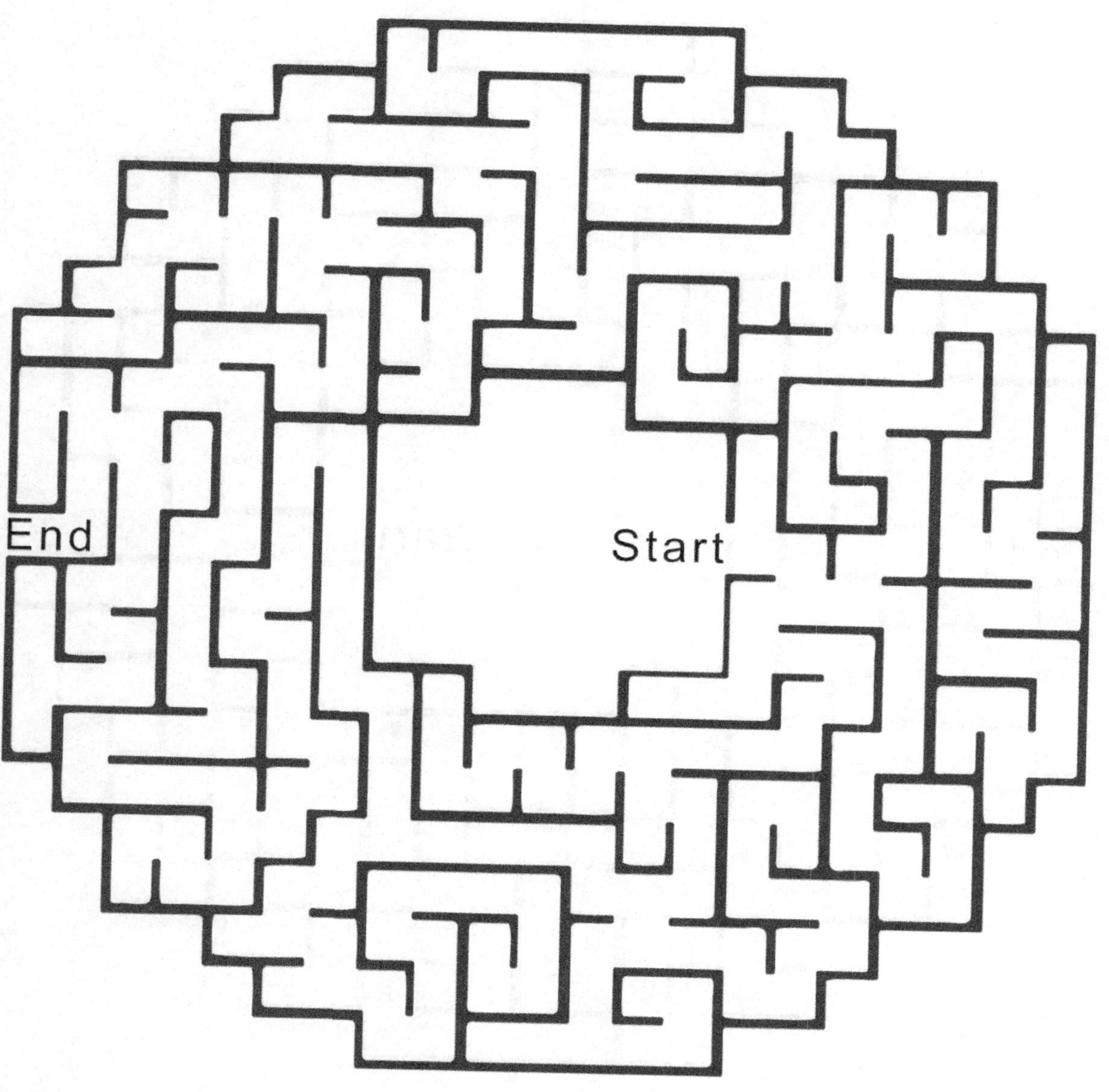

Start time: __________ End time: __________

Total time, maze 1: __________

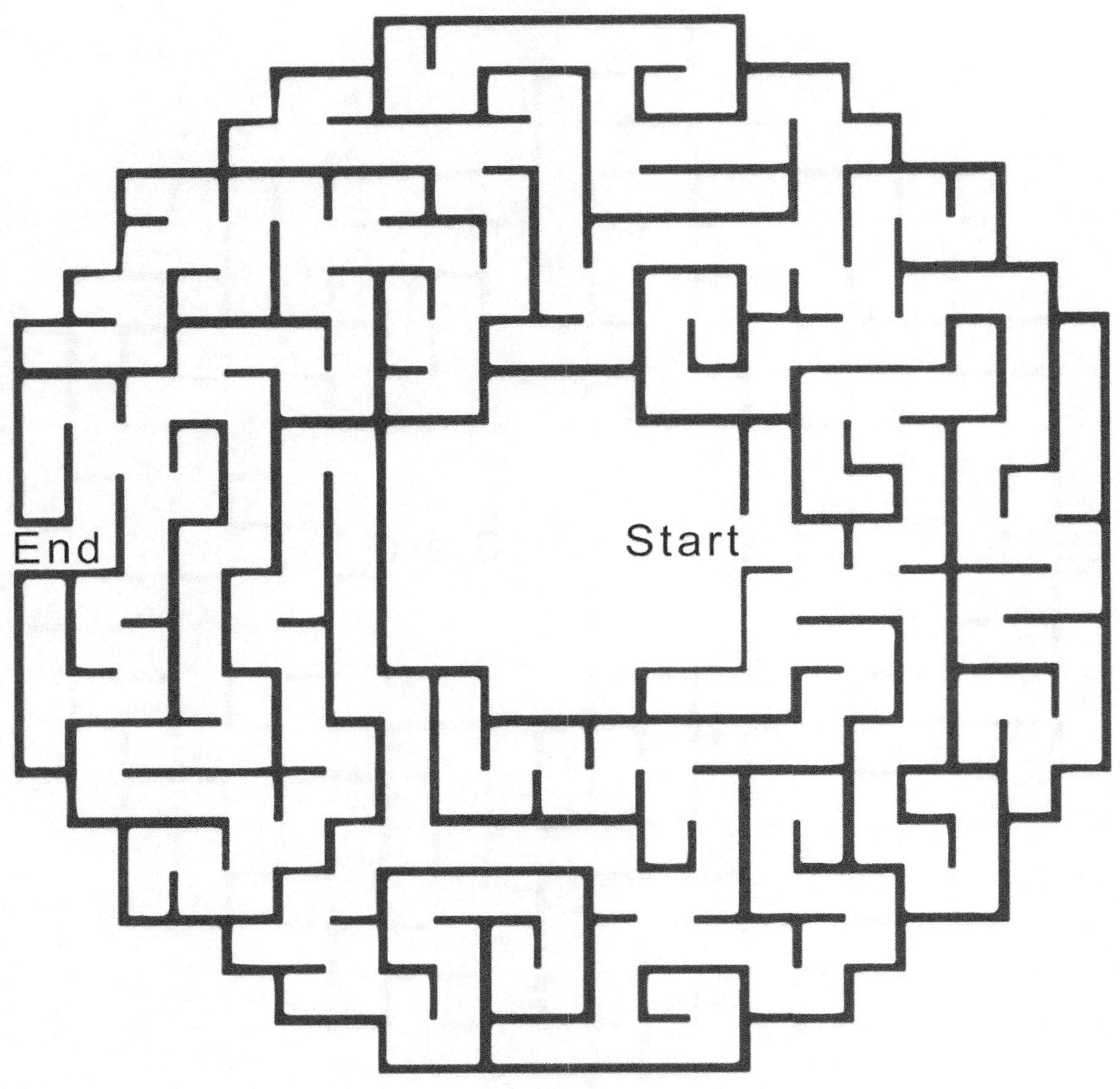

Start time: __________ End time: __________

Total time, maze 2: __________

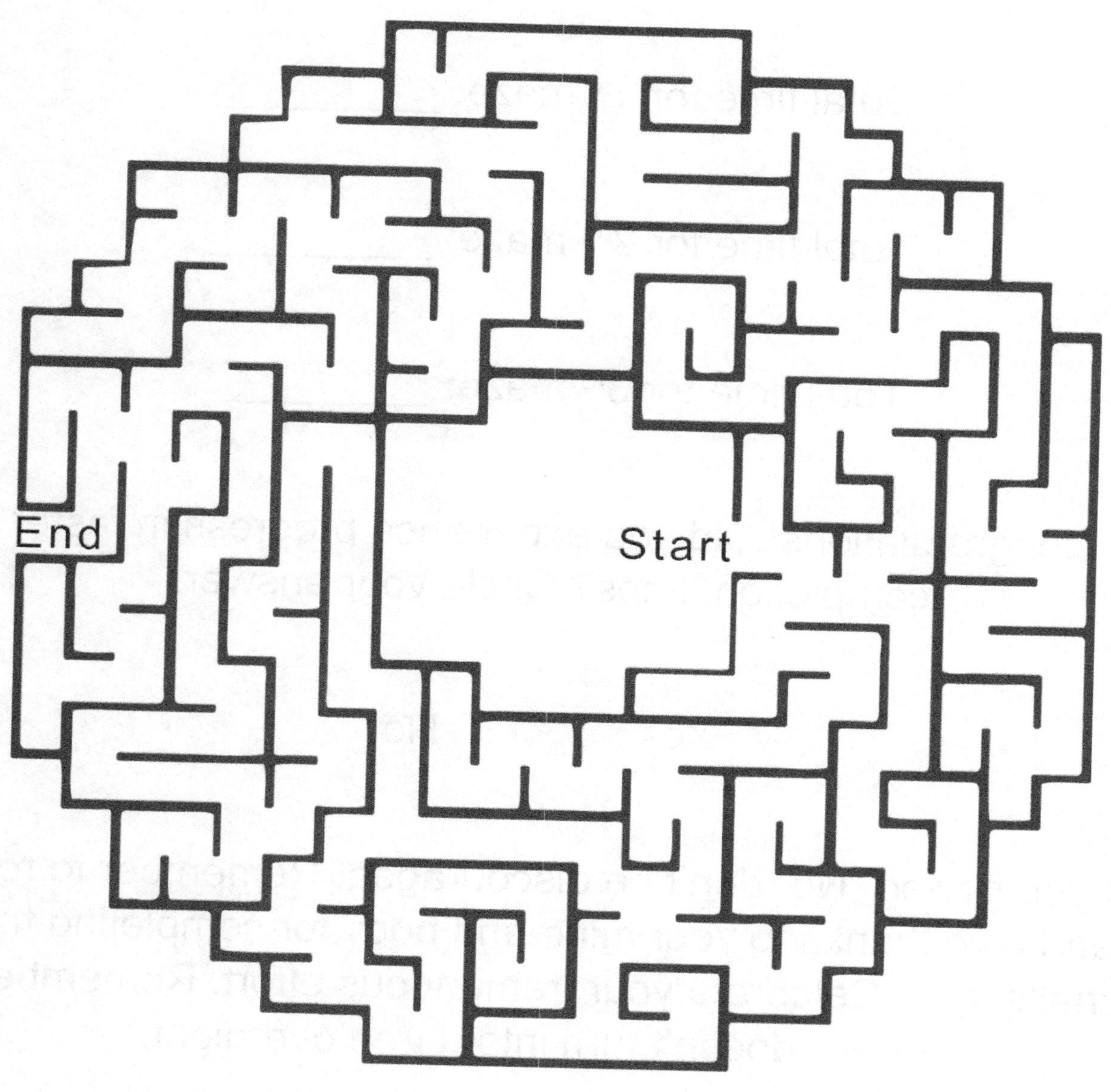

Start time: __________ End time: __________

Total time, maze 3: __________

Total time for 1st maze: __________

Total time for 2nd maze: __________

Total time for 3rd maze: __________

Congratulations! Did you experience progress in faster completion times? Circle your answer.

Yes No

If you circled "No" don't be discouraged. Remember to rest and give thanks to your mind and body for completing the challenges. Celebrate your tremendous effort. Remember, a seed doesn't turn into a tree overnight.

A man can get discouraged many times but he is not a failure until he begins to blame somebody else and stops trying.

—*John Burroughs*

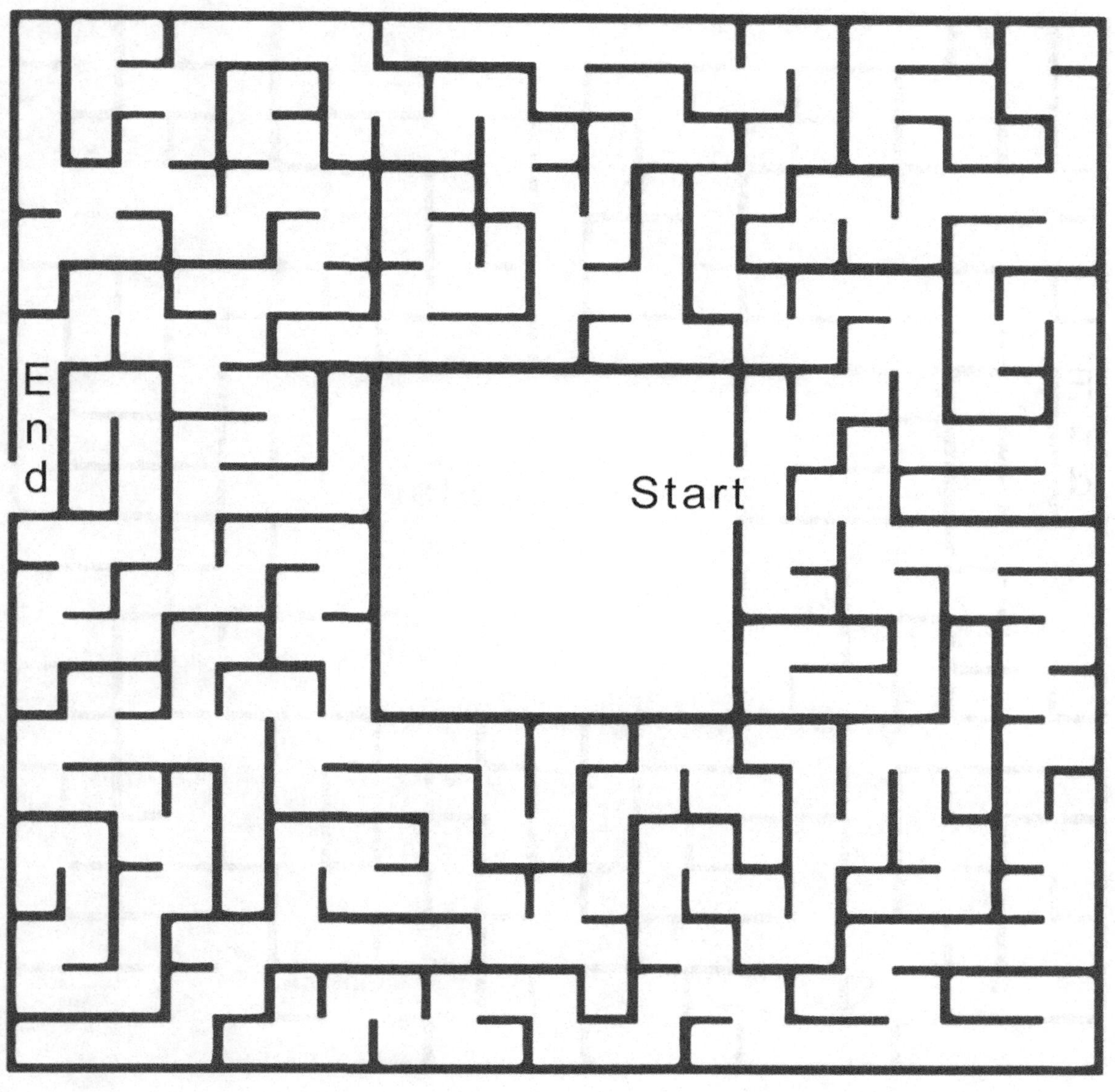

Start time: __________ End time: __________

Total time, maze 1: __________

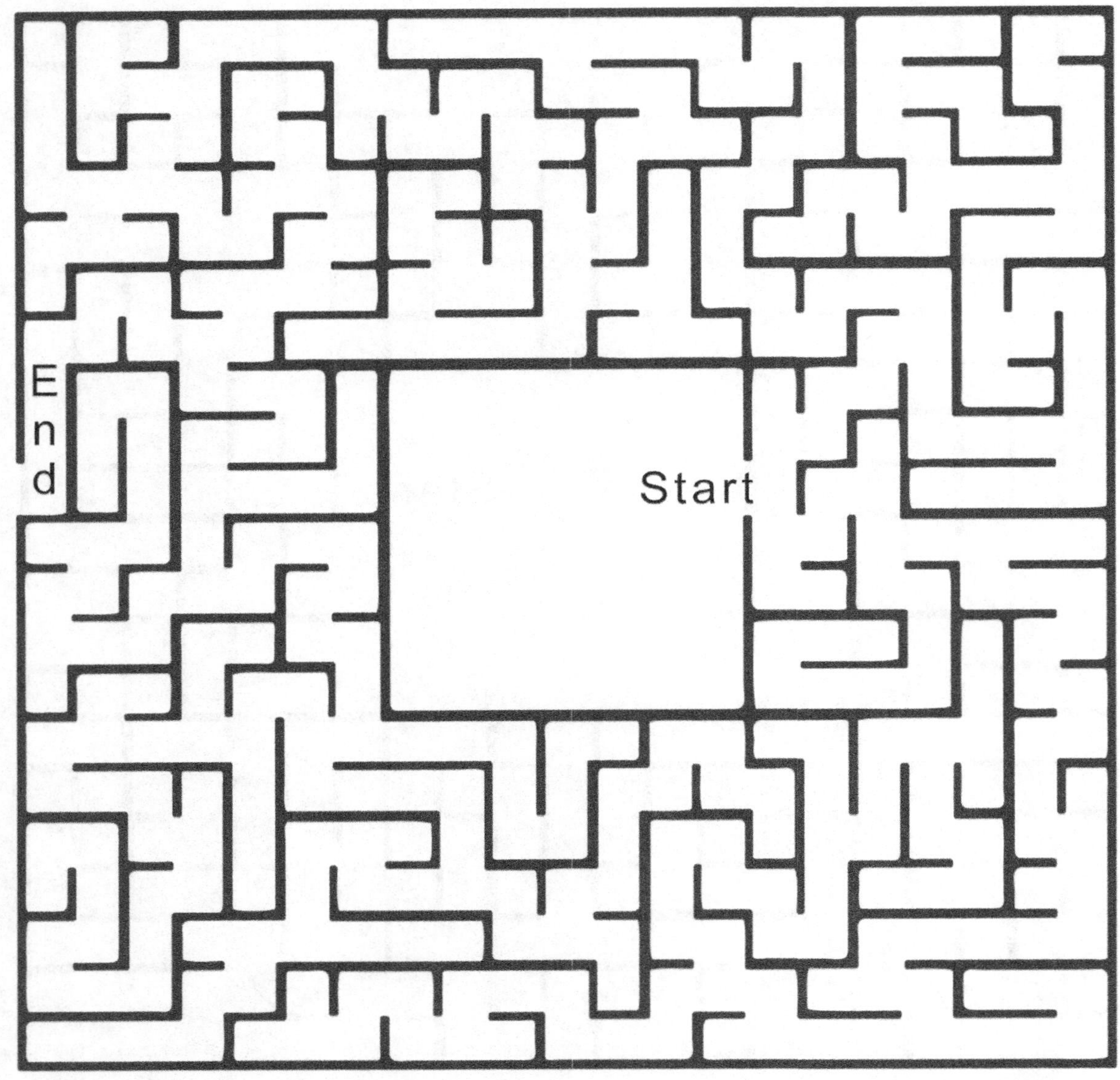

Start time: __________ End time: __________

Total time, maze 2: __________

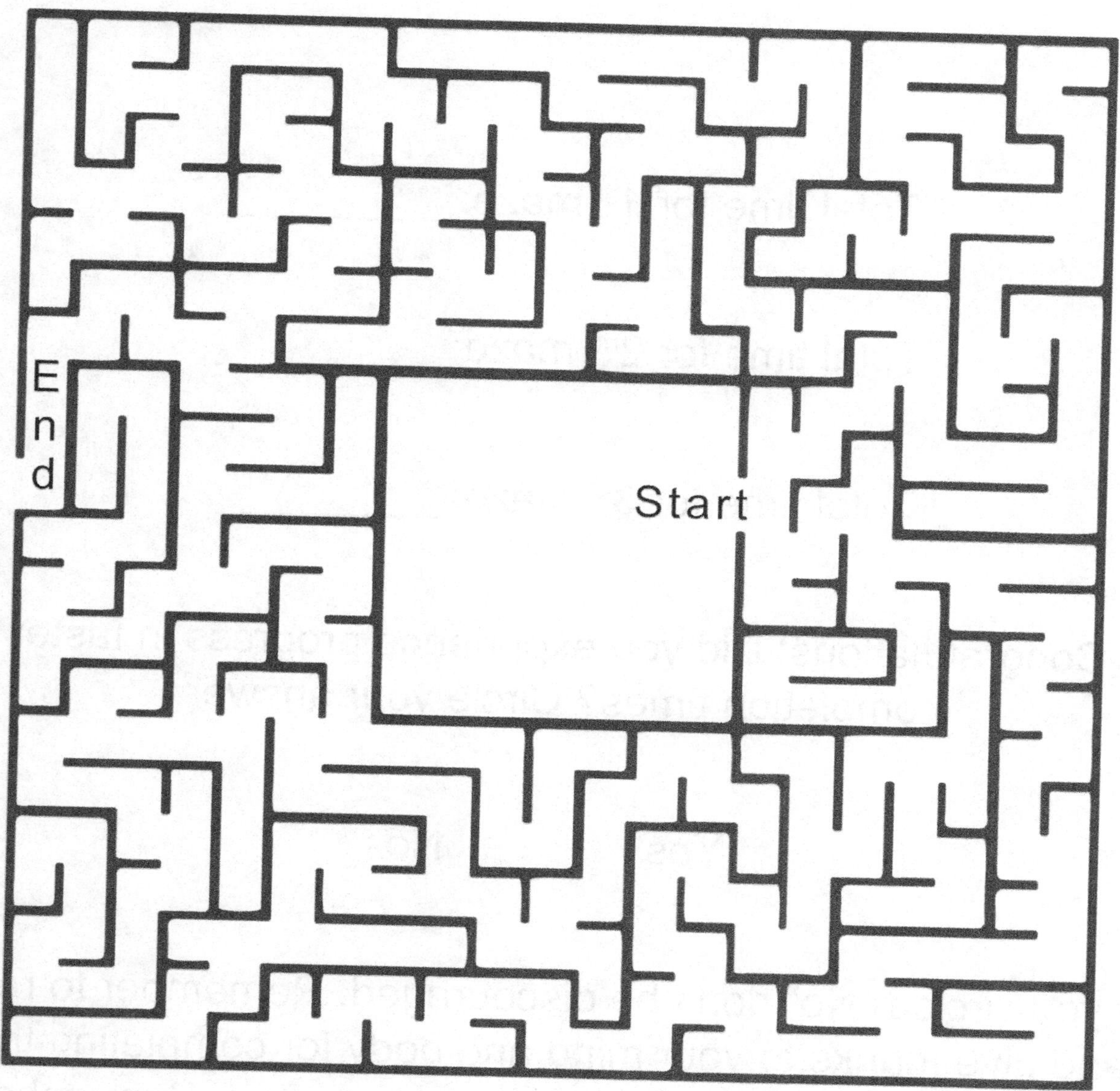

Start time: __________ End time: __________

Total time, maze 3: __________

Total time for 1st maze: __________

Total time for 2nd maze: __________

Total time for 3rd maze: __________

Congratulations! Did you experience progress in faster completion times? Circle your answer.

Yes No

If you circled “No” don’t be discouraged. Remember to rest and give thanks to your mind and body for completing the challenges. Celebrate your tremendous effort. Remember, a seed doesn’t turn into a tree overnight.

Keep watering, keep planting, keep cultivating, and one day your garden will bloom.

Chapter 3.

25 ADVANCED PUZZLES (in Triplicate to Track your Progress)

The End is the Beginning

Your dream is on the making, my dear.
It is a beautiful creation that of yours.
Don't despair, the end is almost here,
it will come as the most amazing beginning.
You have earned it and we are proud of you...

—Roxana Jones

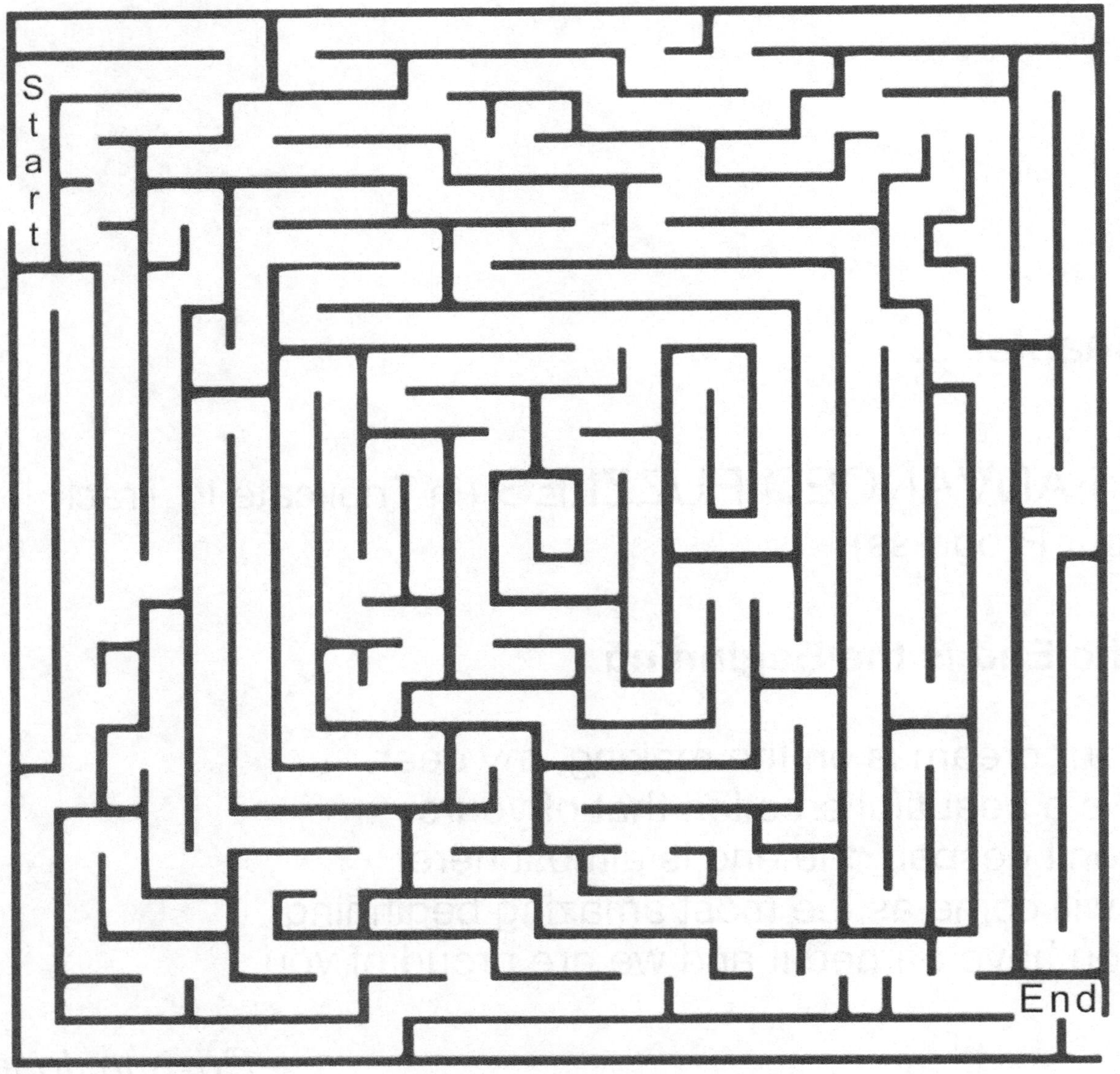

Start time: __________ End time: __________

Total time, maze 1: __________

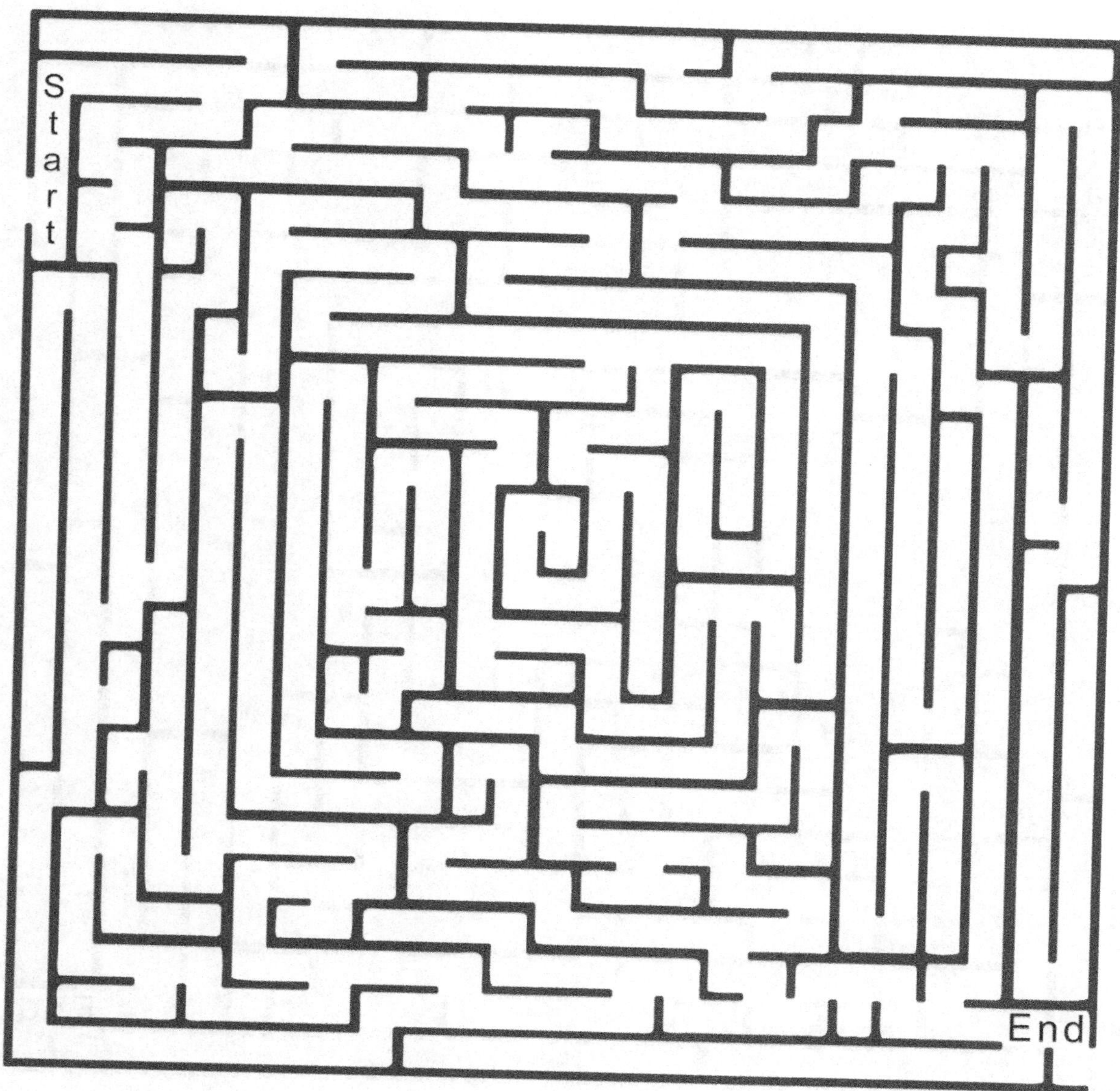

Start time: __________ End time: __________

Total time, maze 2: __________

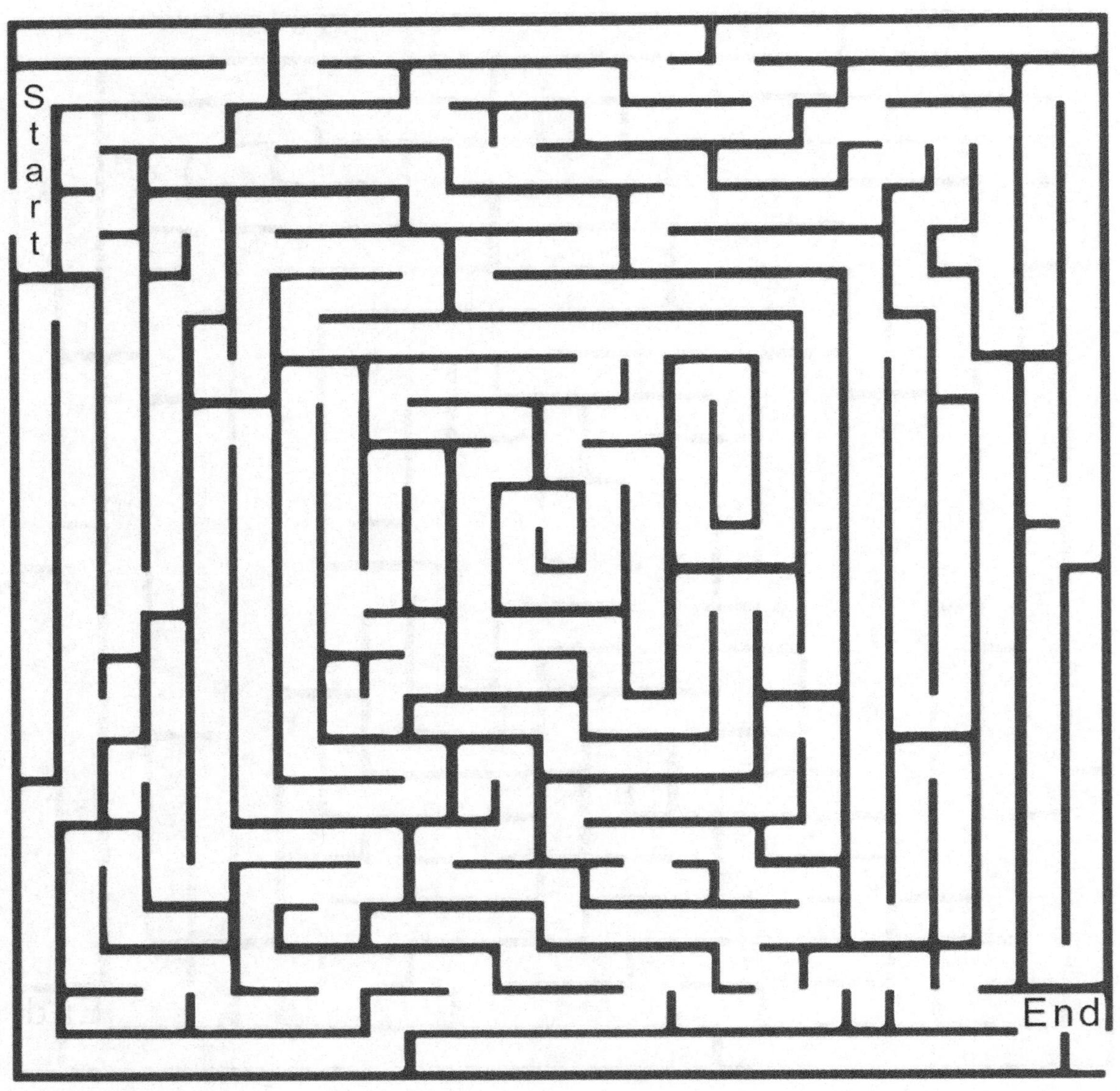

Start time: __________ End time: __________

Total time, maze 3: __________

Total time for 1st maze: __________

Total time for 2nd maze: __________

Total time for 3rd maze: __________

Congratulations! Did you experience progress in faster completion times? Circle your answer.

Yes No

If you circled "No" don't be discouraged. Remember to rest and give thanks to your mind and body for completing the challenges. Celebrate your tremendous effort. Remember, a seed doesn't turn into a tree overnight.

Continuous, unflagging effort, persistence and determination will win. Let not the man be discouraged who has these.

—*James Whitcomb Riley*

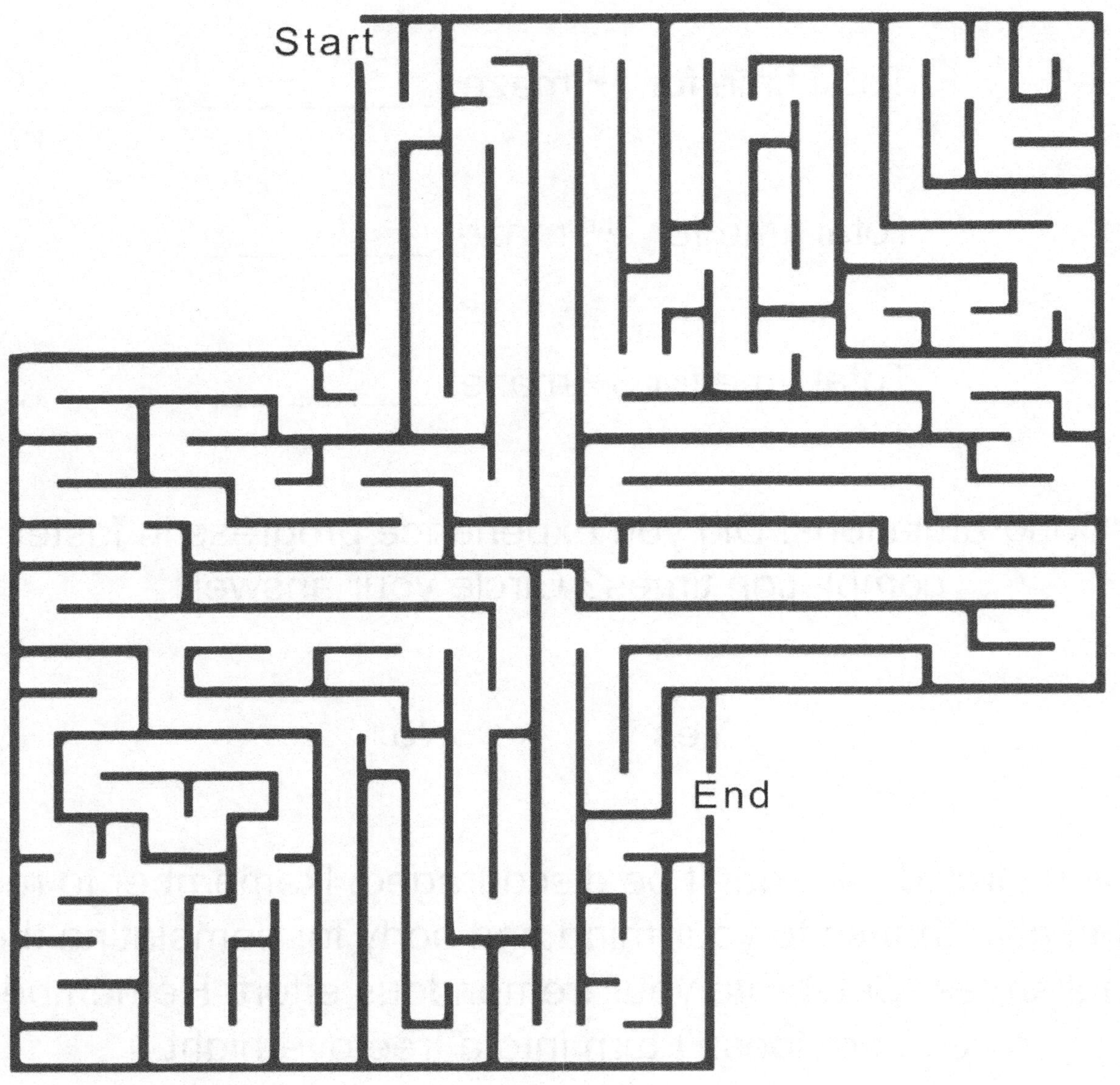

Start time: __________ End time: __________

Total time, maze 1: __________

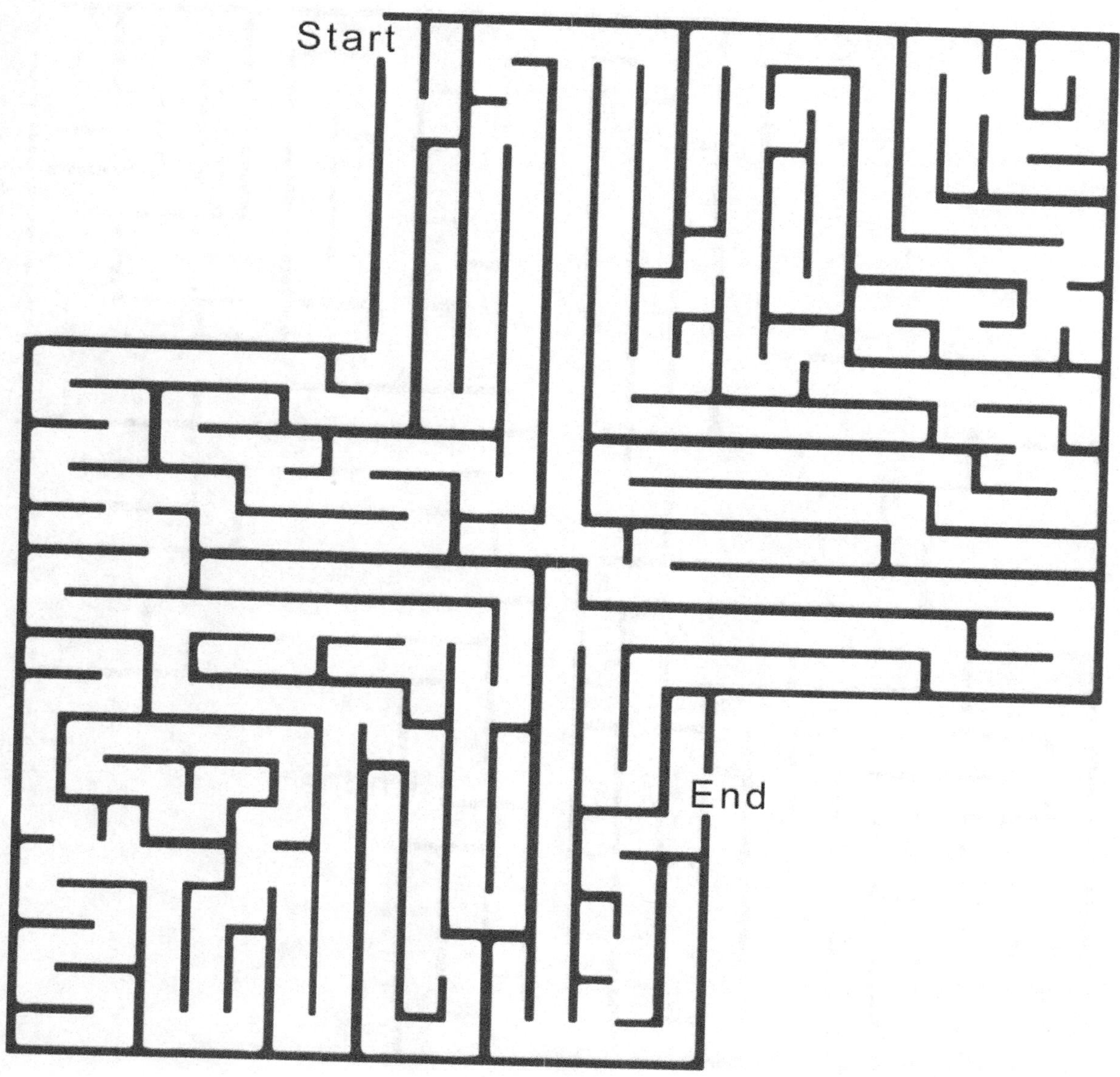

Start time: __________ End time: __________

Total time, maze 2: __________

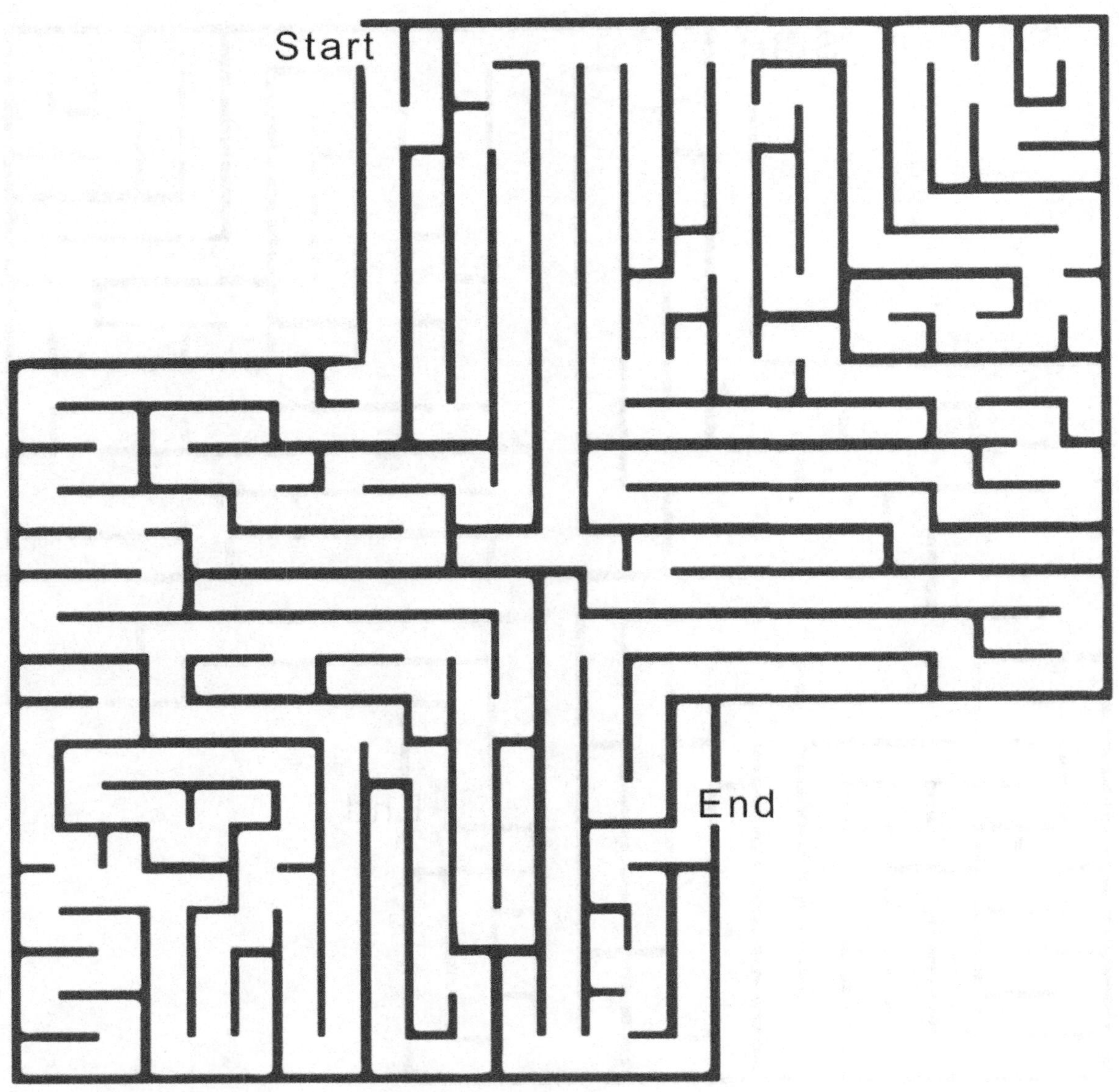

Start time: __________ End time: __________

Total time, maze 3: __________

Total time for 1st maze: __________

Total time for 2nd maze: __________

Total time for 3rd maze: __________

Congratulations! Did you experience progress in faster completion times? Circle your answer.

Yes No

If you circled “No” don’t be discouraged. Remember to rest and give thanks to your mind and body for completing the challenges. Celebrate your tremendous effort. Remember, a seed doesn’t turn into a tree overnight.

What is important is to believe in something so strongly that you're never discouraged.

—*Salma Hayek*

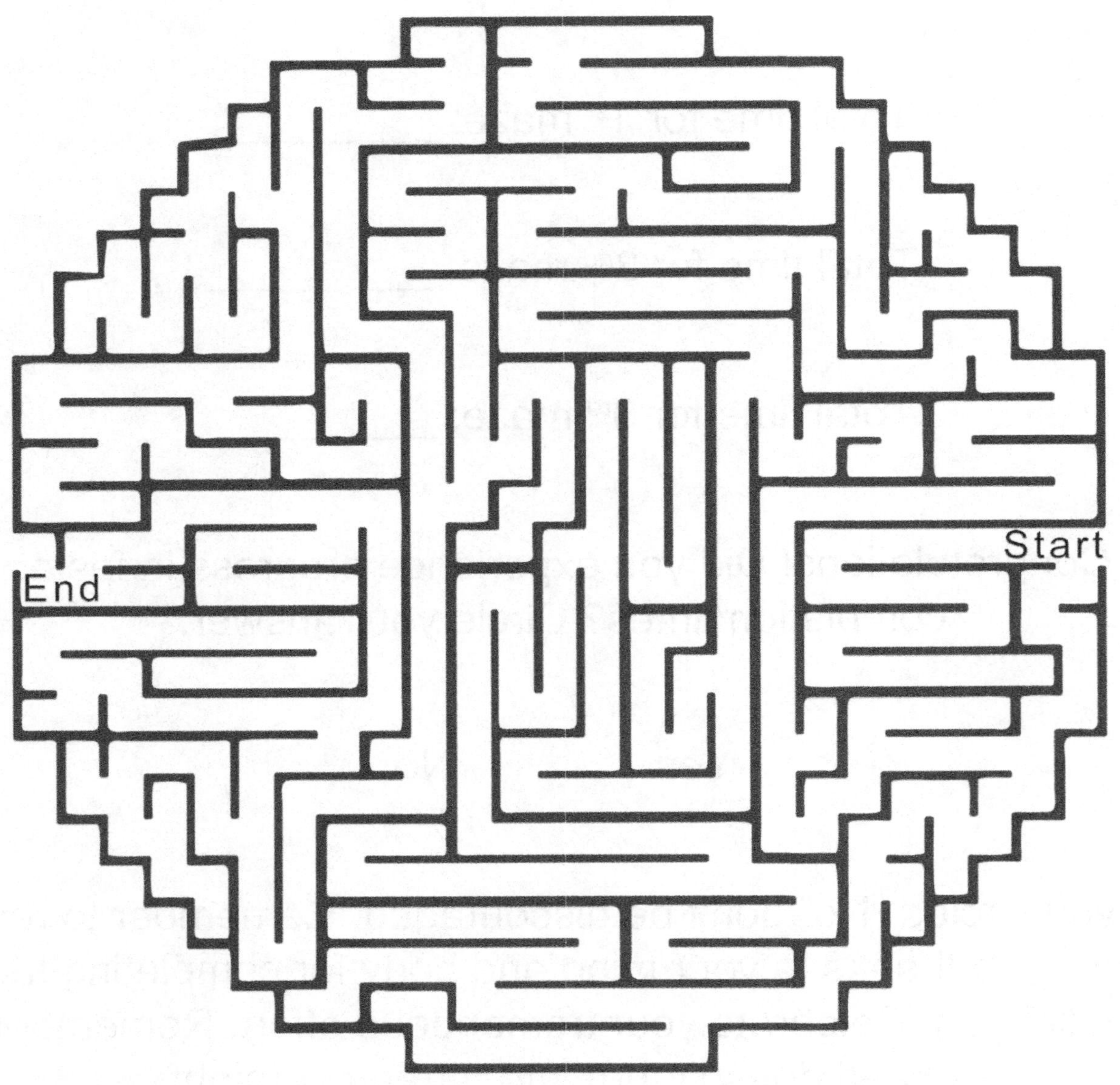

Start time: __________ End time: __________

Total time, maze 1: __________

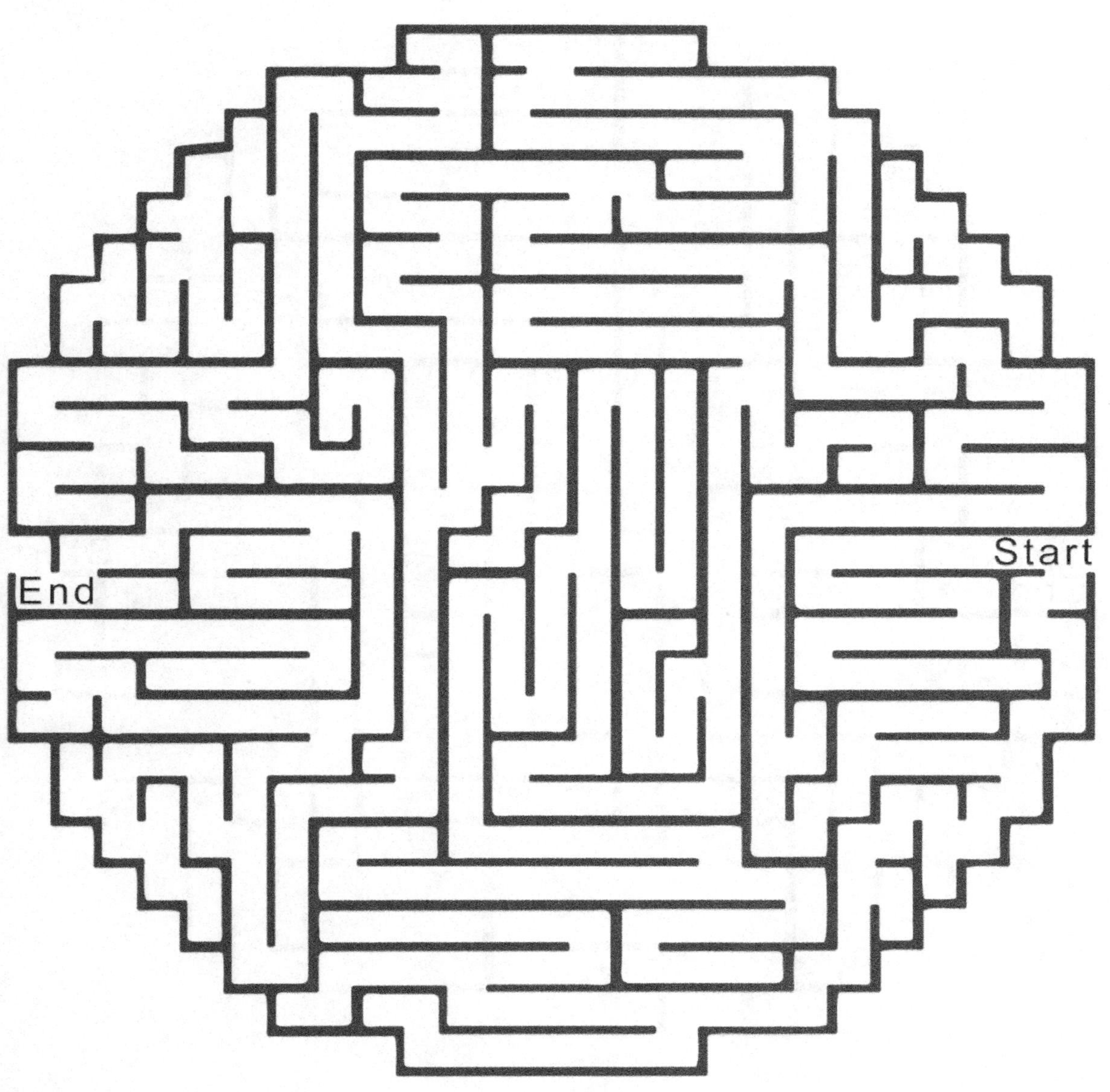

Start time: __________ End time: __________

Total time, maze 2: __________

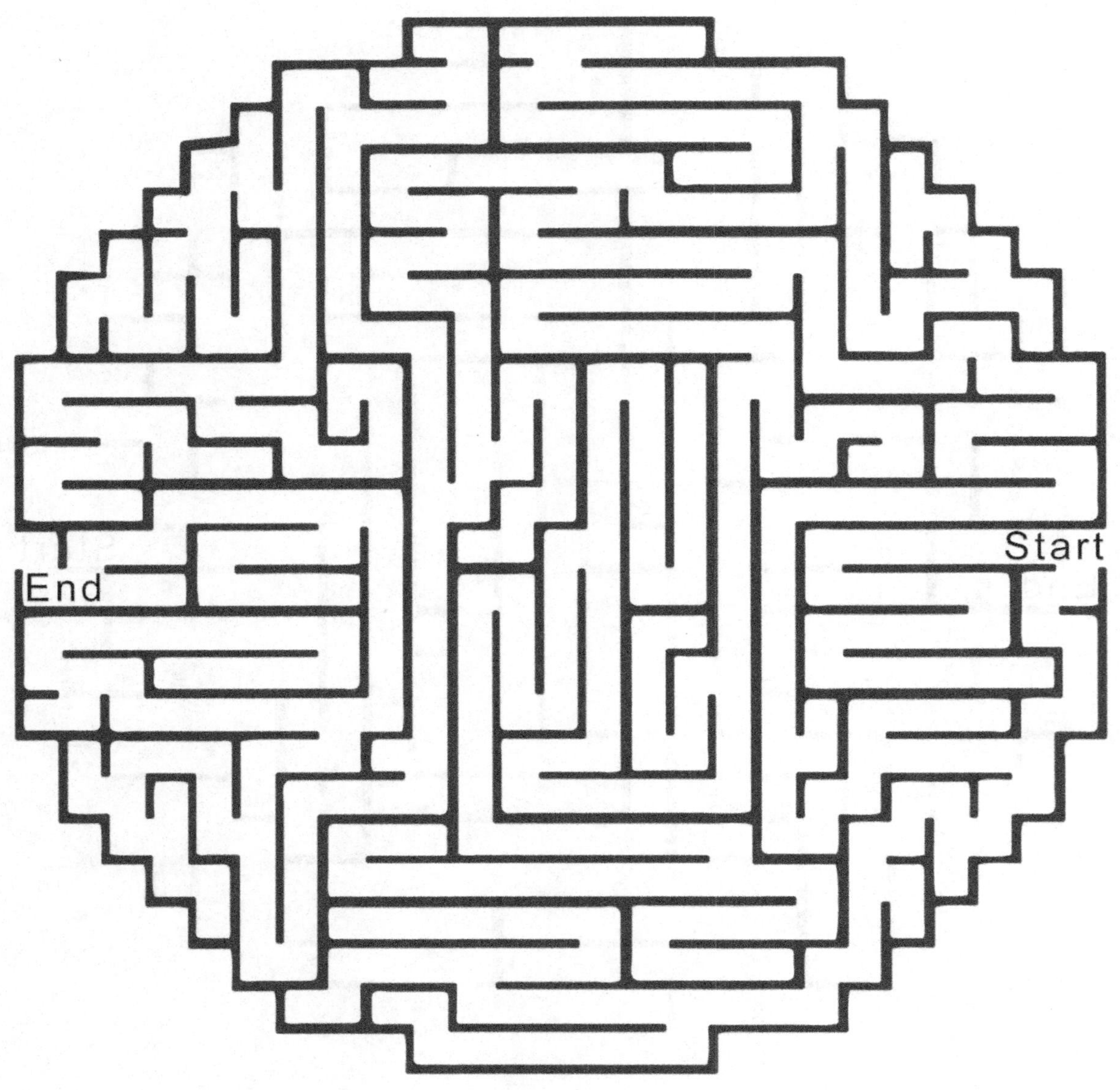

Start time: __________ End time: __________

Total time, maze 3: __________

Total time for 1st maze: __________

Total time for 2nd maze: __________

Total time for 3rd maze: __________

Congratulations! Did you experience progress in faster completion times? Circle your answer.

Yes No

If you circled "No" don't be discouraged. Remember to rest and give thanks to your mind and body for completing the challenges. Celebrate your tremendous effort. Remember, a seed doesn't turn into a tree overnight.

Stop beating yourself up. You are a work in progress - which means you get there a little at a time, not all at once.

—*Unknown*

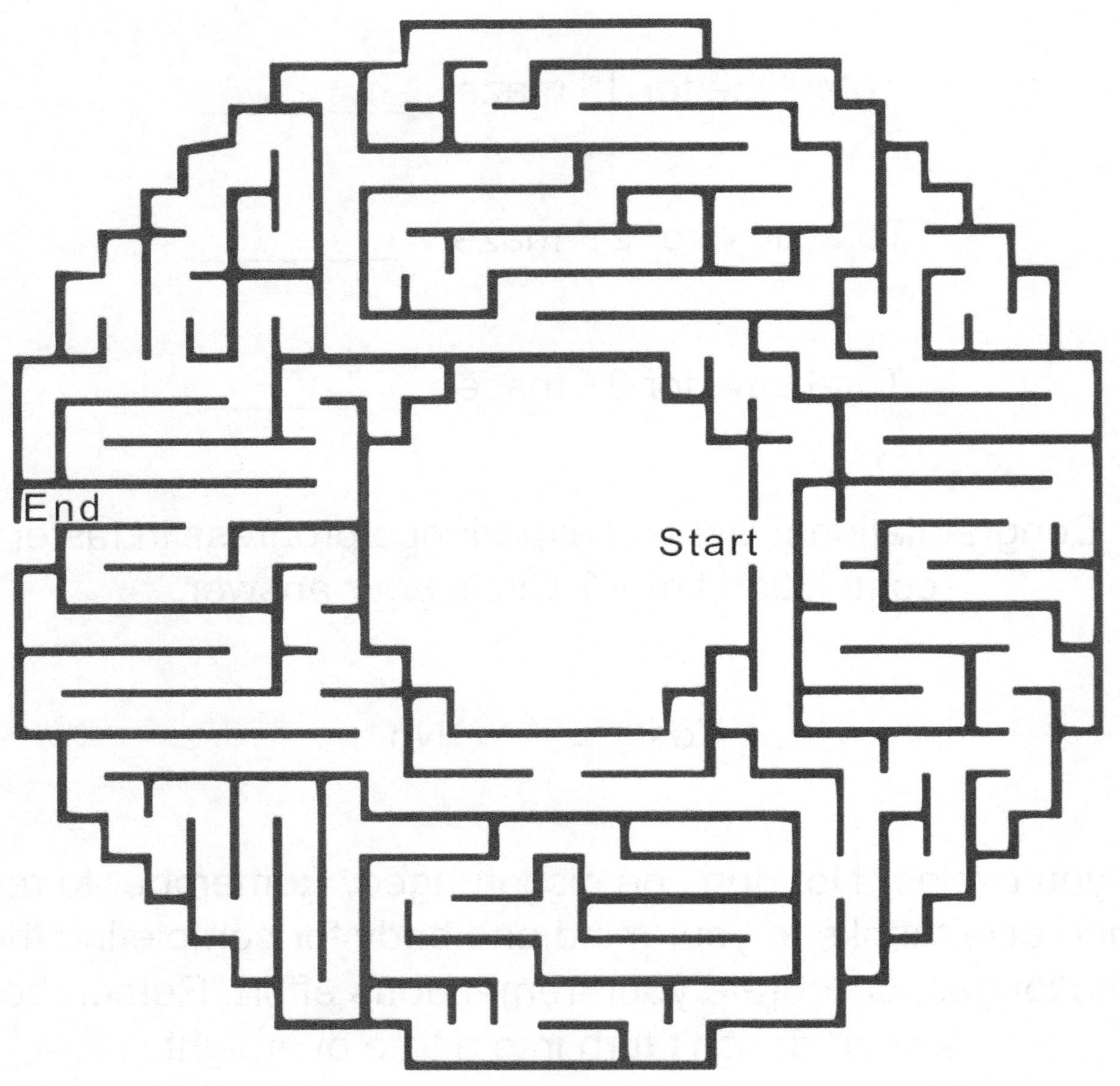

Start time: __________ End time: __________

Total time, maze 1: __________

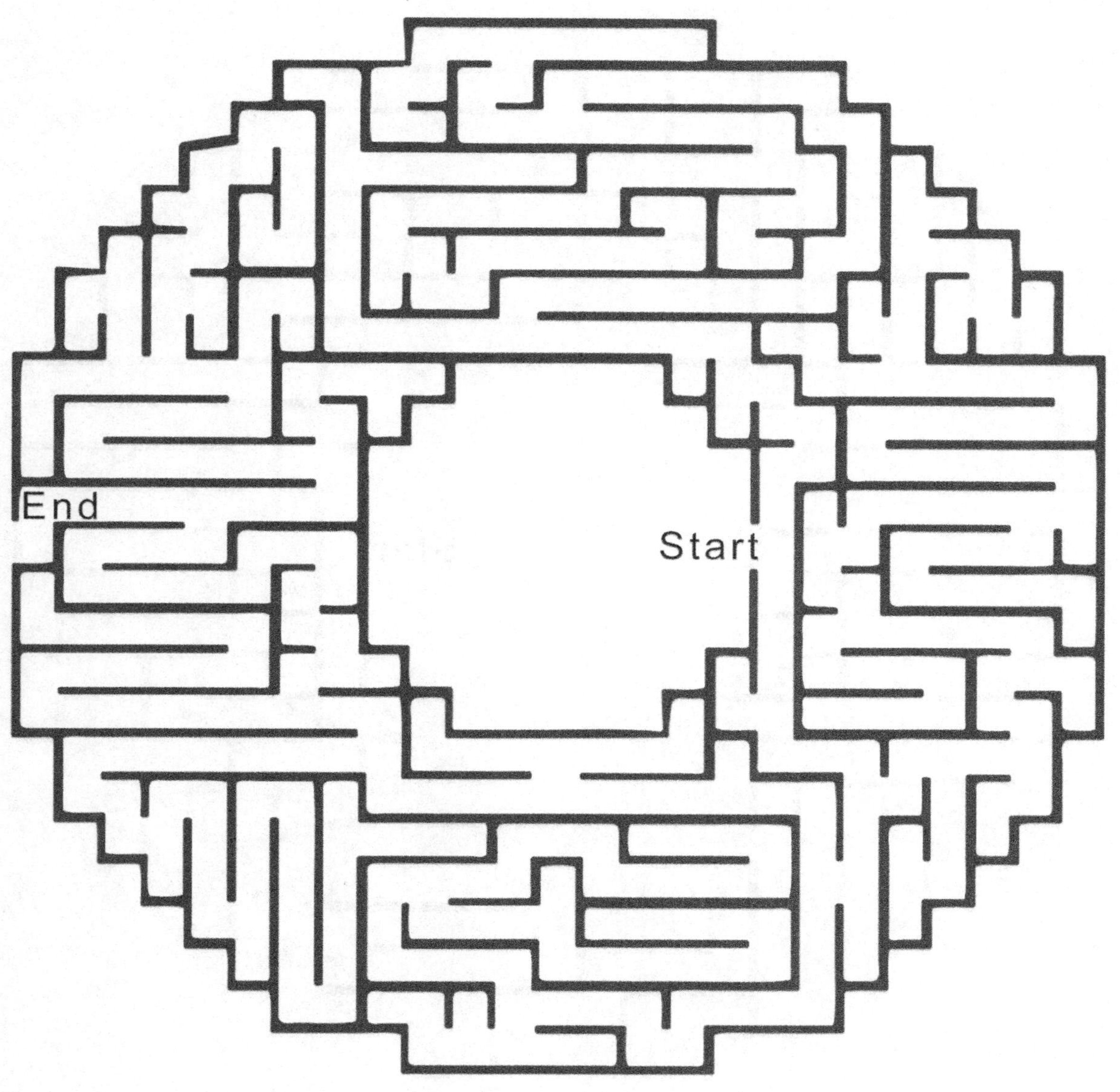

Start time: ___________ End time: ___________

Total time, maze 2: ___________

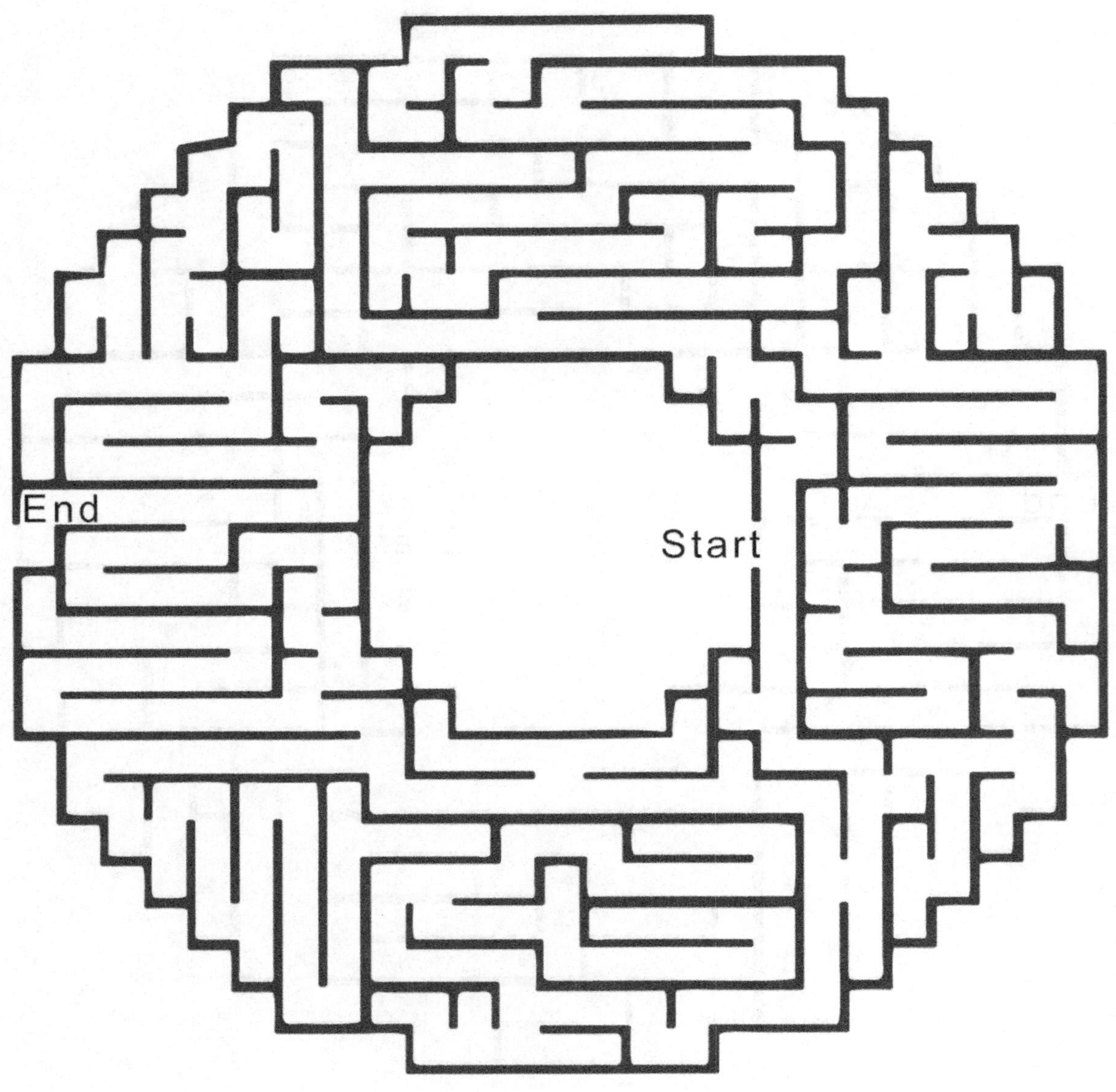

Start time: __________ End time: __________

Total time, maze 3: __________

Total time for 1st maze: __________

Total time for 2nd maze: __________

Total time for 3rd maze: __________

Congratulations! Did you experience progress in faster completion times? Circle your answer.

Yes No

If you circled "No" don't be discouraged. Remember to rest and give thanks to your mind and body for completing the challenges. Celebrate your tremendous effort. Remember, a seed doesn't turn into a tree overnight.

Yesterday I was clever so I wanted to change the world. Today I am wise, so I am changing myself.

—*Rumi*

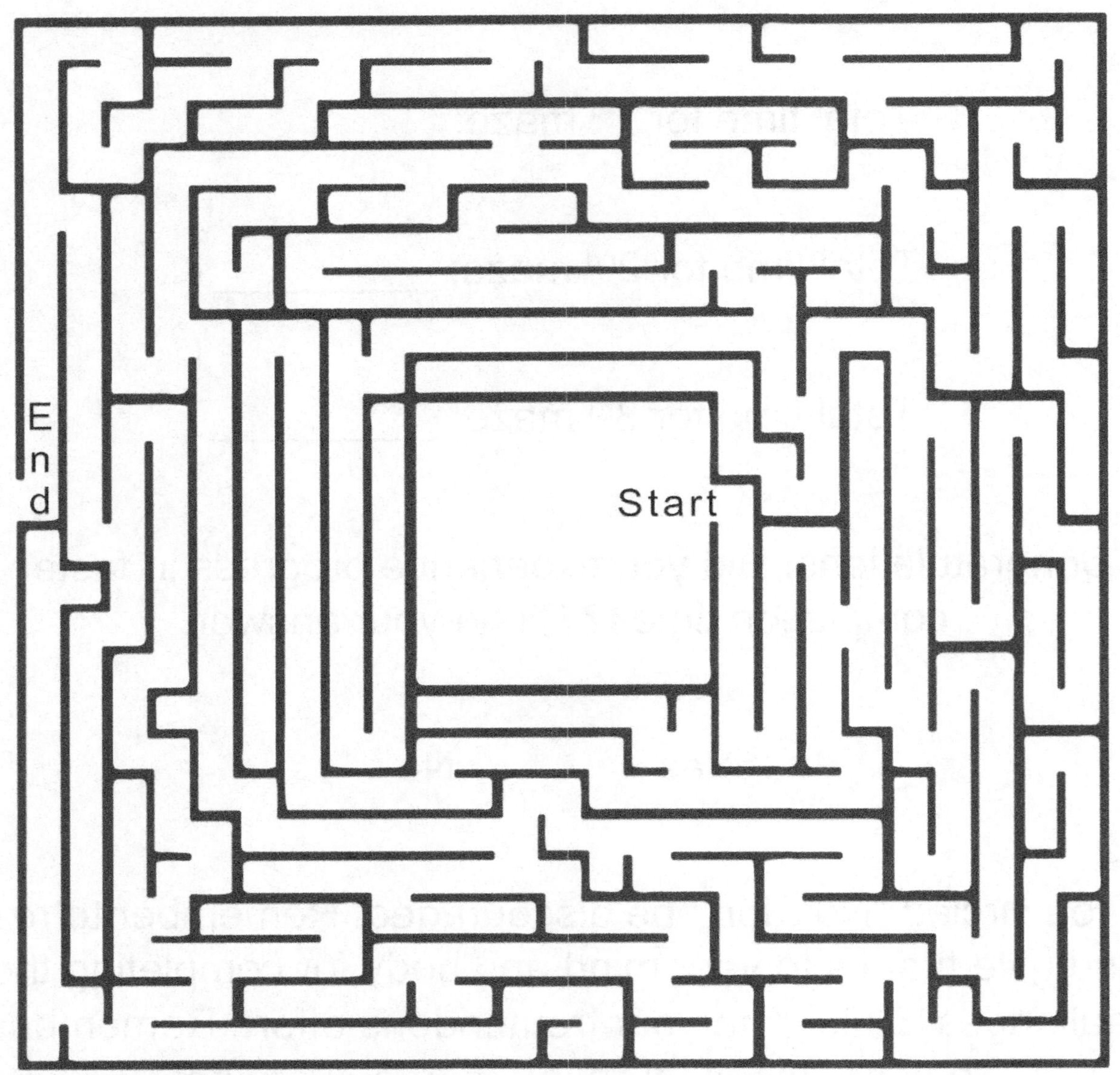

Start time: __________ End time: __________

Total time, maze 3: __________

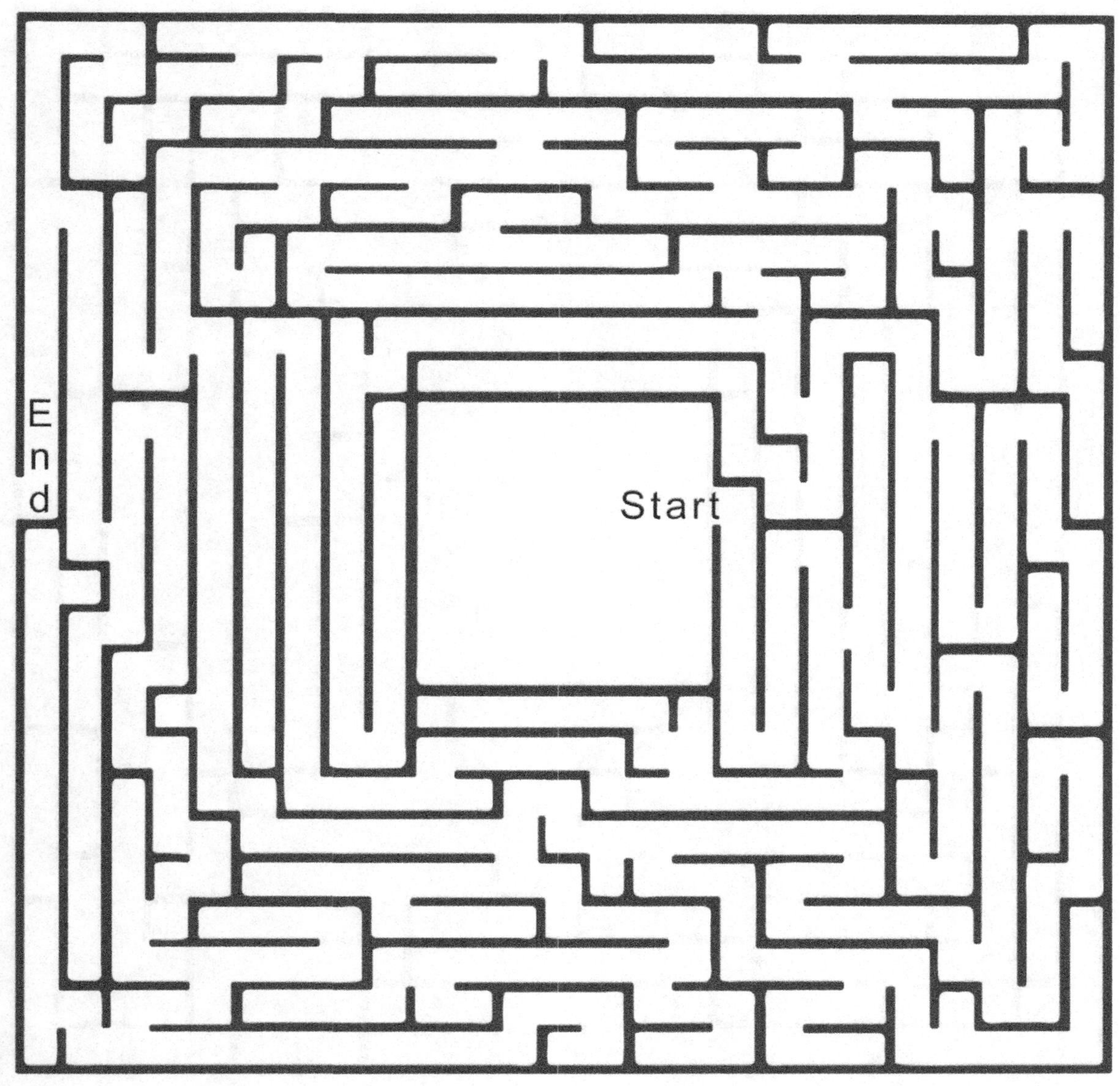

Start time: __________ End time: __________

Total time, maze 3: __________

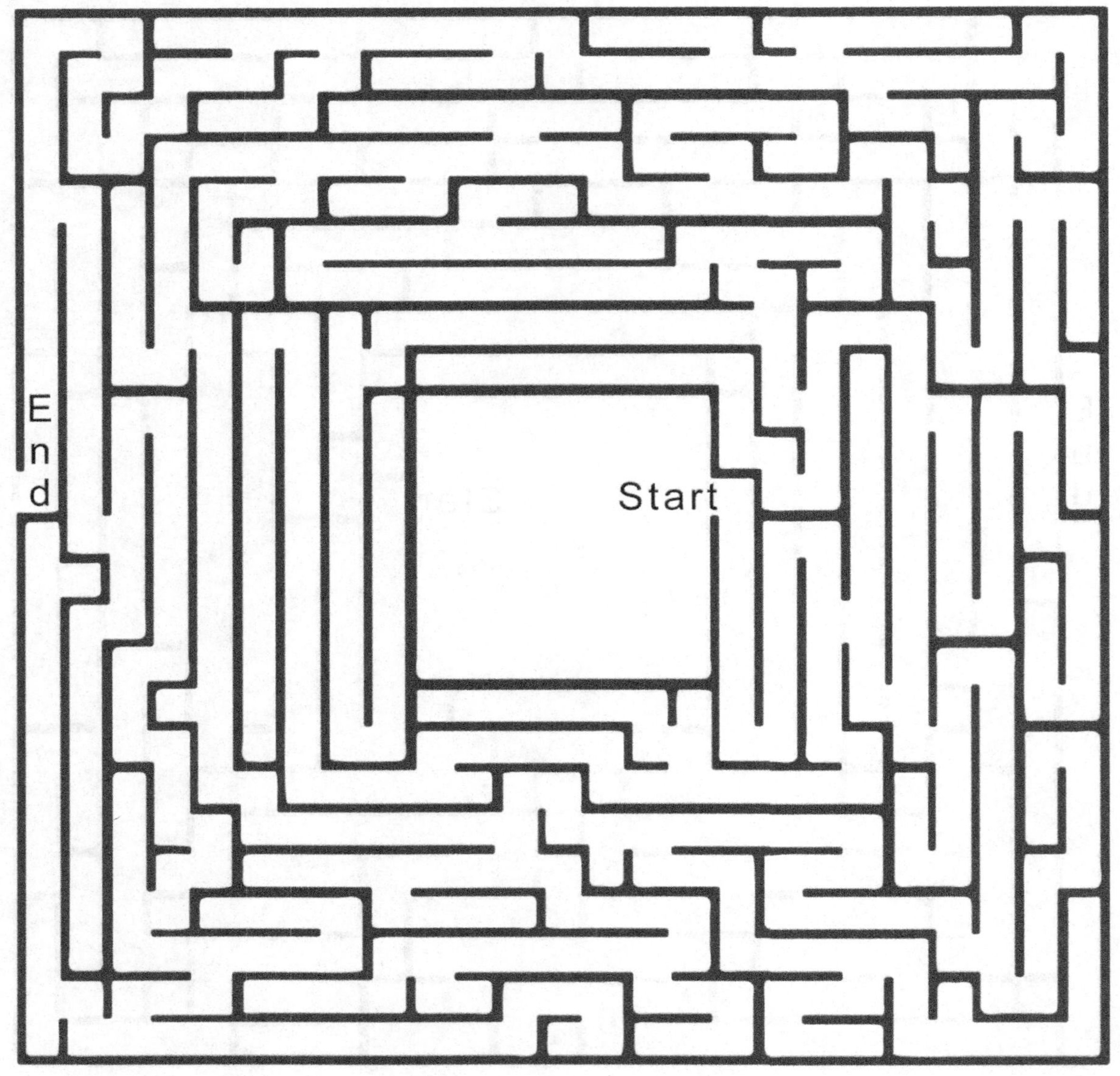

Start time: __________ End time: __________

Total time, maze 3: __________

Total time for 1st maze: __________

Total time for 2nd maze: __________

Total time for 3rd maze: __________

Congratulations! Did you experience progress in faster completion times? Circle your answer.

Yes No

If you circled "No" don't be discouraged. Remember to rest and give thanks to your mind and body for completing the challenges. Celebrate your tremendous effort. Remember, a seed doesn't turn into a tree overnight.

If you really want to do something, you'll find a way. If you don't, you'll find an excuse.

—*Jim Rohn*

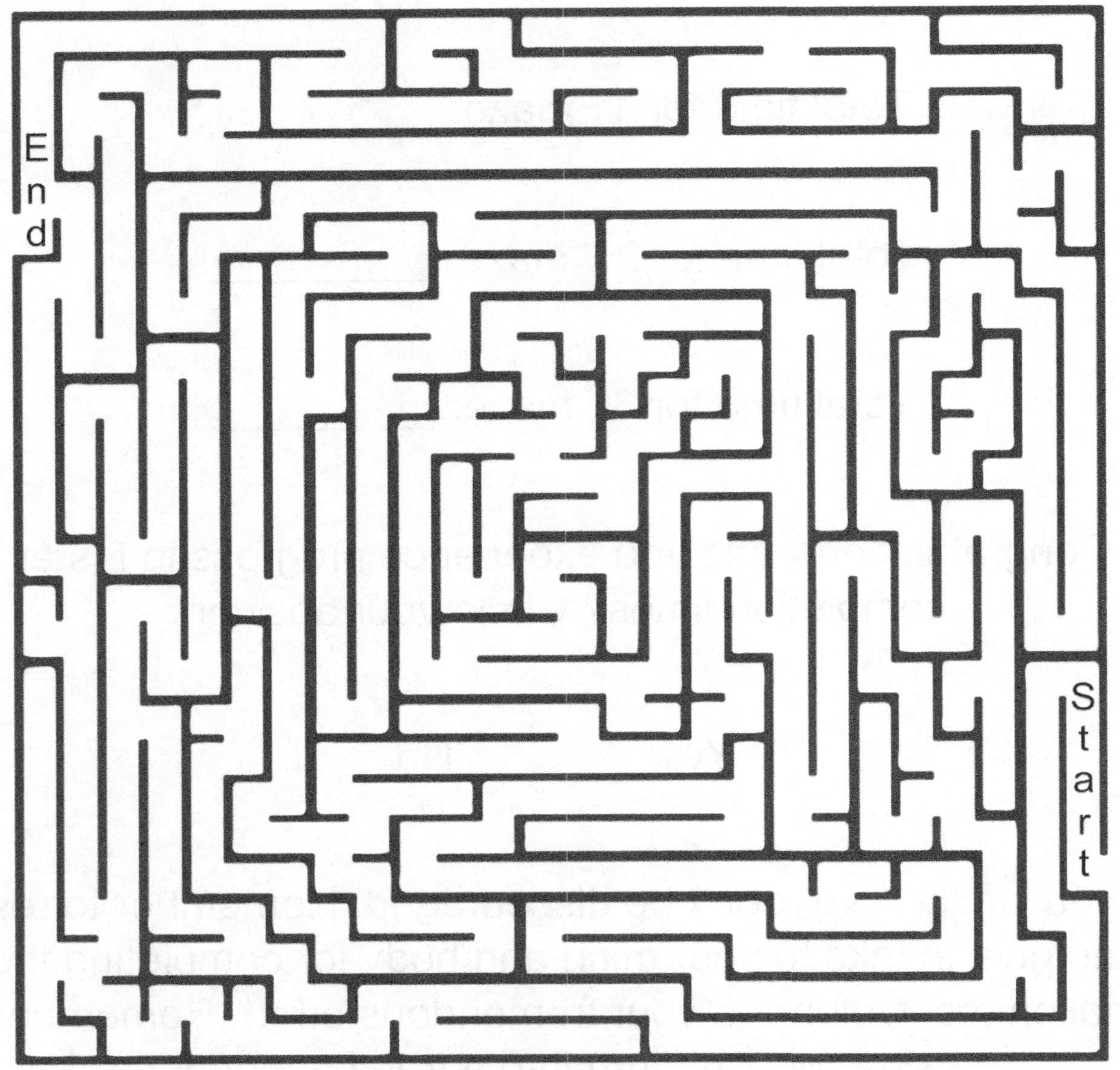

Start time: __________ End time: __________

Total time, maze 1: __________

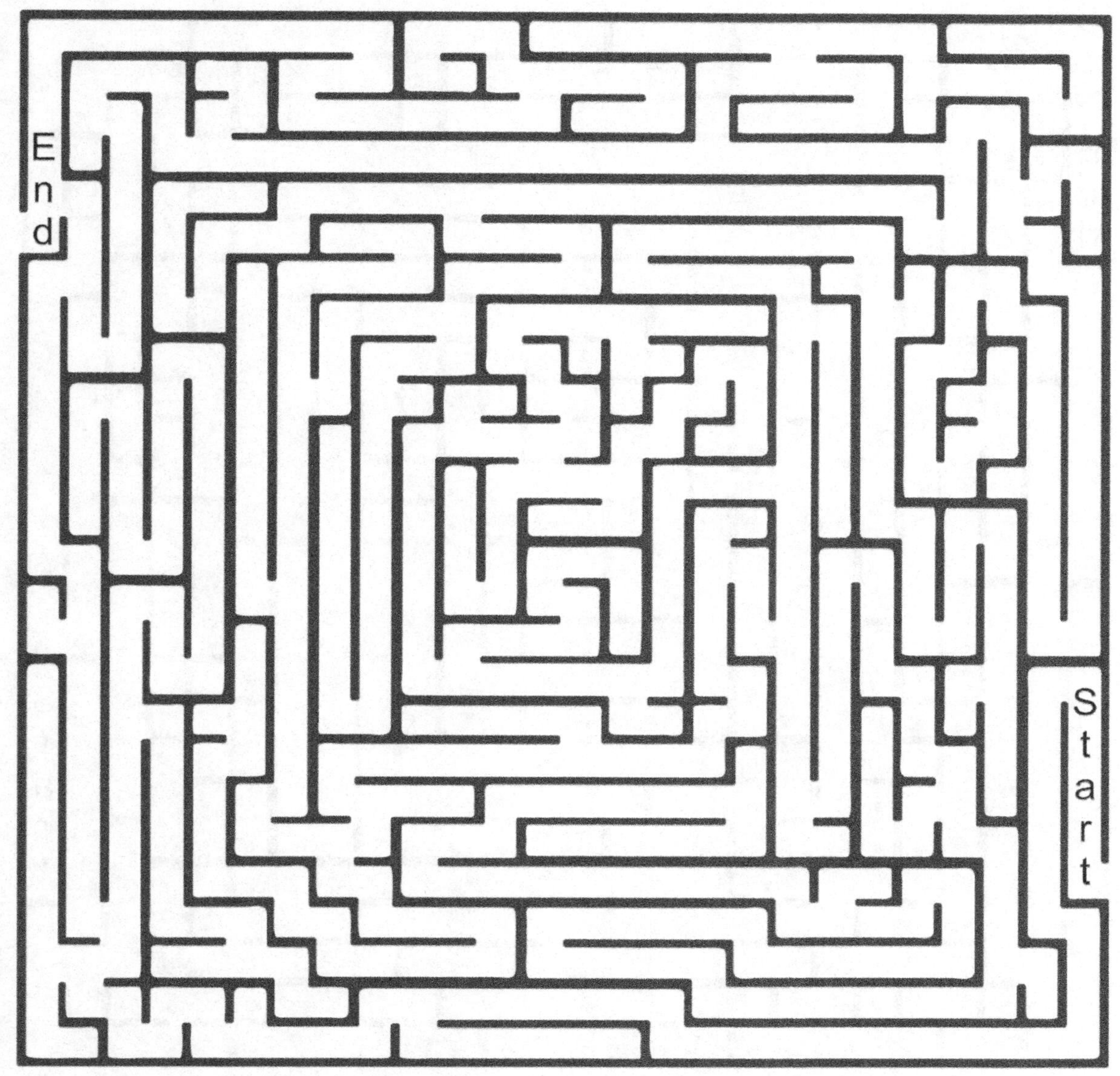

Start time: ___________ End time: ___________

Total time, maze 2: ___________

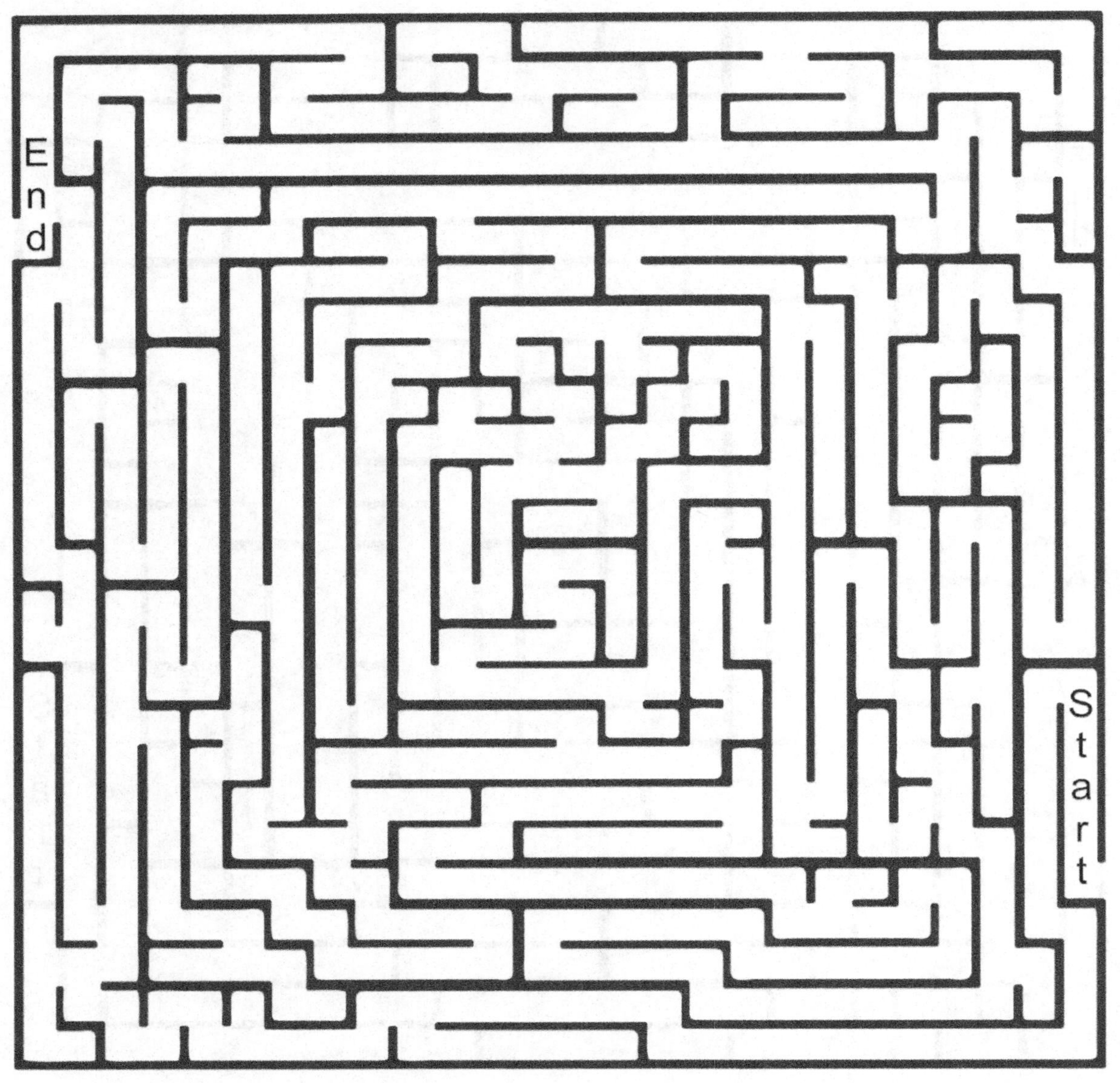

Start time: __________ End time: __________

Total time, maze 3: __________

Total time for 1st maze: __________

Total time for 2nd maze: __________

Total time for 3rd maze: __________

Congratulations! Did you experience progress in faster completion times? Circle your answer.

Yes No

If you circled "No" don't be discouraged. Remember to rest and give thanks to your mind and body for completing the challenges. Celebrate your tremendous effort. Remember, a seed doesn't turn into a tree overnight.

F.E.A.R: has two meanings: 1). Forget Everything And Run or 2). Face Everything And Rise; the choice is yours!

—Zig Ziglar

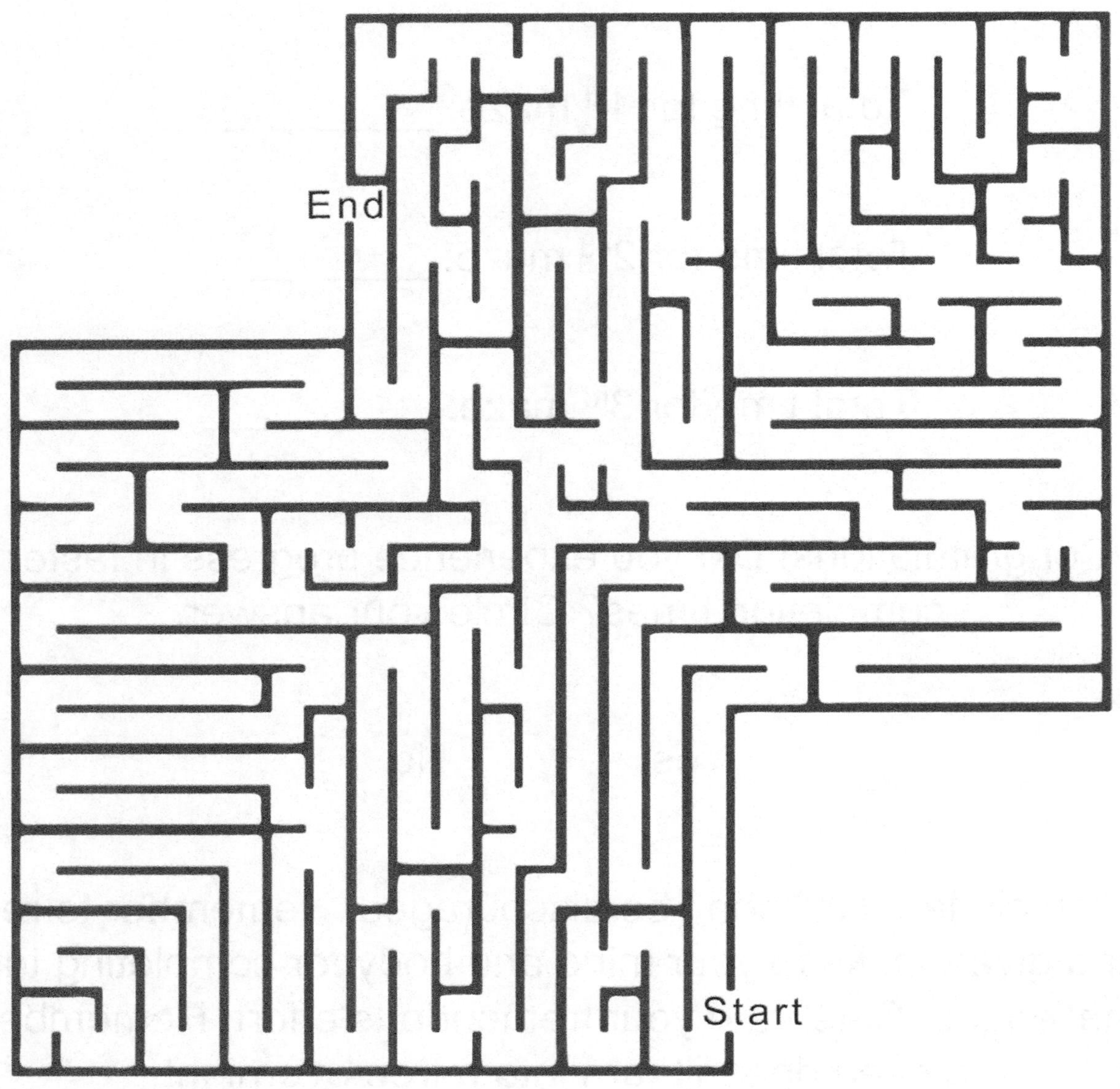

Start time: __________ End time: __________

Total time, maze 1: __________

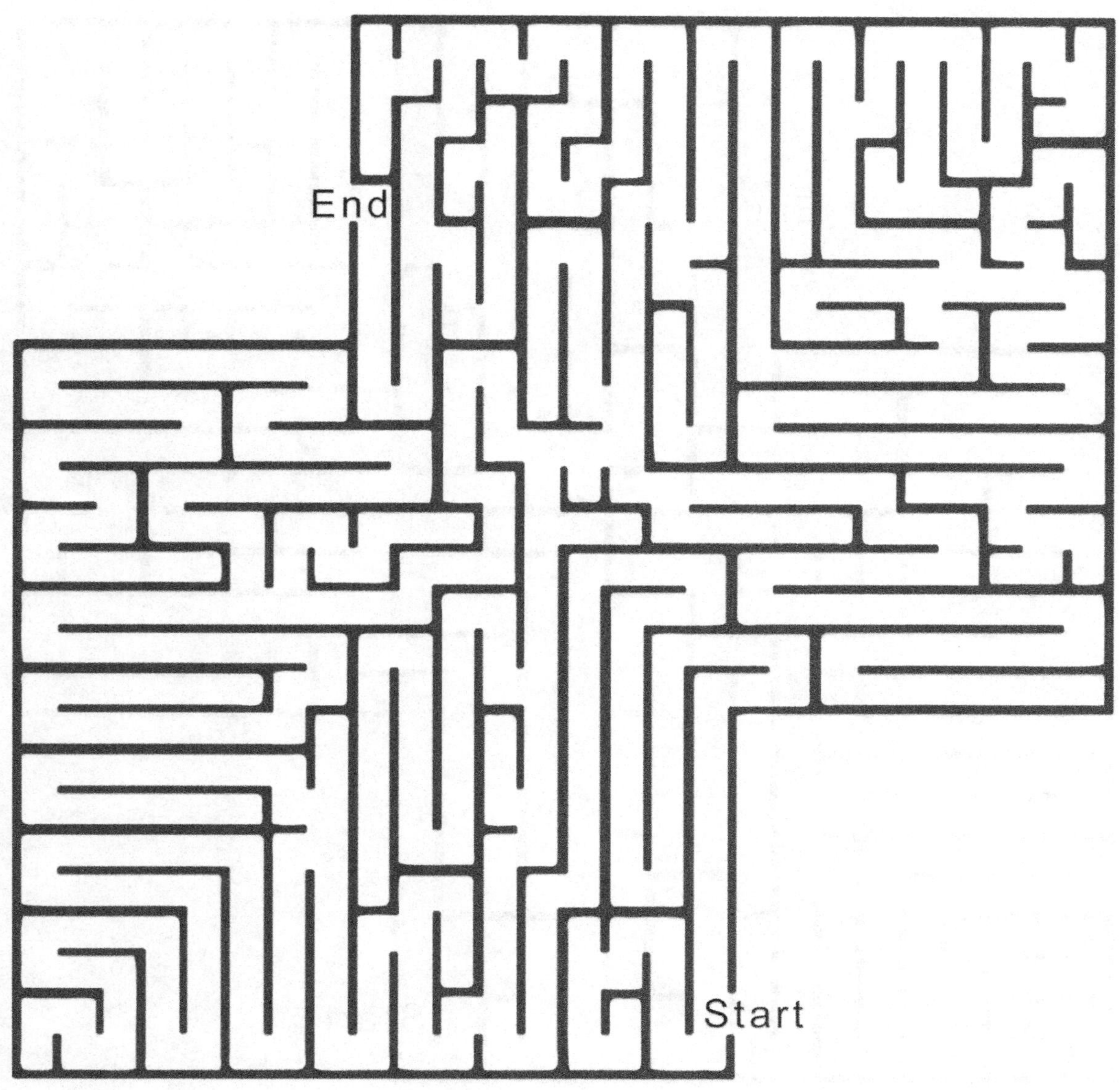

Start time: __________ End time: __________

Total time, maze 2: __________

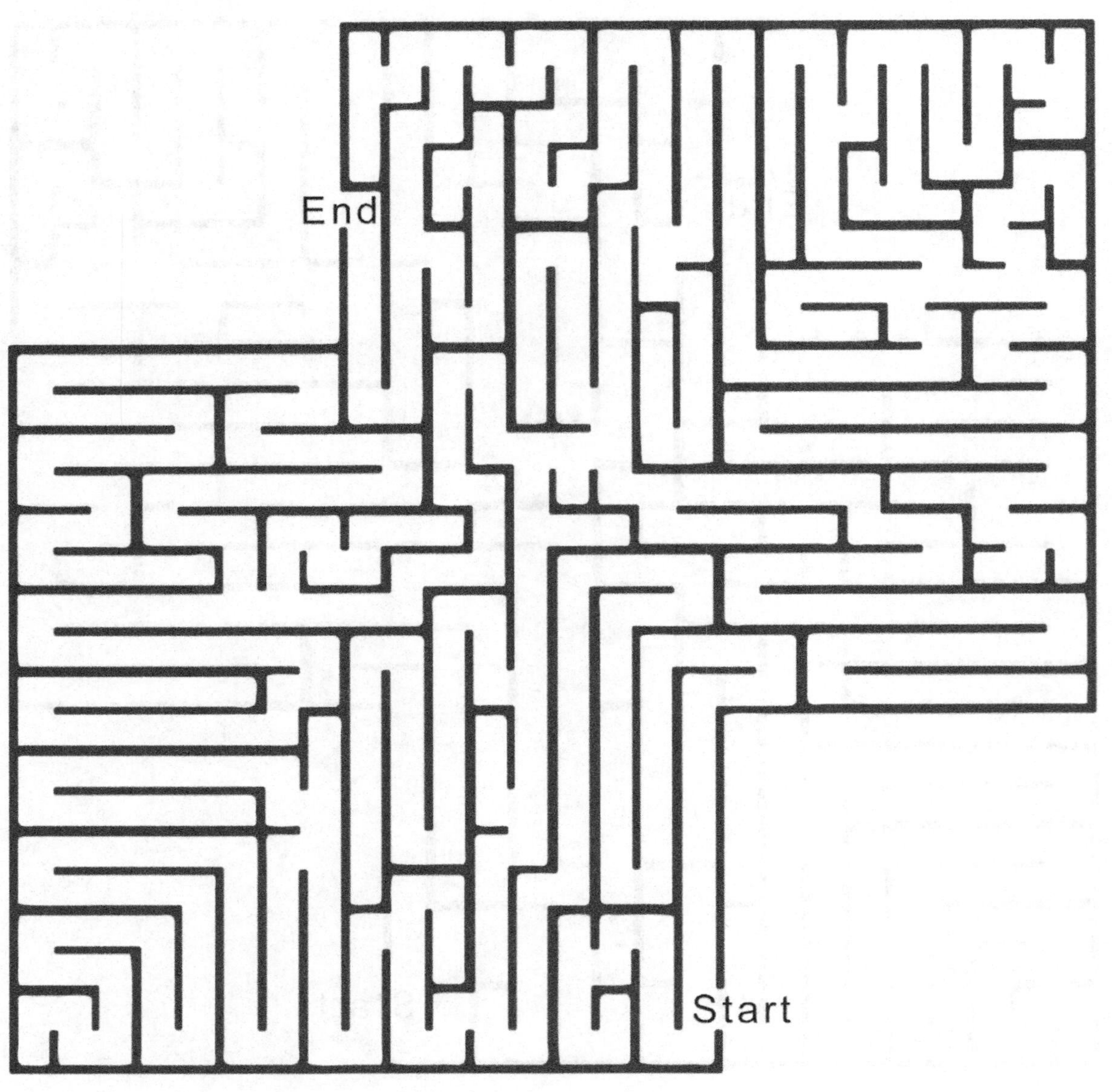

Start time: __________ End time: __________

Total time, maze 3: __________

Total time for 1st maze: __________

Total time for 2nd maze: __________

Total time for 3rd maze: __________

Congratulations! Did you experience progress in faster completion times? Circle your answer.

Yes No

If you circled "No" don't be discouraged. Remember to rest and give thanks to your mind and body for completing the challenges. Celebrate your tremendous effort. Remember, a seed doesn't turn into a tree overnight.

Life is like a camera... Focus on what's important, Capture the good times, Develop from the negatives, and if things don't work out, take another shot.

—Unknown

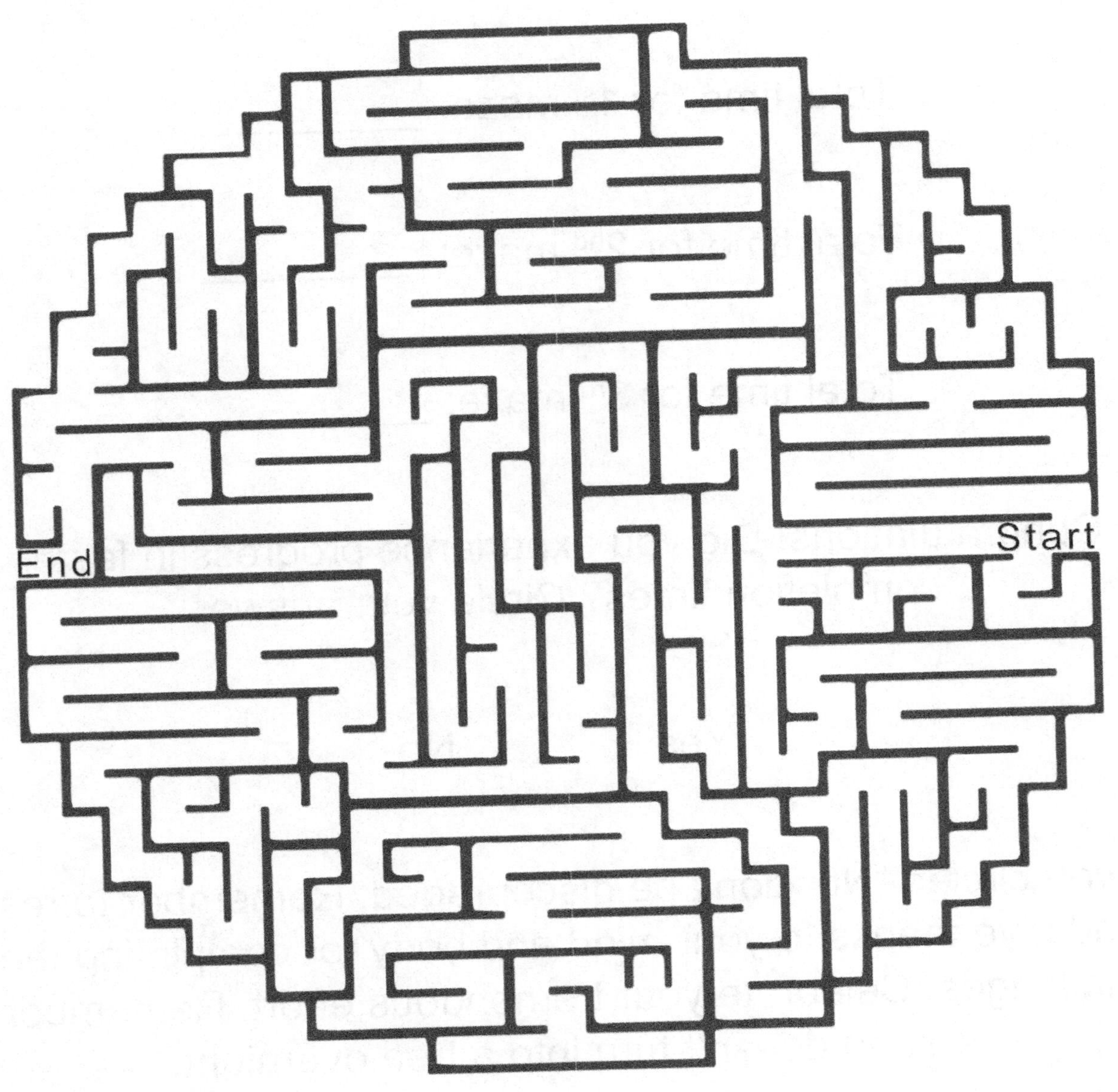

Start time: __________ End time: __________

Total time, maze 1: __________

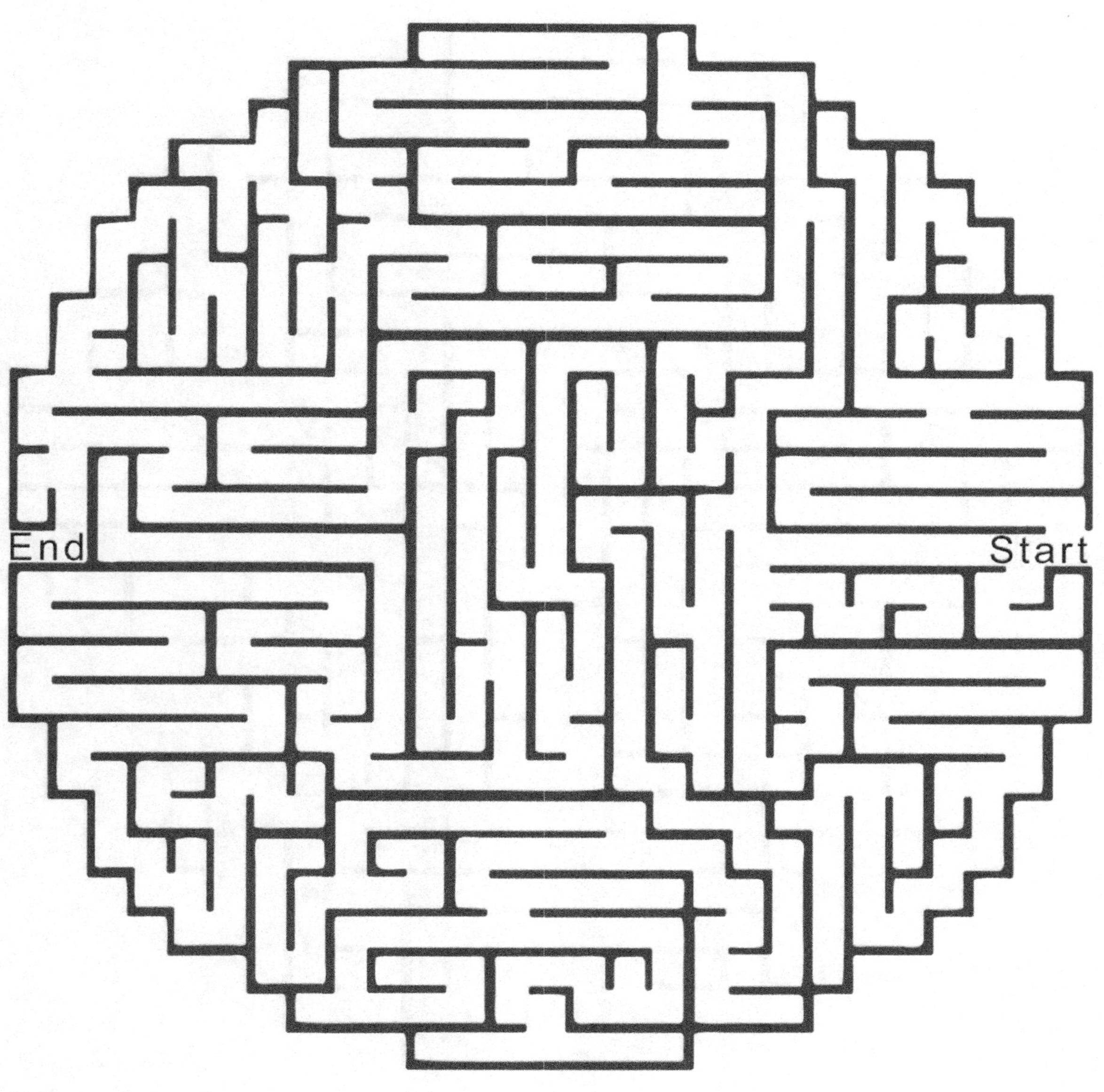

Start time: __________ End time: __________

Total time, maze 2: __________

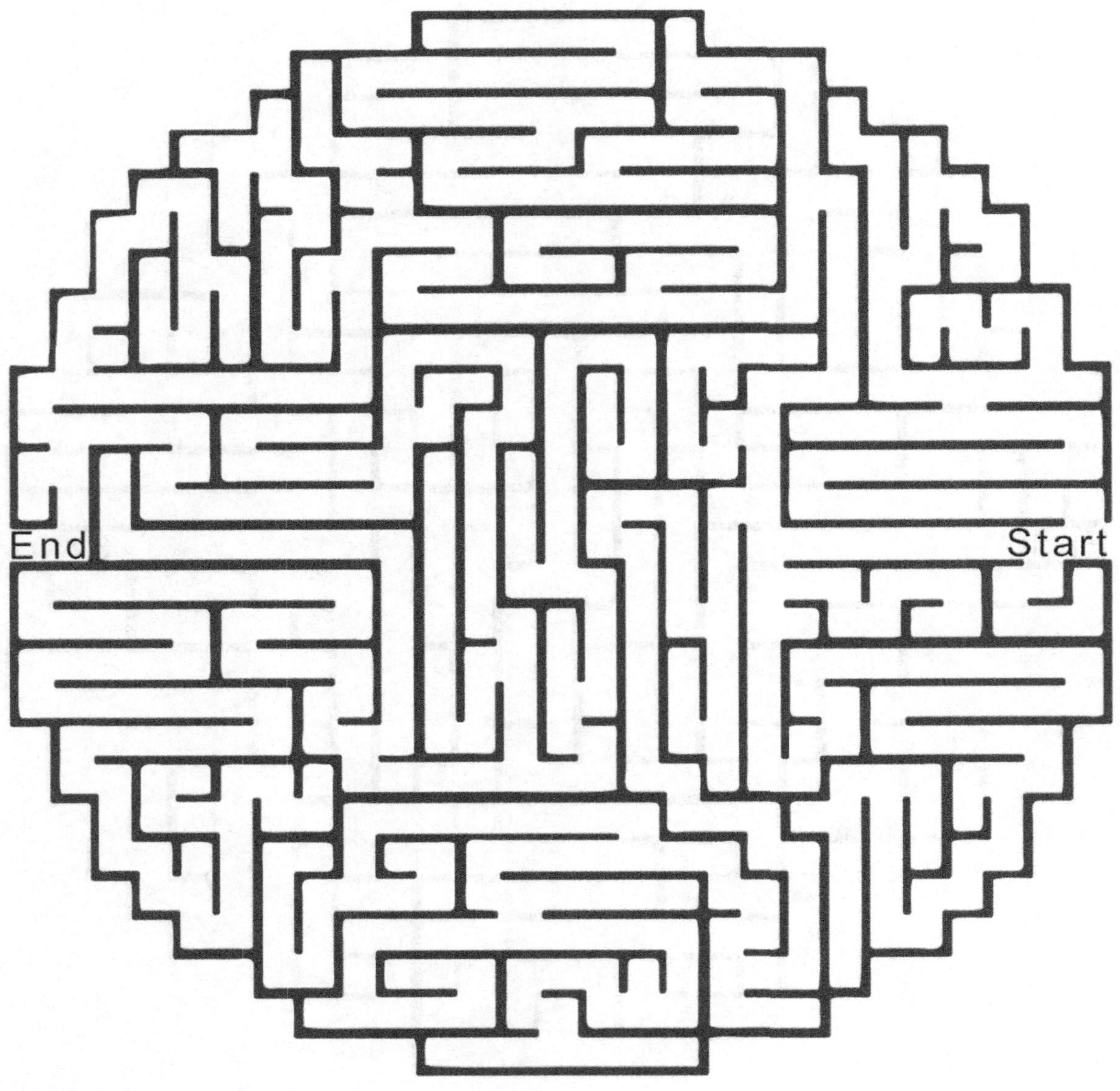

Start time: __________ End time: __________

Total time, maze 3: __________

Total time for 1st maze: __________

Total time for 2nd maze: __________

Total time for 3rd maze: __________

Congratulations! Did you experience progress in faster completion times? Circle your answer.

Yes No

If you circled "No" don't be discouraged. Remember to rest and give thanks to your mind and body for completing the challenges. Celebrate your tremendous effort. Remember, a seed doesn't turn into a tree overnight.

Keep watering, keep planting, keep cultivating, and one day your garden will bloom.

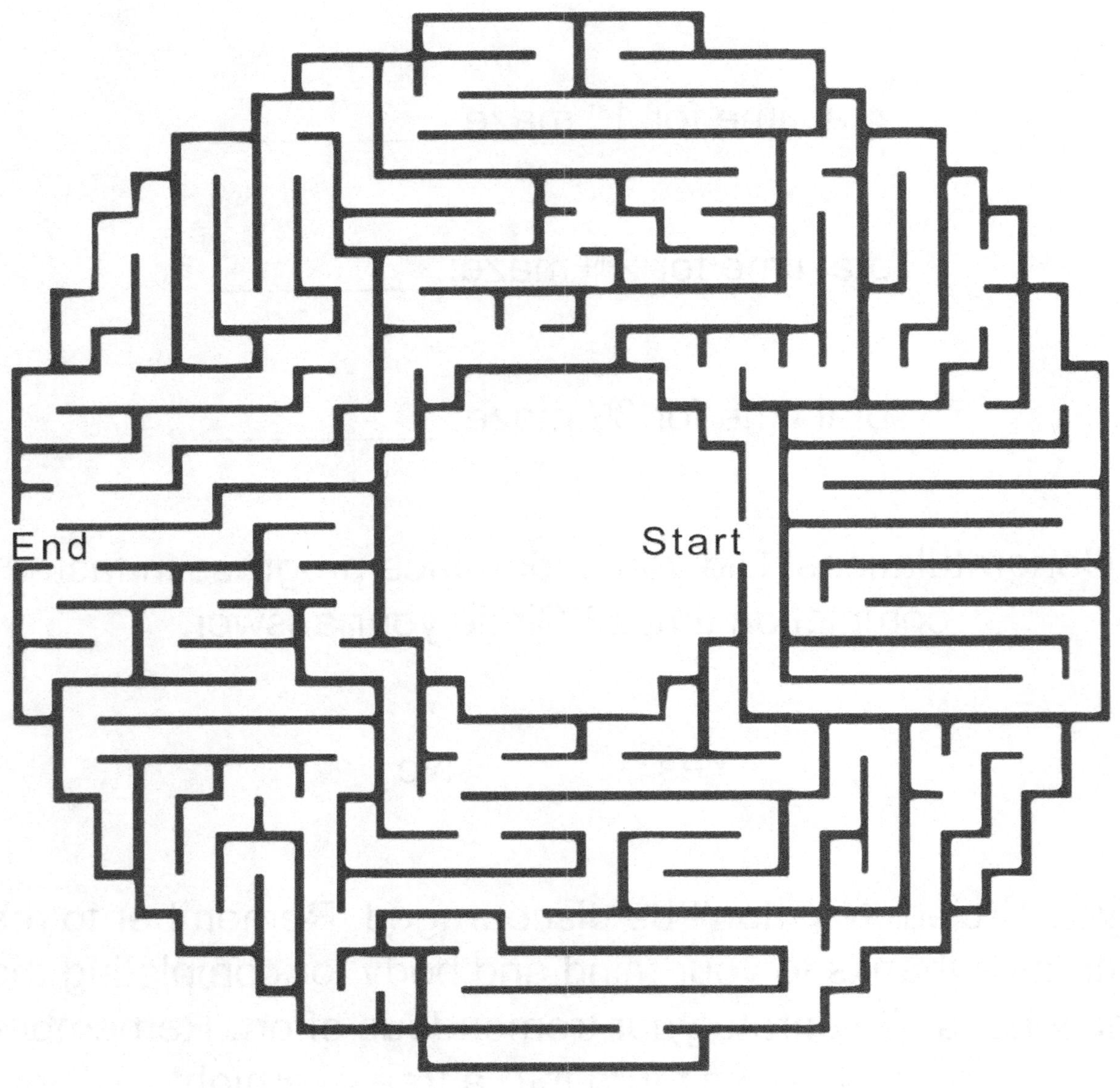

Start time: __________ End time: __________

Total time, maze 1: __________

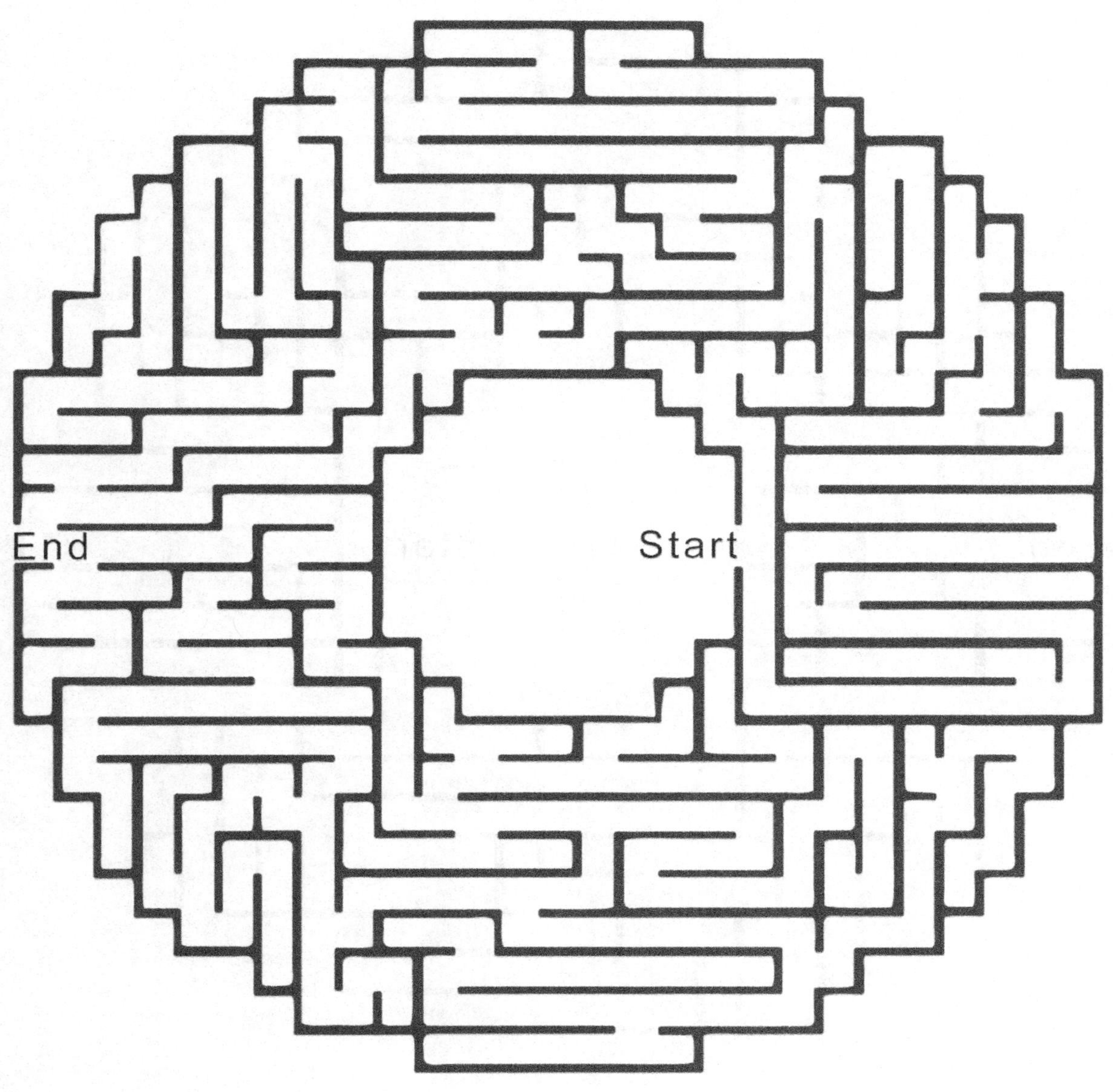

Start time: __________ End time: __________

Total time, maze 2: __________

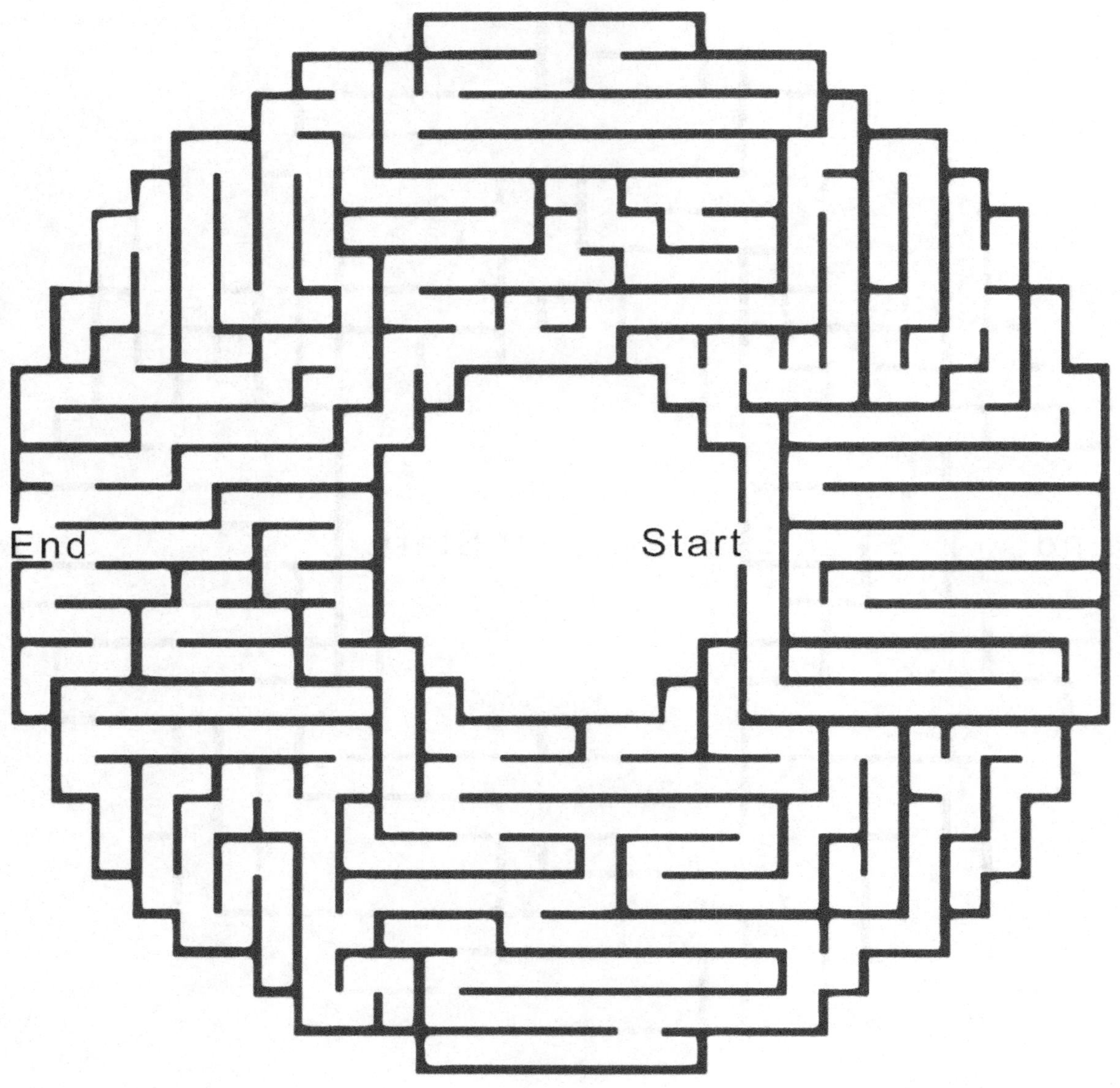

Start time: __________ End time: __________

Total time, maze 3: __________

Total time for 1st maze: __________

Total time for 2nd maze: __________

Total time for 3rd maze: __________

Congratulations! Did you experience progress in faster completion times? Circle your answer.

Yes No

If you circled "No" don't be discouraged. Remember to rest and give thanks to your mind and body for completing the challenges. Celebrate your tremendous effort. Remember, a seed doesn't turn into a tree overnight.

One of the things I learned the hard way was that it doesn't pay to get discouraged. Keeping busy and making optimism a way of life can restore your faith in yourself.

—Lucille Ball

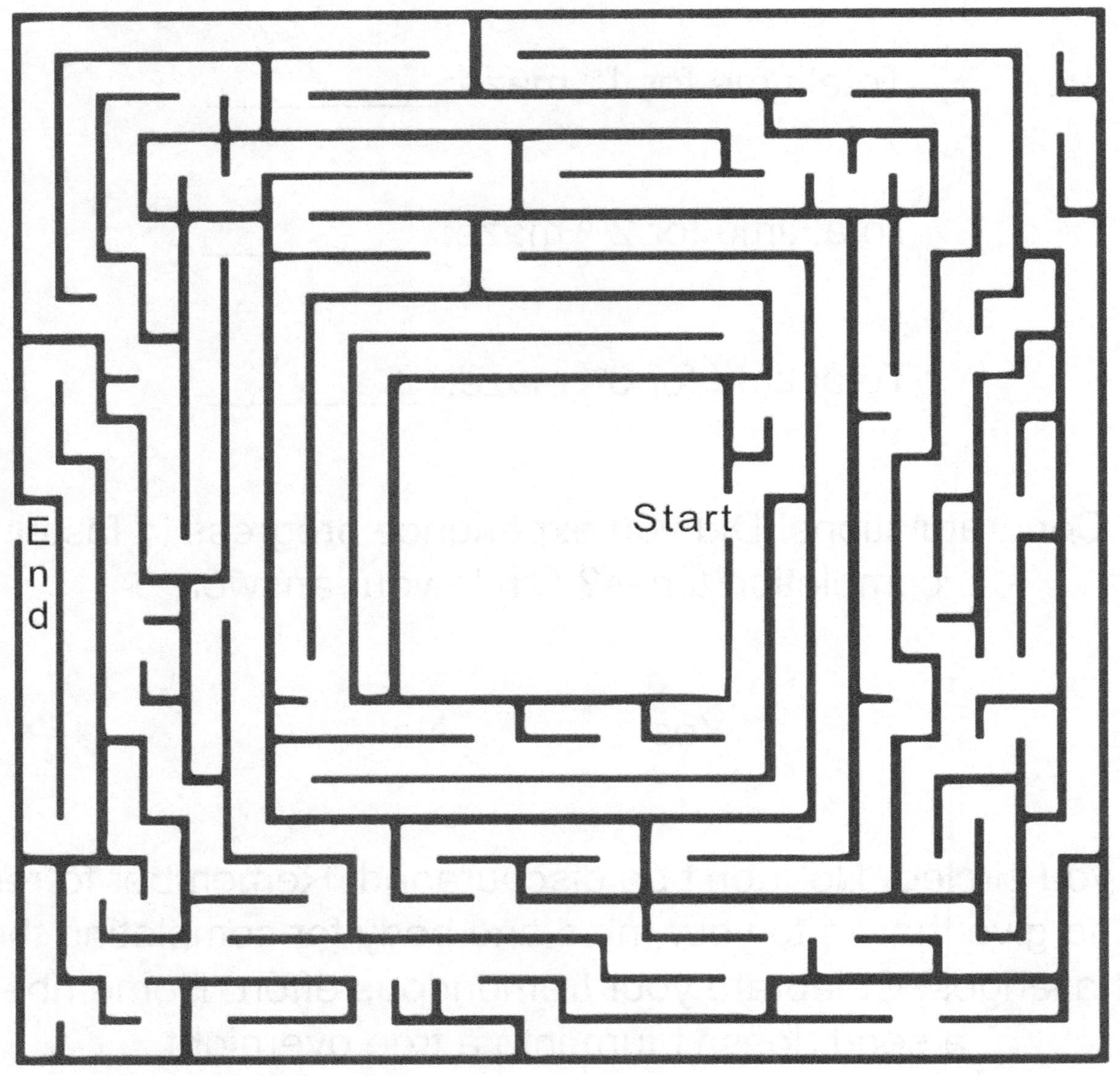

Start time: __________ End time: __________

Total time, maze 1: __________

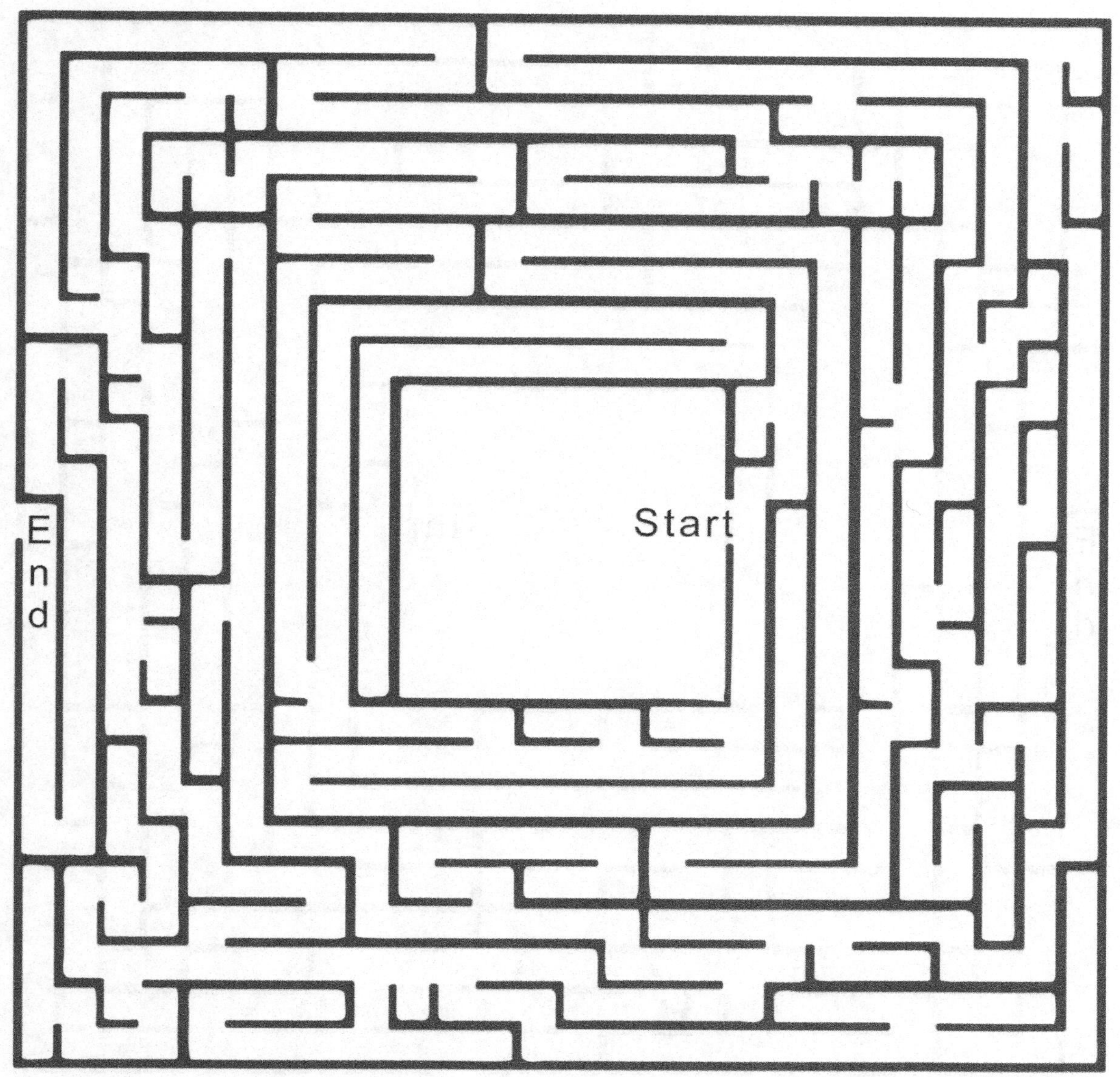

Start time: __________ End time: __________

Total time, maze 2: __________

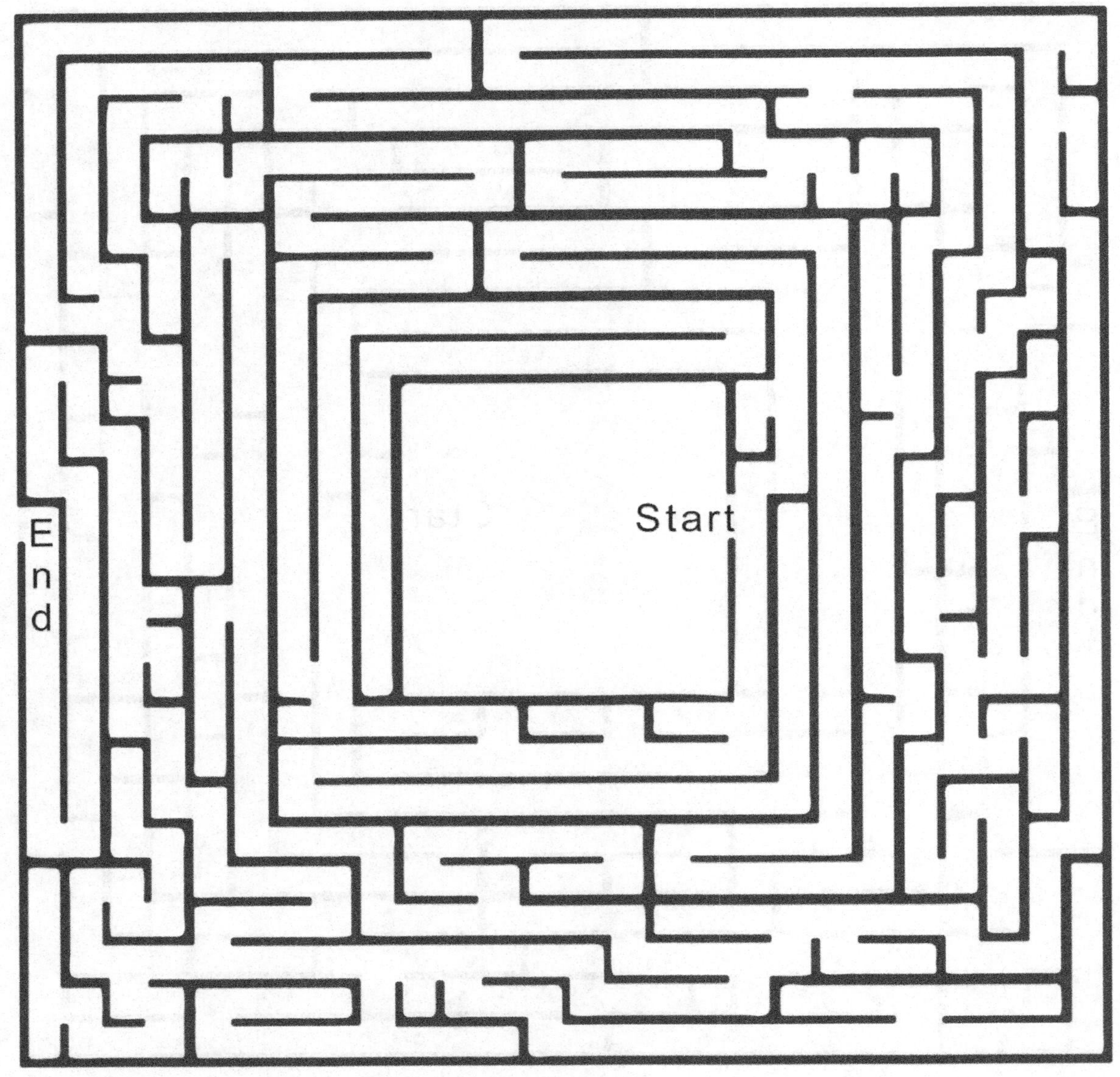

Start time: __________ End time: __________

Total time, maze 3: __________

Total time for 1st maze: __________

Total time for 2nd maze: __________

Total time for 3rd maze: __________

Congratulations! Did you experience progress in faster completion times? Circle your answer.

Yes No

If you circled "No" don't be discouraged. Remember to rest and give thanks to your mind and body for completing the challenges. Celebrate your tremendous effort. Remember, a seed doesn't turn into a tree overnight.

Edison failed 10,000 times before he made the electric light. Do not be discouraged if you fail a few times.

—*Napoleon Hill*

Often what feels like the end of the world
is really a challenging pathway to a far better place.

—*Karen Salmansohn*

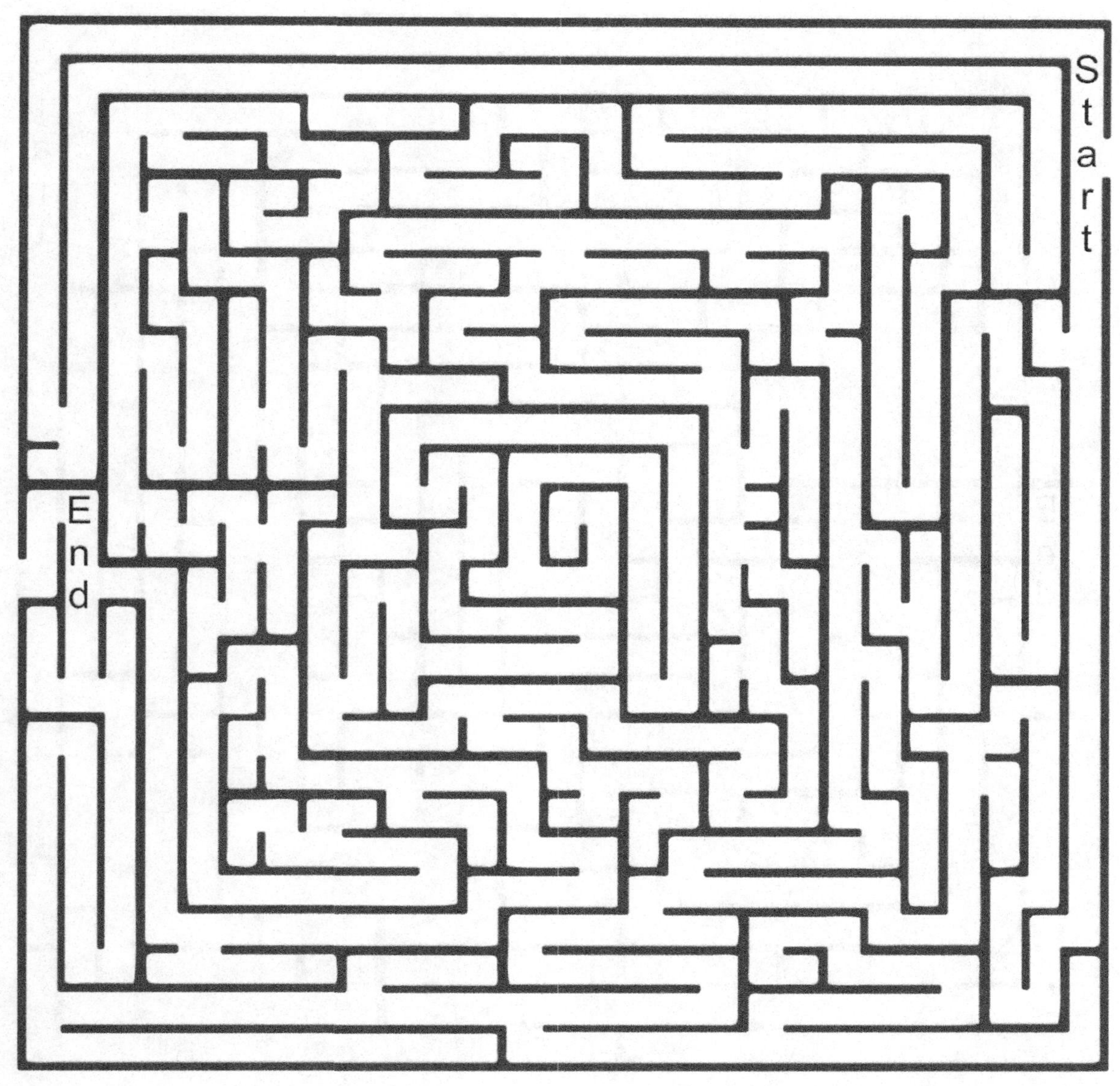

Start time: __________ End time: __________

Total time, maze 1: __________

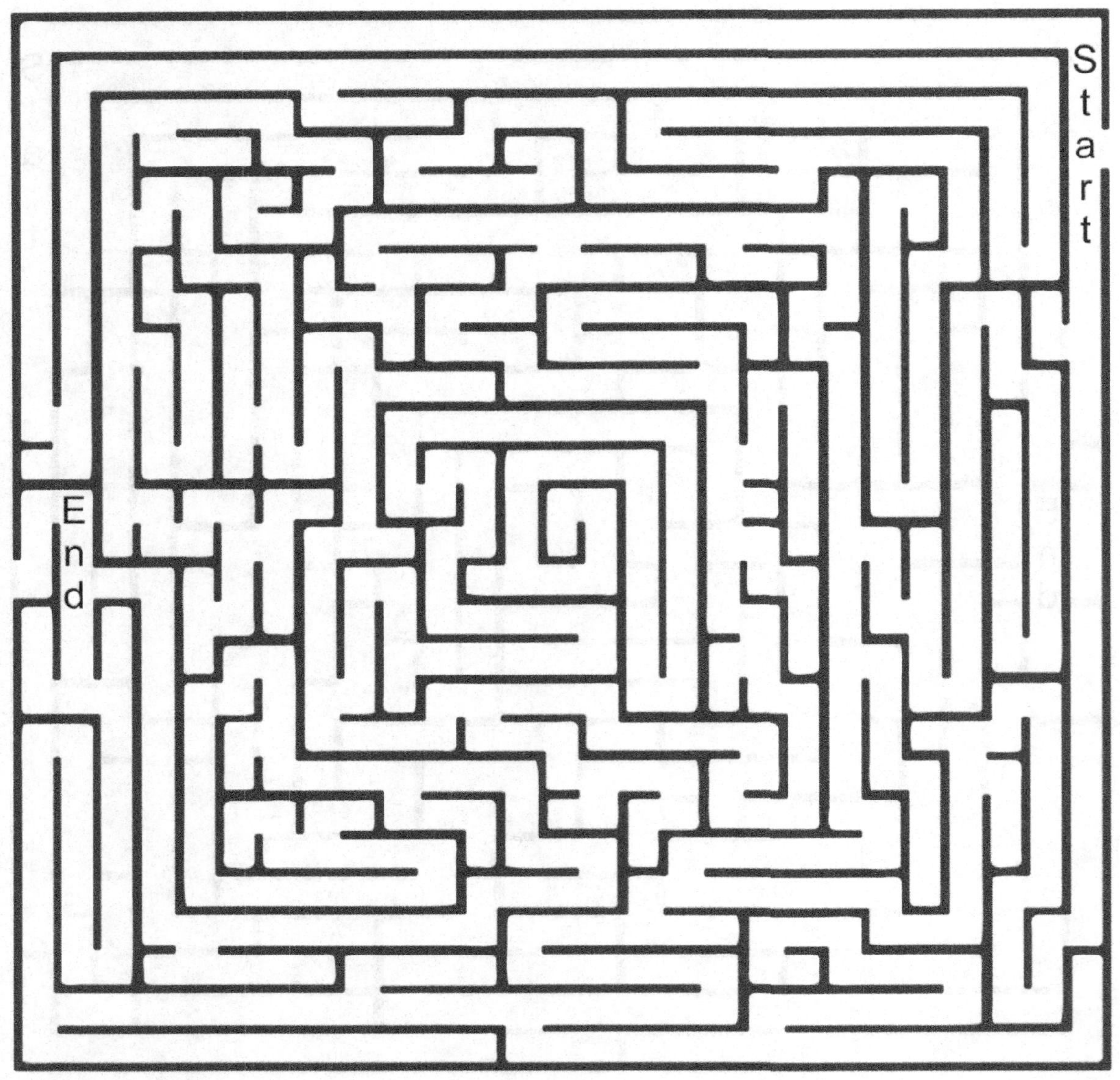

Start time: __________ End time: __________

Total time, maze 2: __________

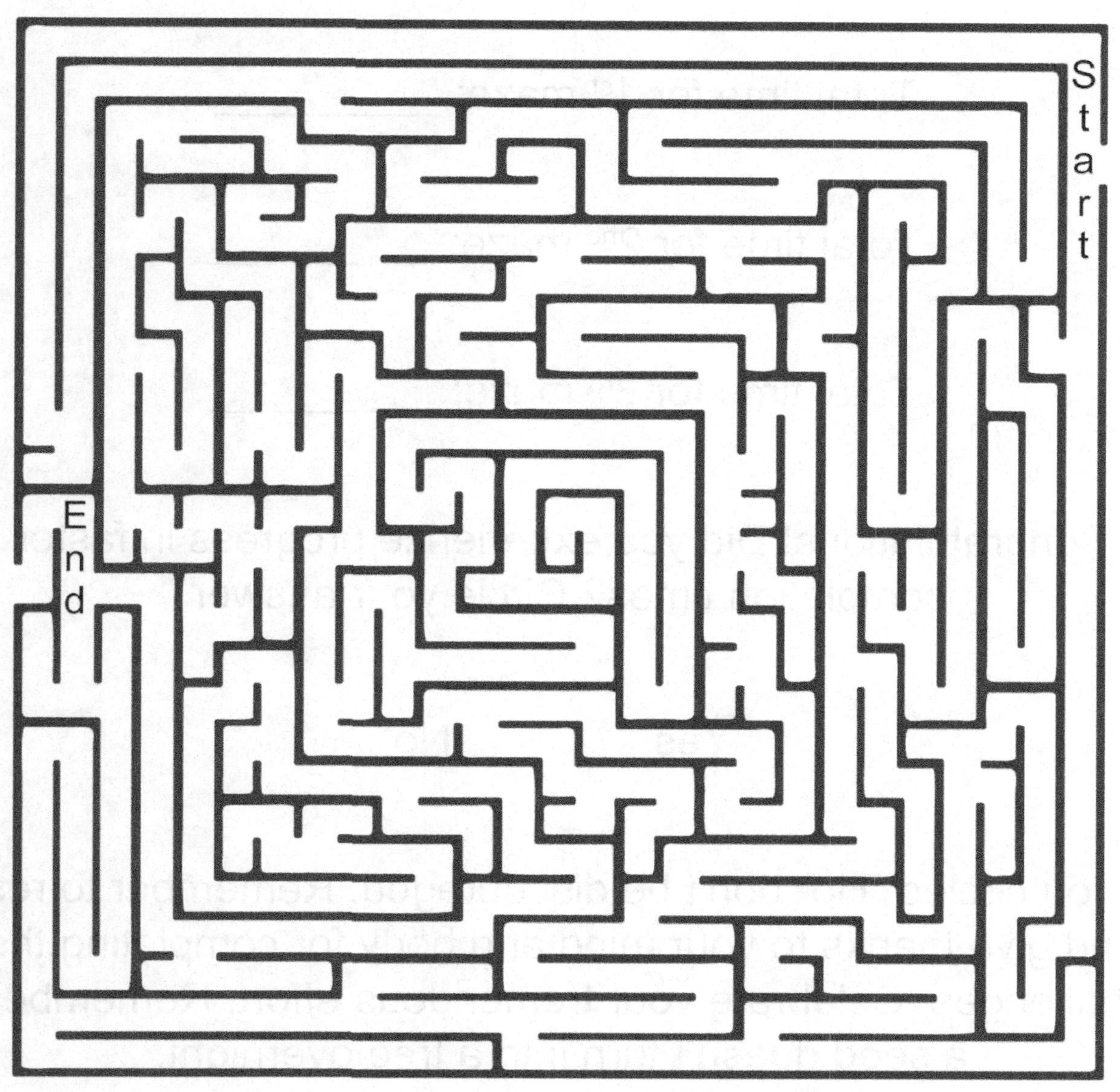

Start time: __________ End time: __________

Total time, maze 3: __________

Total time for 1st maze: __________

Total time for 2nd maze: __________

Total time for 3rd maze: __________

Congratulations! Did you experience progress in faster completion times? Circle your answer.

Yes No

If you circled “No” don’t be discouraged. Remember to rest and give thanks to your mind and body for completing the challenges. Celebrate your tremendous effort. Remember, a seed doesn’t turn into a tree overnight.

A man can get discouraged many times but he is not a failure until he begins to blame somebody else and stops trying.

—John Burroughs

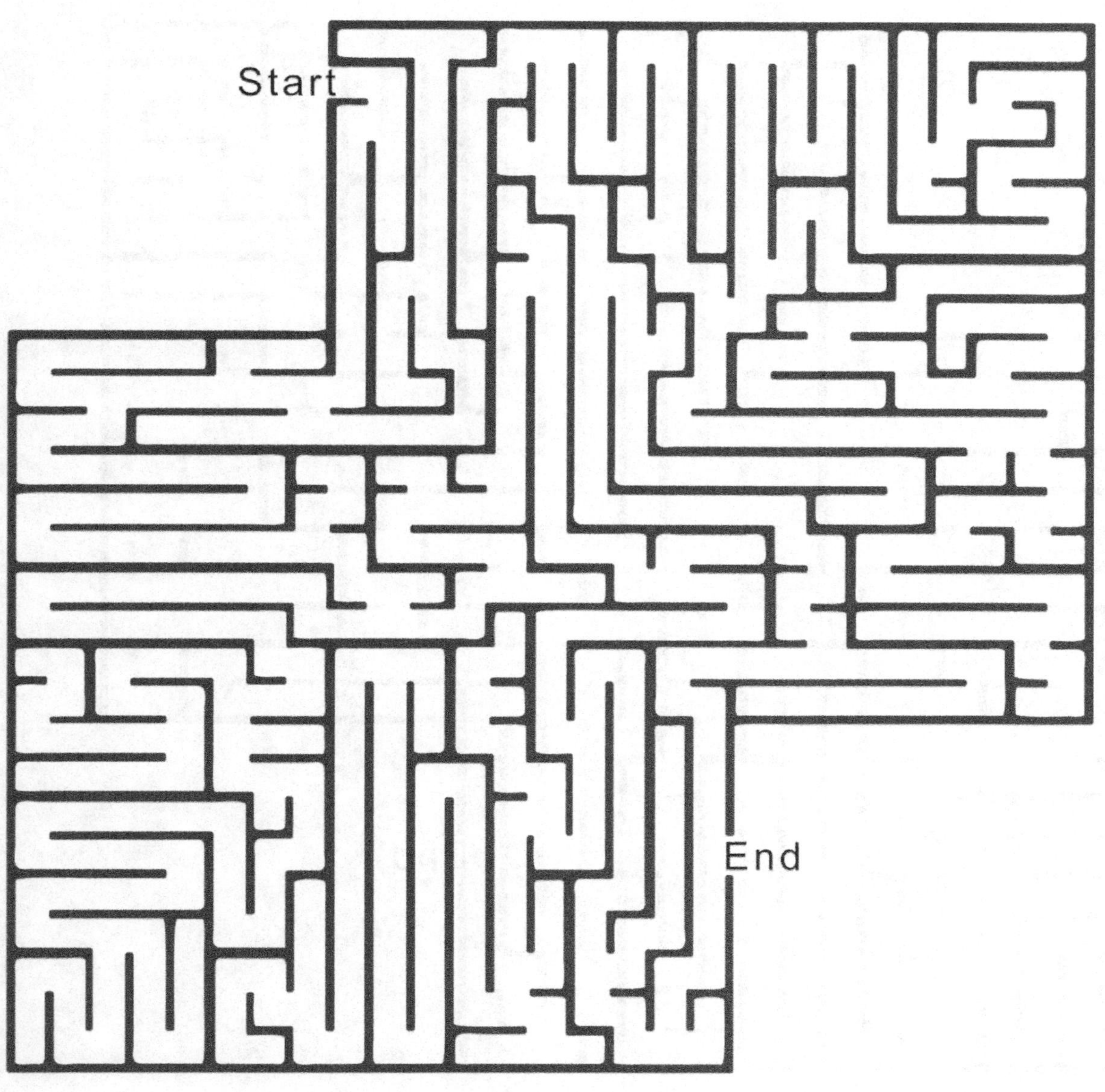

Start time: __________ End time: __________

Total time, maze 1: __________

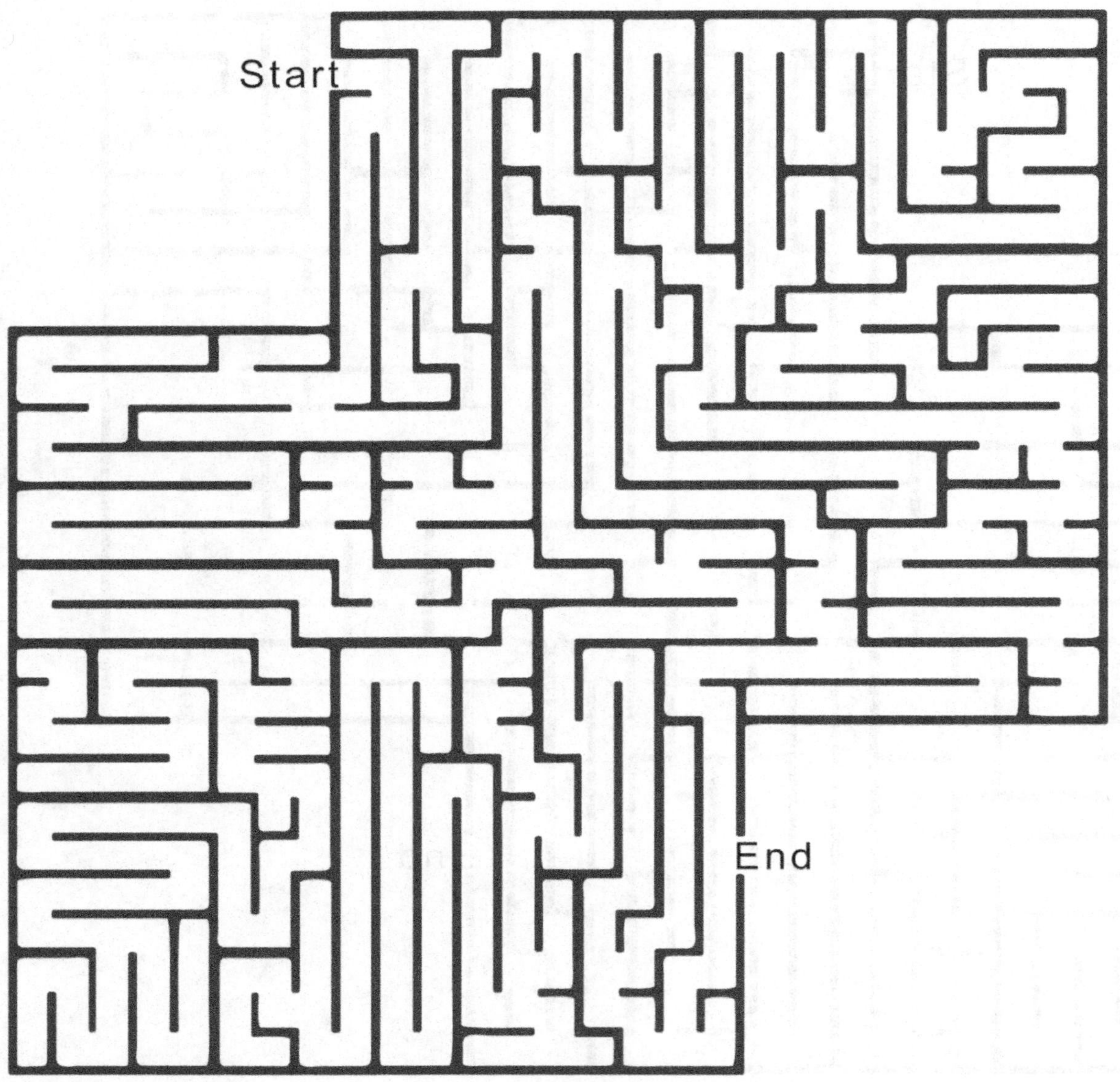

Start time: __________ End time: __________

Total time, maze 2: __________

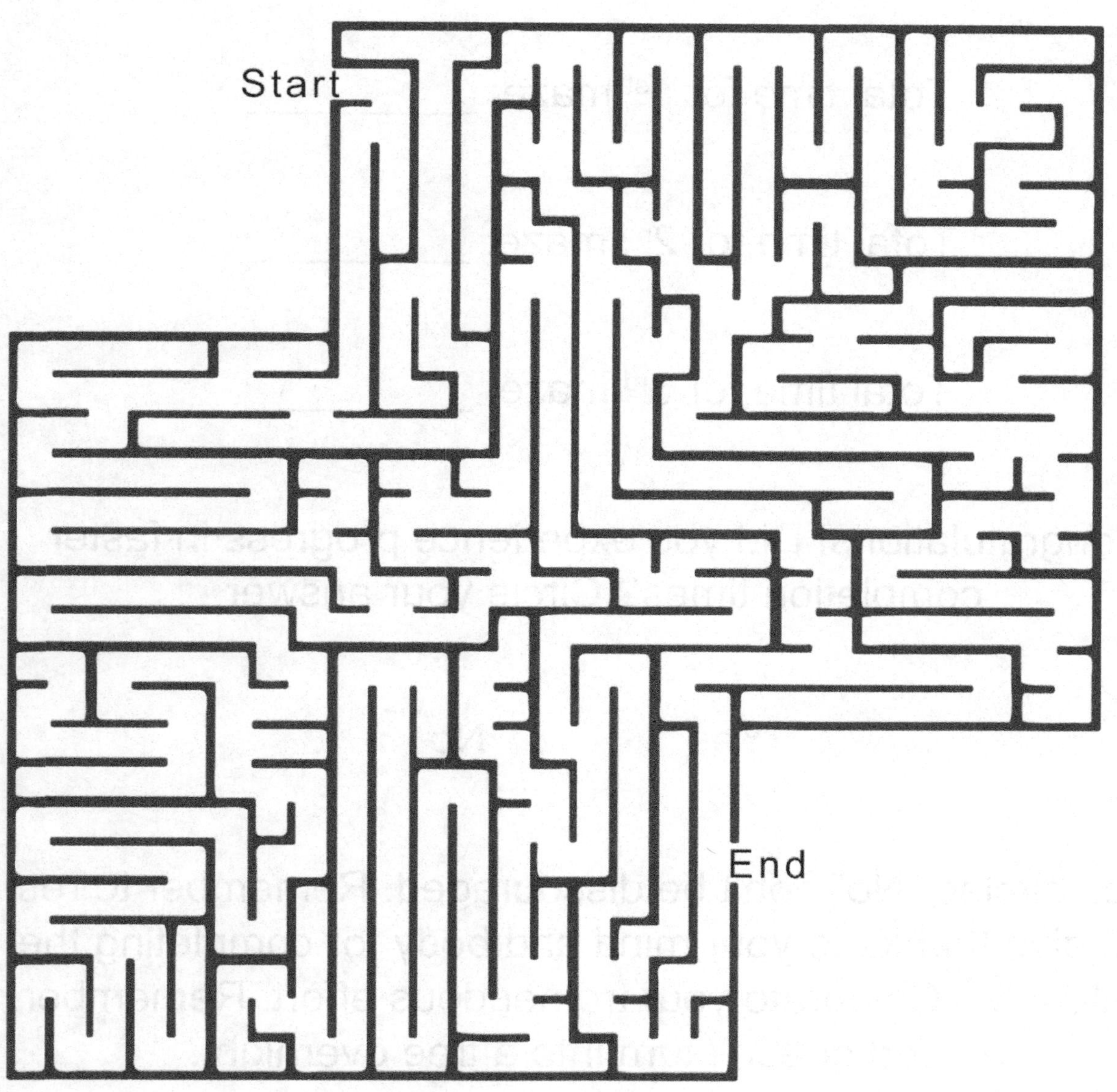

Start time: __________ End time: __________

Total time, maze 3: __________

Total time for 1st maze: __________

Total time for 2nd maze: __________

Total time for 3rd maze: __________

Congratulations! Did you experience progress in faster completion times? Circle your answer.

Yes No

If you circled "No" don't be discouraged. Remember to rest and give thanks to your mind and body for completing the challenges. Celebrate your tremendous effort. Remember, a seed doesn't turn into a tree overnight.

Continuous, unflagging effort, persistence and determination will win. Let not the man be discouraged who has these.

—James Whitcomb Riley

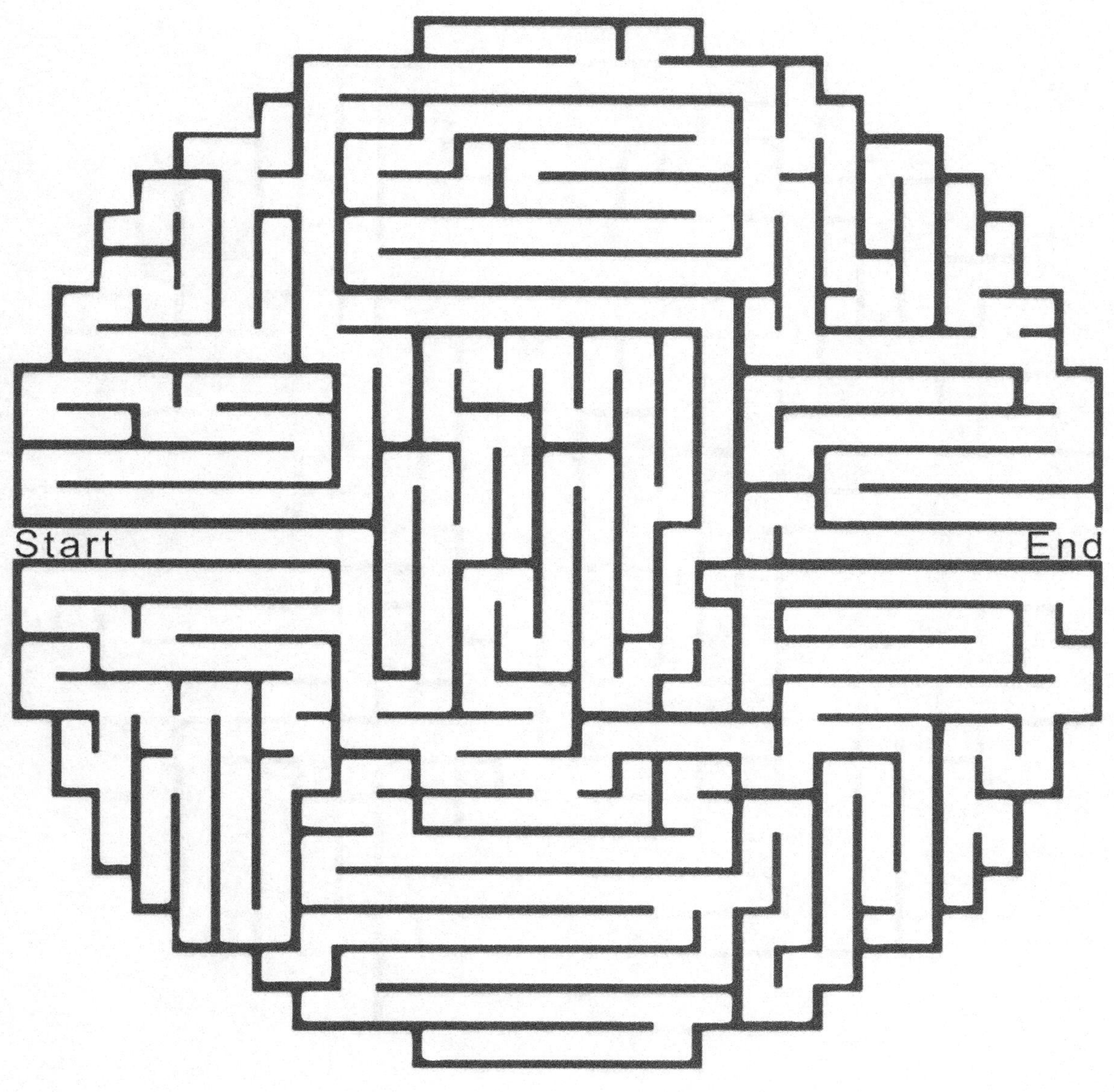

Start time: __________ End time: __________

Total time, maze 1: __________

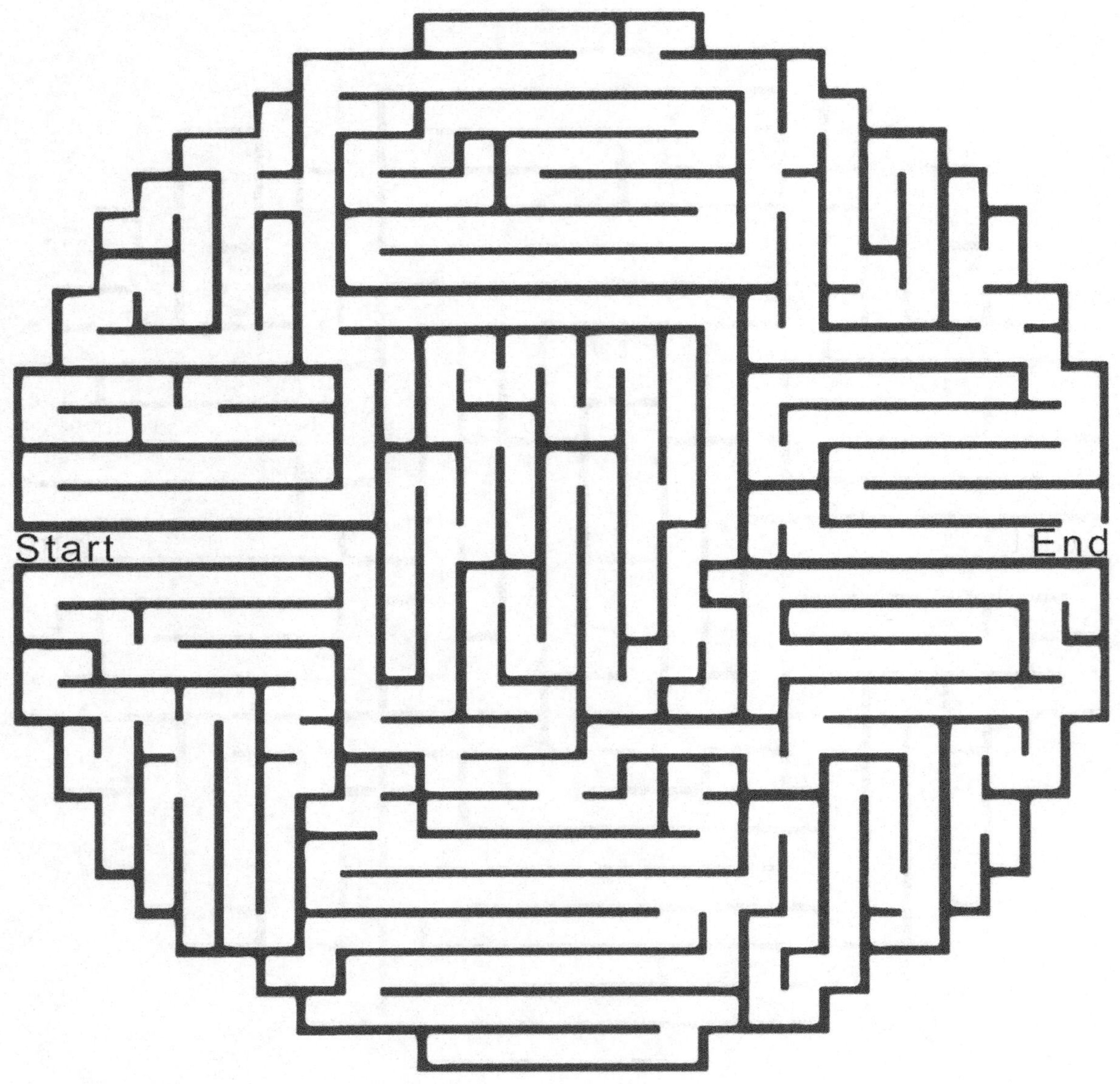

Start time: __________ End time: __________

Total time, maze 2: __________

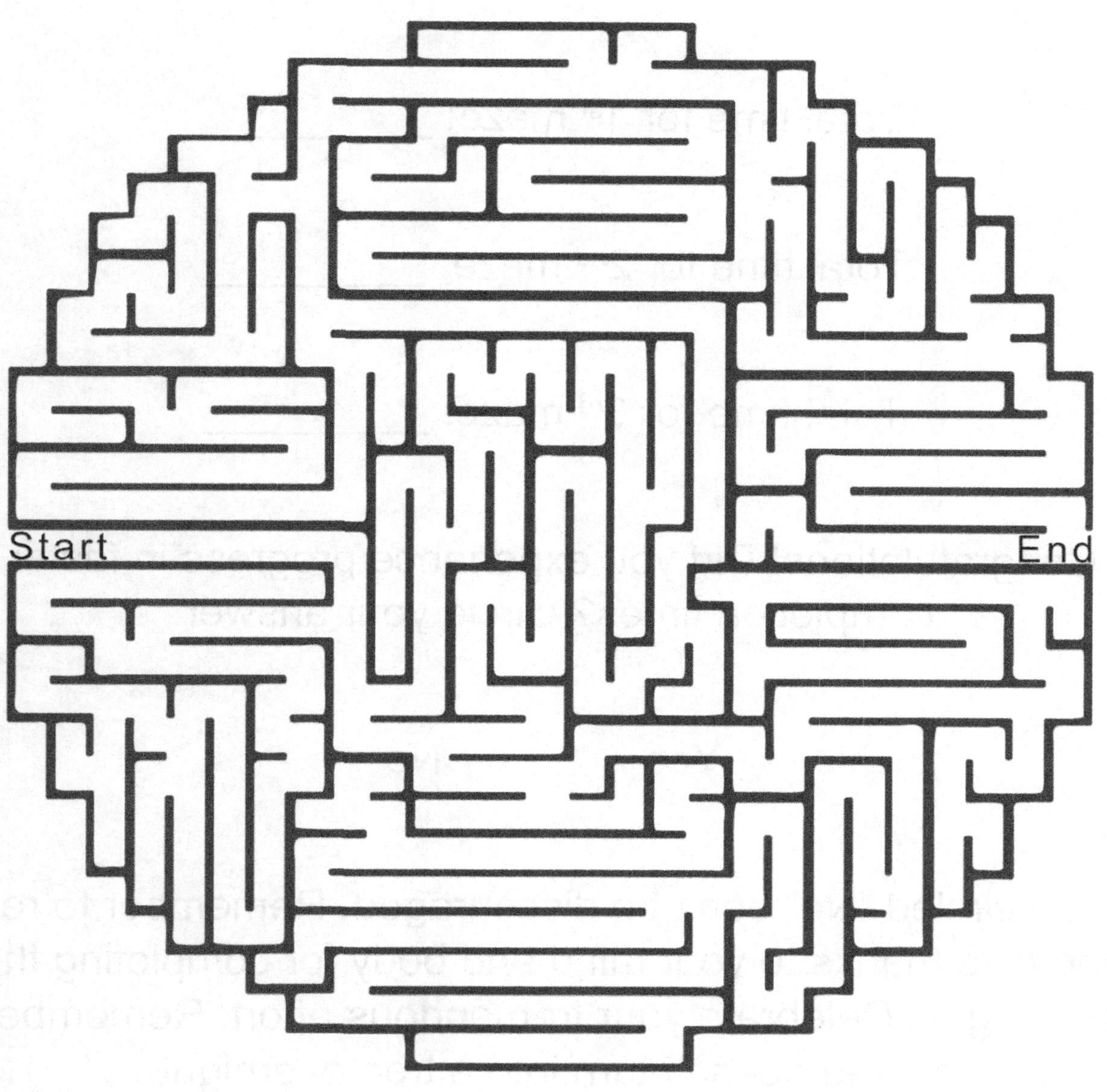

Start time: __________ End time: __________

Total time, maze 3: __________

Total time for 1st maze: __________

Total time for 2nd maze: __________

Total time for 3rd maze: __________

Congratulations! Did you experience progress in faster completion times? Circle your answer.

Yes No

If you circled "No" don't be discouraged. Remember to rest and give thanks to your mind and body for completing the challenges. Celebrate your tremendous effort. Remember, a seed doesn't turn into a tree overnight.

What is important is to believe in something so strongly that you're never discouraged.

—*Salma Hayek*

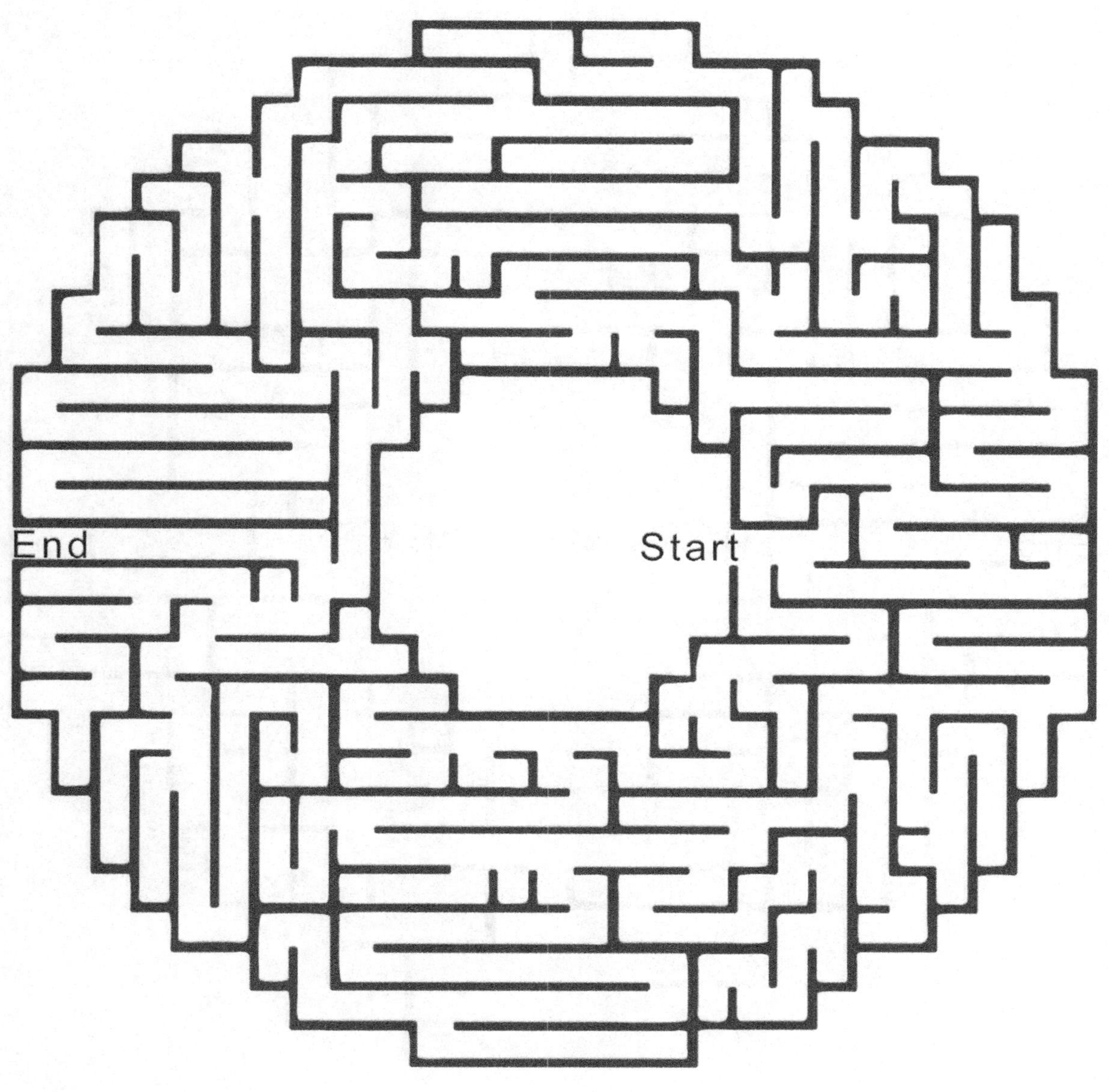

Start time: __________ End time: __________

Total time, maze 1: __________

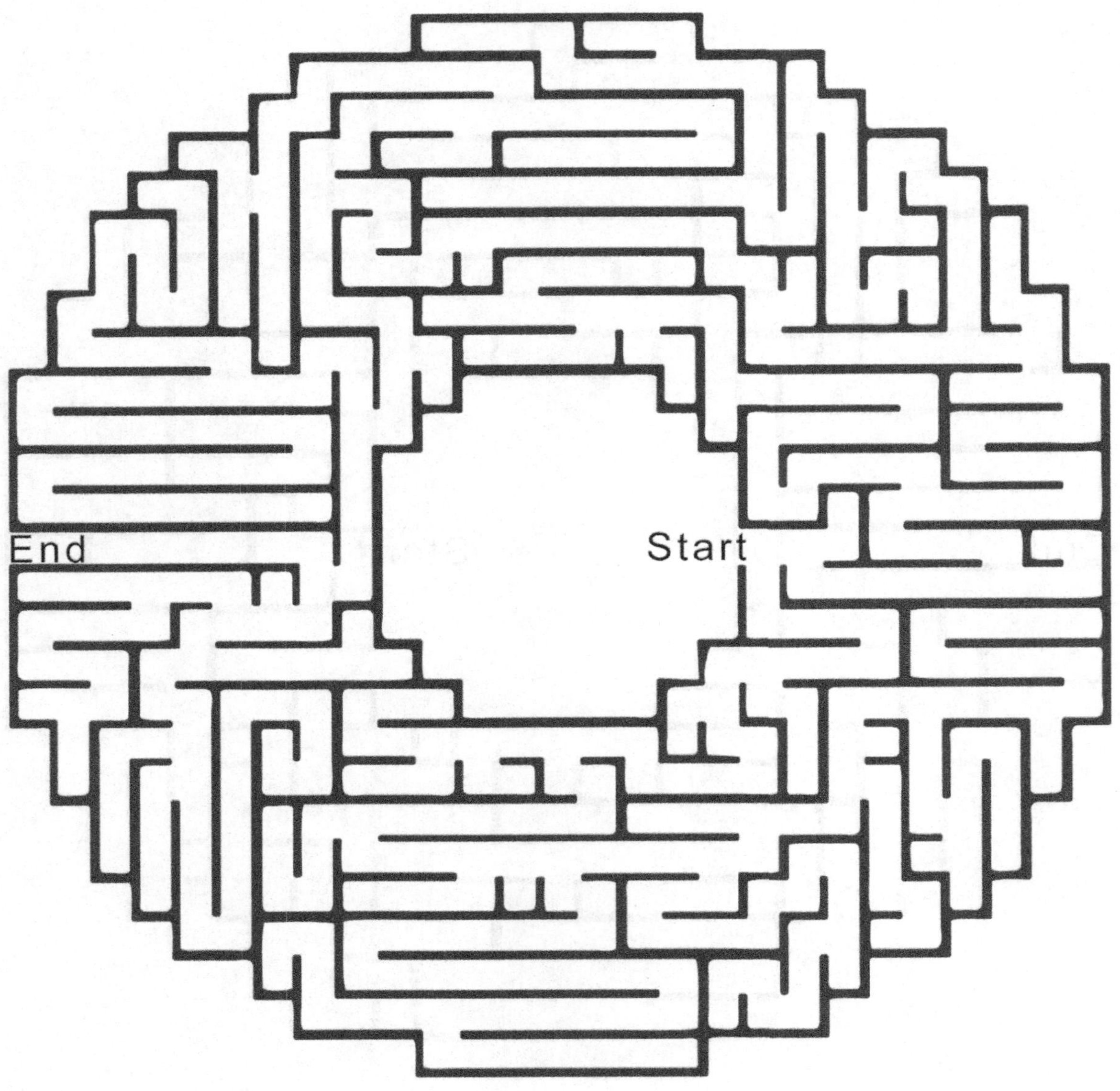

Start time: __________ End time: __________

Total time, maze 2: __________

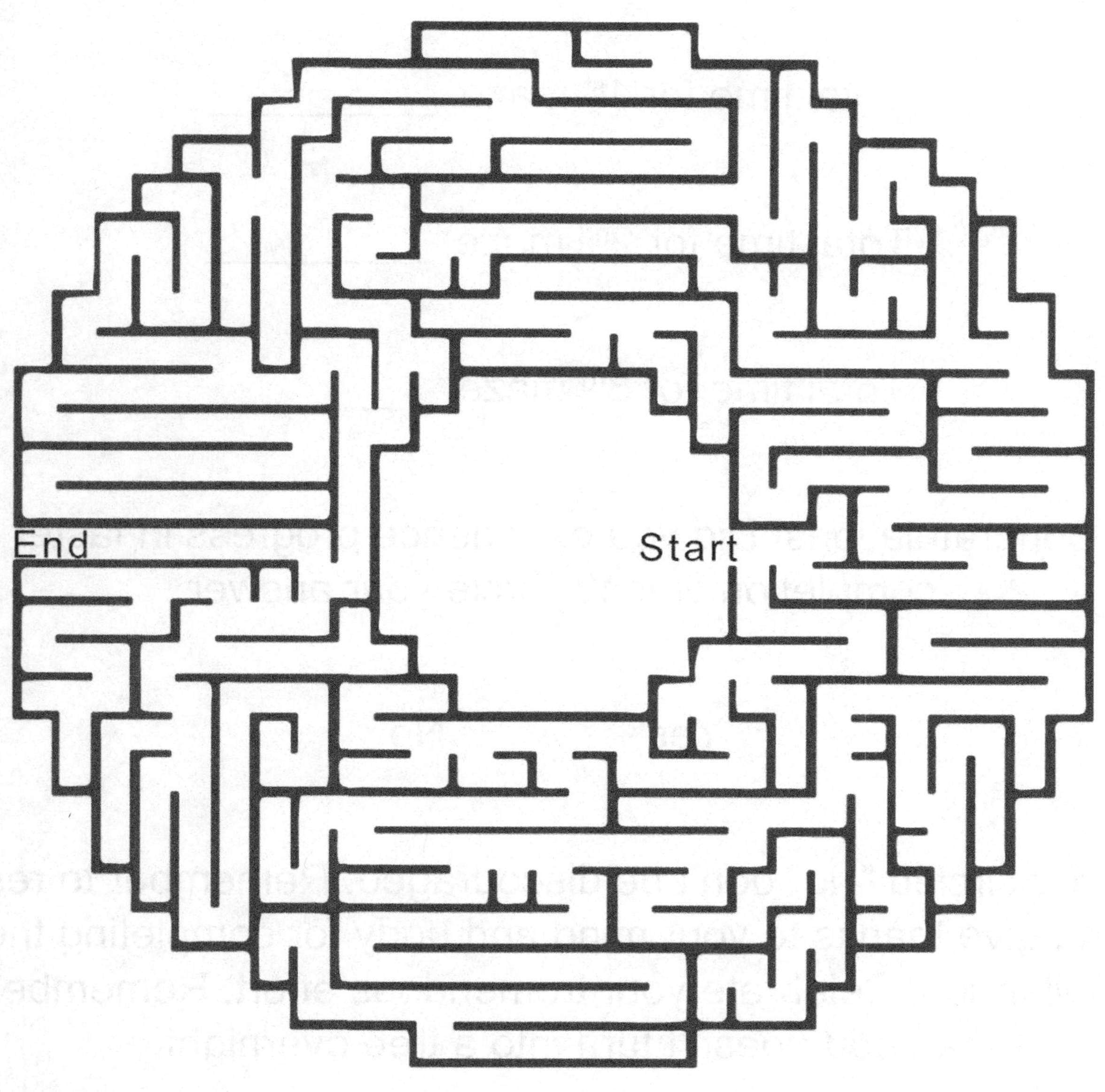

Start time: __________ End time: __________

Total time, maze 3: __________

Total time for 1st maze: __________

Total time for 2nd maze: __________

Total time for 3rd maze: __________

Congratulations! Did you experience progress in faster completion times? Circle your answer.

Yes No

If you circled "No" don't be discouraged. Remember to rest and give thanks to your mind and body for completing the challenges. Celebrate your tremendous effort. Remember, a seed doesn't turn into a tree overnight.

Stop beating yourself up. You are a work in progress - which means you get there a little at a time, not all at once.

—*Unknown*

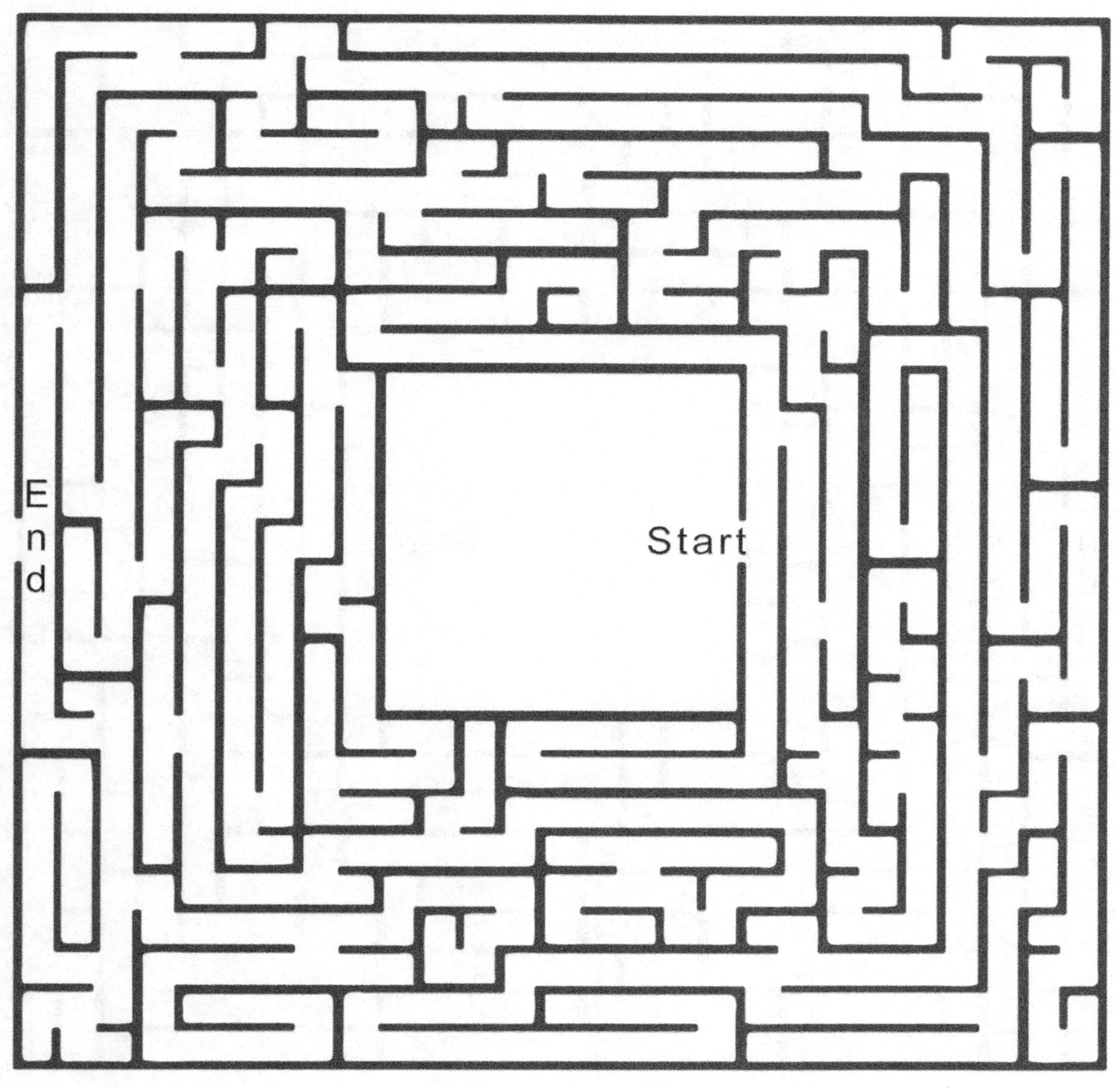

Start time: __________ End time: __________

Total time, maze 1: __________

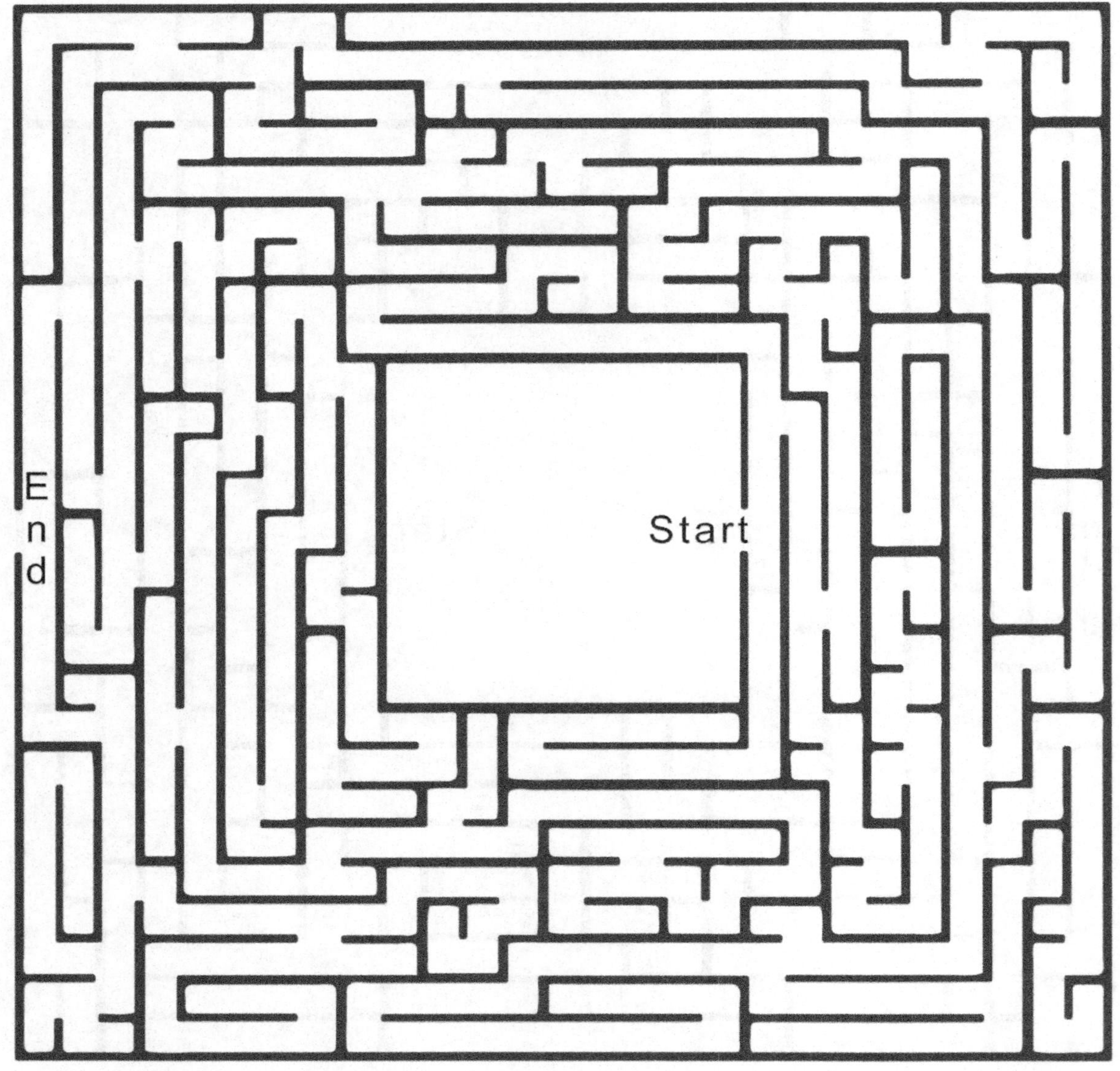

Start time: __________ End time: __________

Total time, maze 2: __________

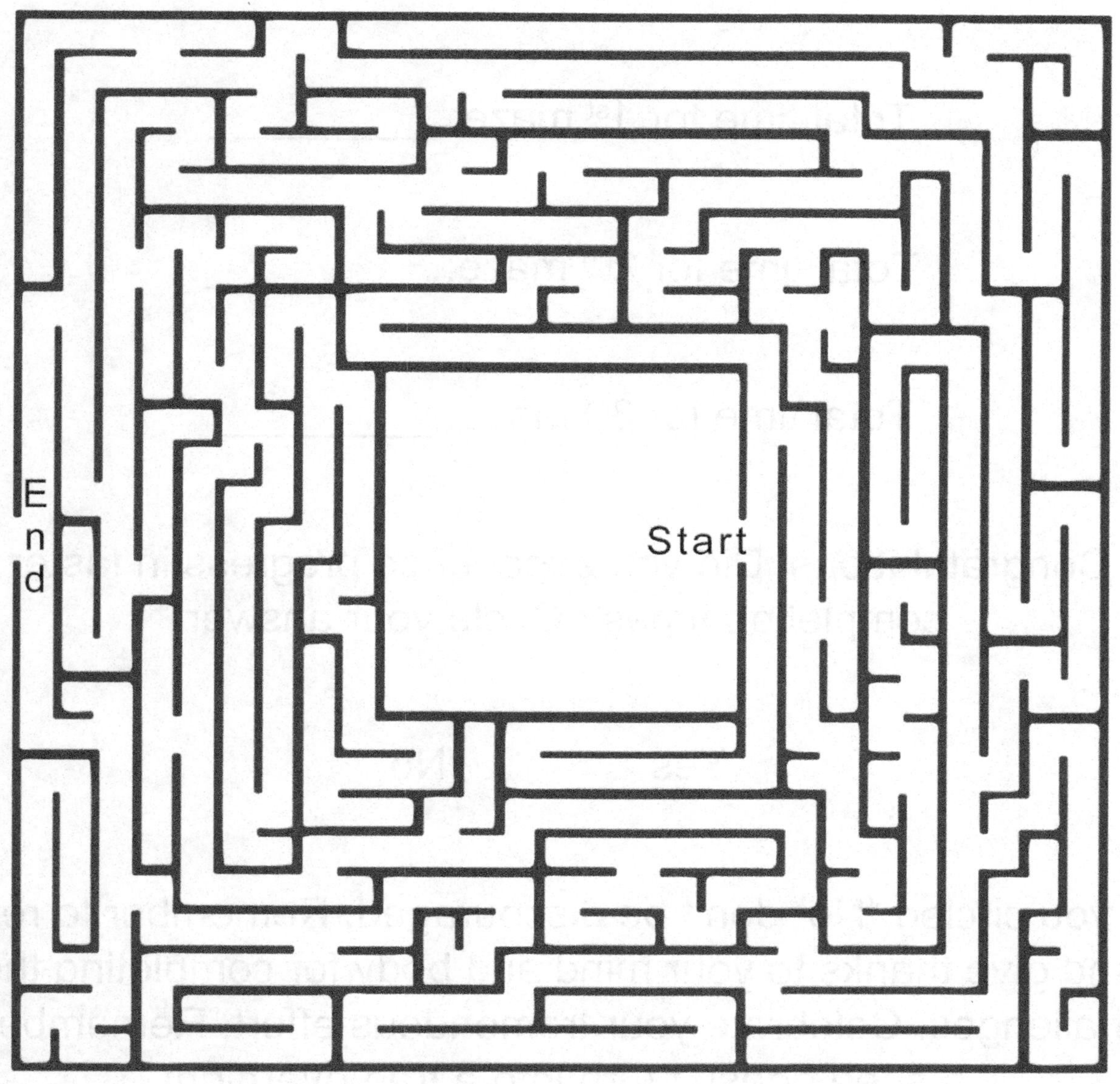

Start time: __________ End time: __________

Total time, maze 3: __________

Total time for 1st maze: __________

Total time for 2nd maze: __________

Total time for 3rd maze: __________

Congratulations! Did you experience progress in faster completion times? Circle your answer.

Yes No

If you circled "No" don't be discouraged. Remember to rest and give thanks to your mind and body for completing the challenges. Celebrate your tremendous effort. Remember, a seed doesn't turn into a tree overnight.

Yesterday I was clever so I wanted to change the world.
Today I am wise, so I am changing myself.

—*Rumi*

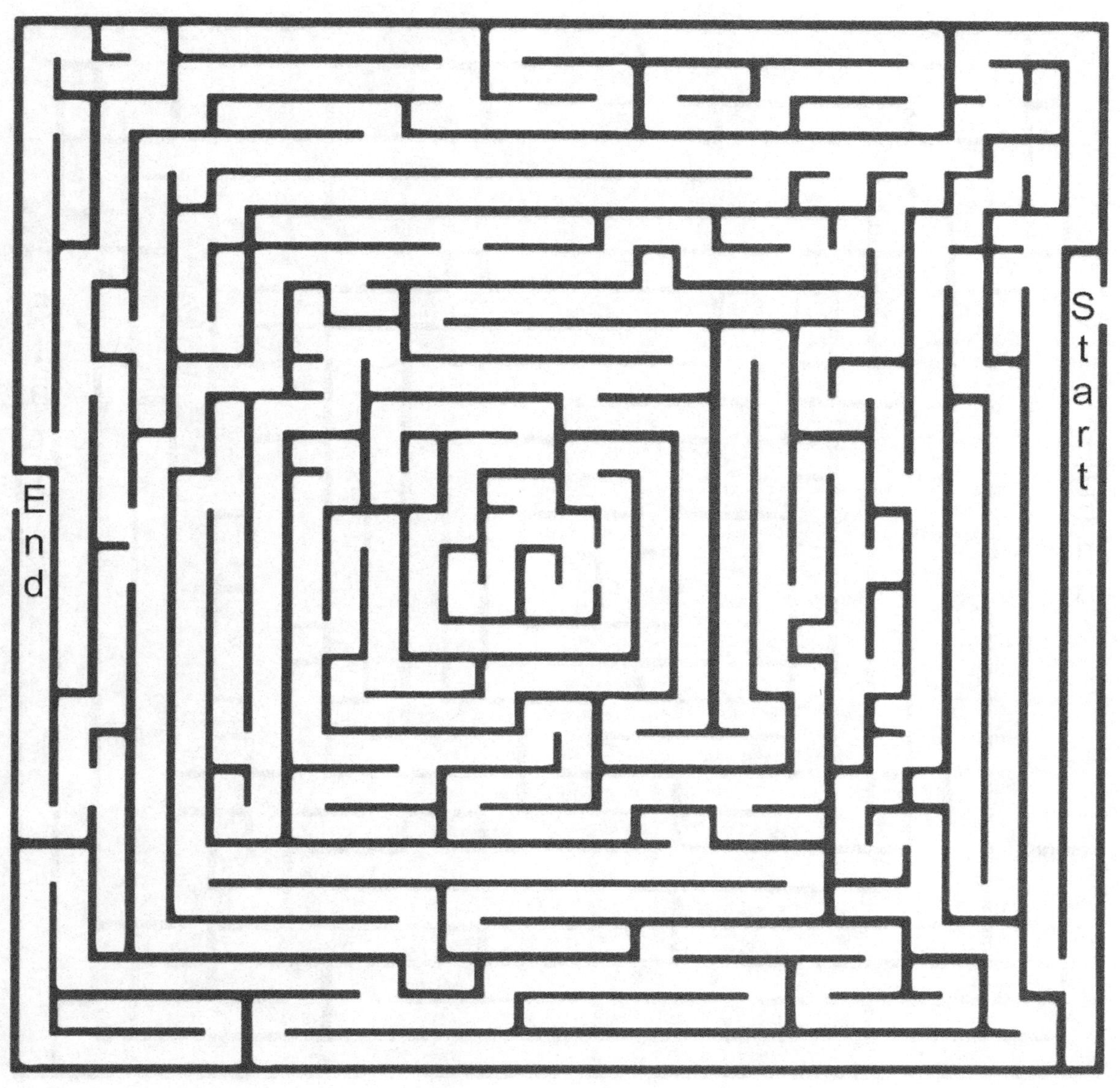

Start time: __________ End time: __________

Total time, maze 1: __________

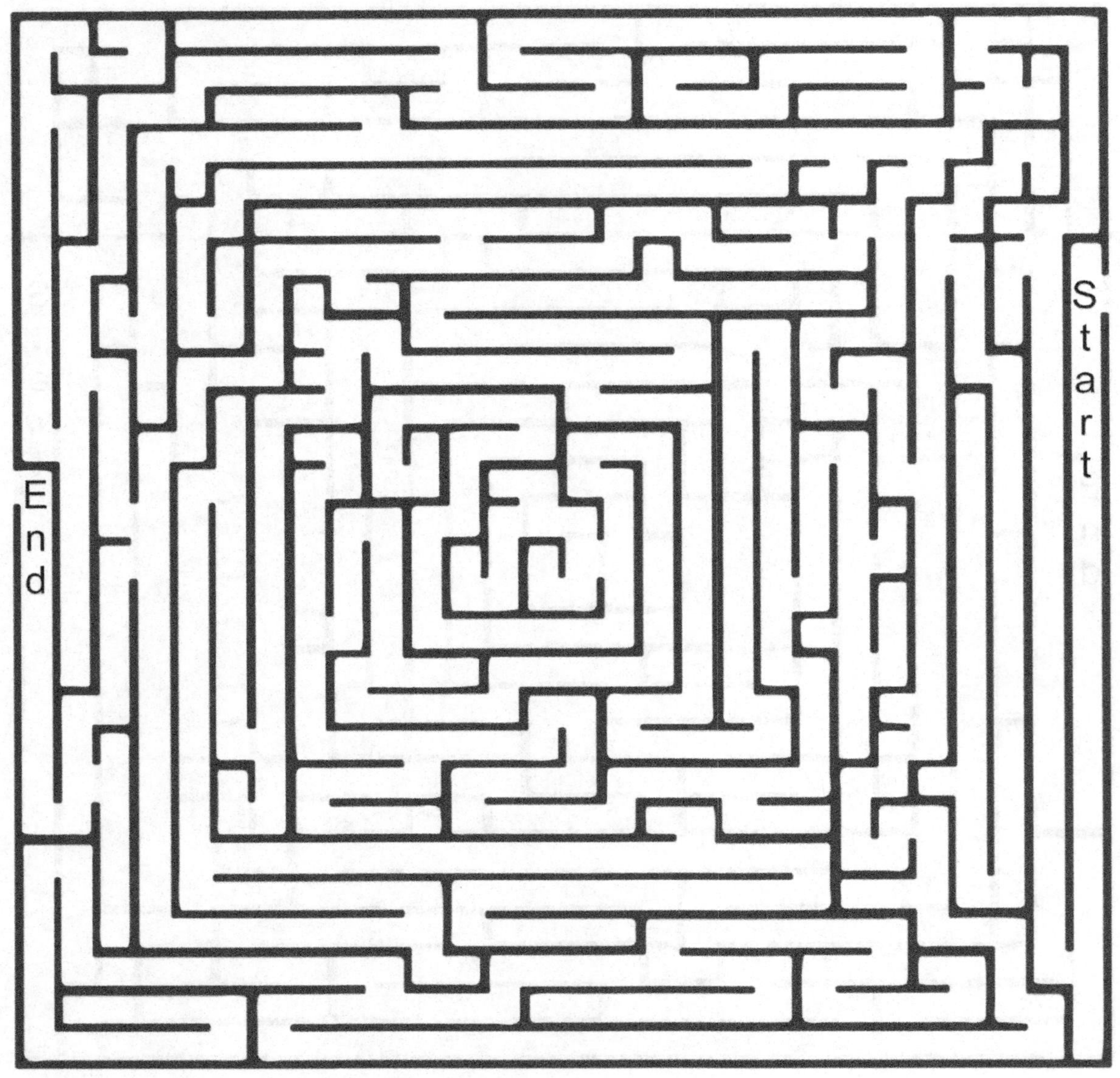

Start time: __________ End time: __________

Total time, maze 2: __________

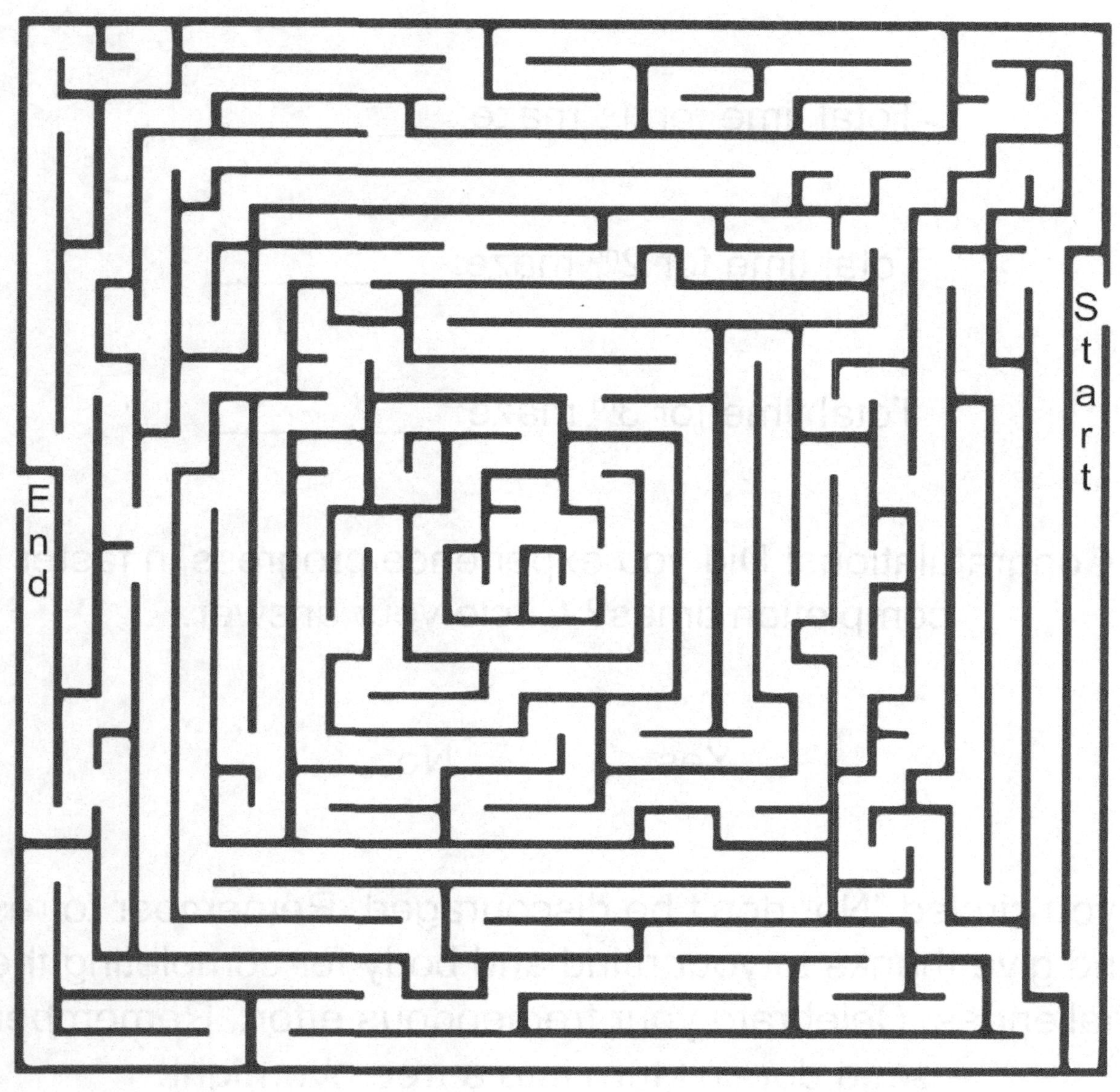

Start time: __________ End time: __________

Total time, maze 3: __________

Total time for 1st maze: __________

Total time for 2nd maze: __________

Total time for 3rd maze: __________

Congratulations! Did you experience progress in faster completion times? Circle your answer.

Yes No

If you circled "No" don't be discouraged. Remember to rest and give thanks to your mind and body for completing the challenges. Celebrate your tremendous effort. Remember, a seed doesn't turn into a tree overnight.

If you really want to do something, you'll find a way. If you don't, you'll find an excuse.

—Jim Rohn

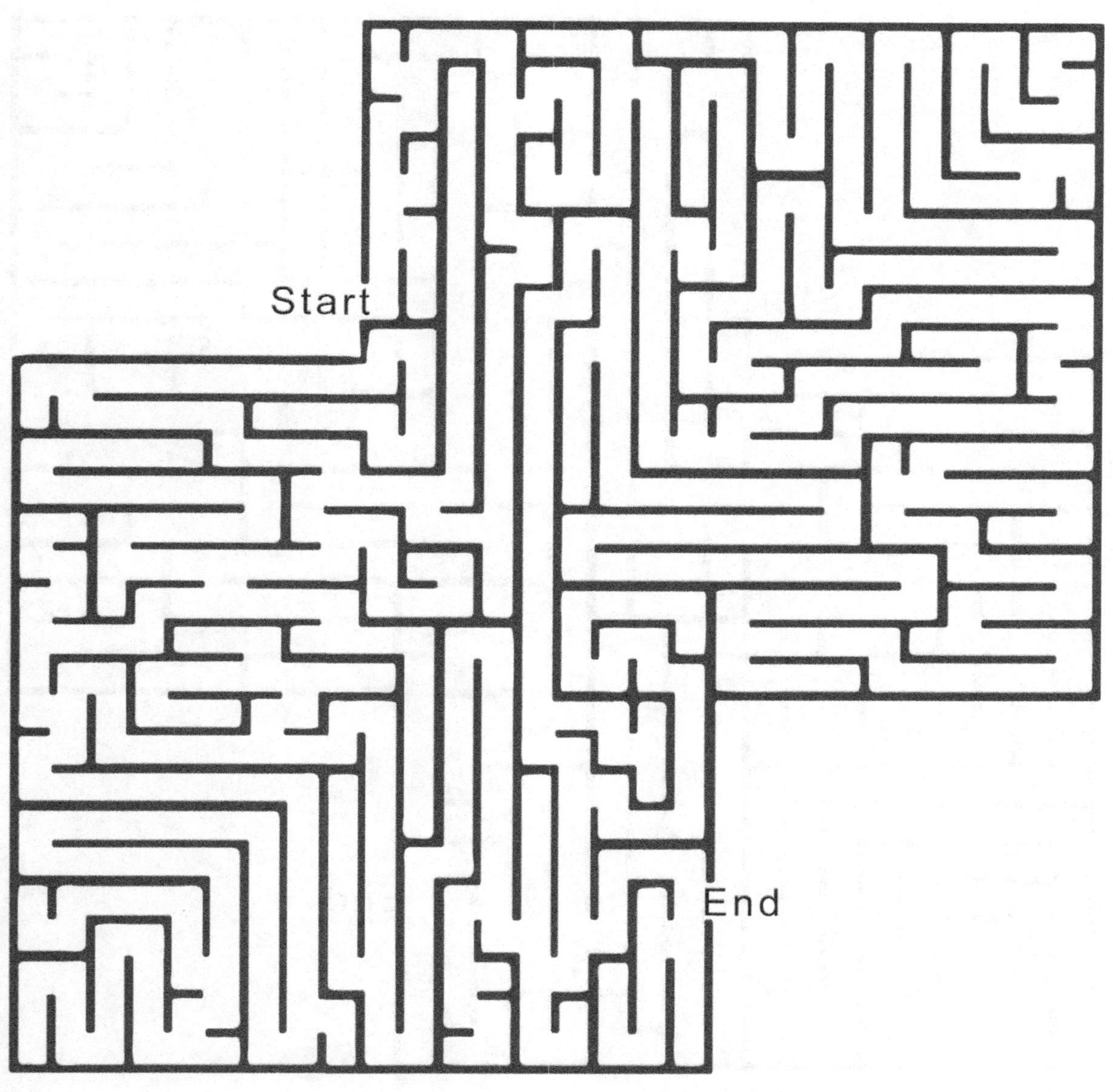

Start time: __________ End time: __________

Total time, maze 1: __________

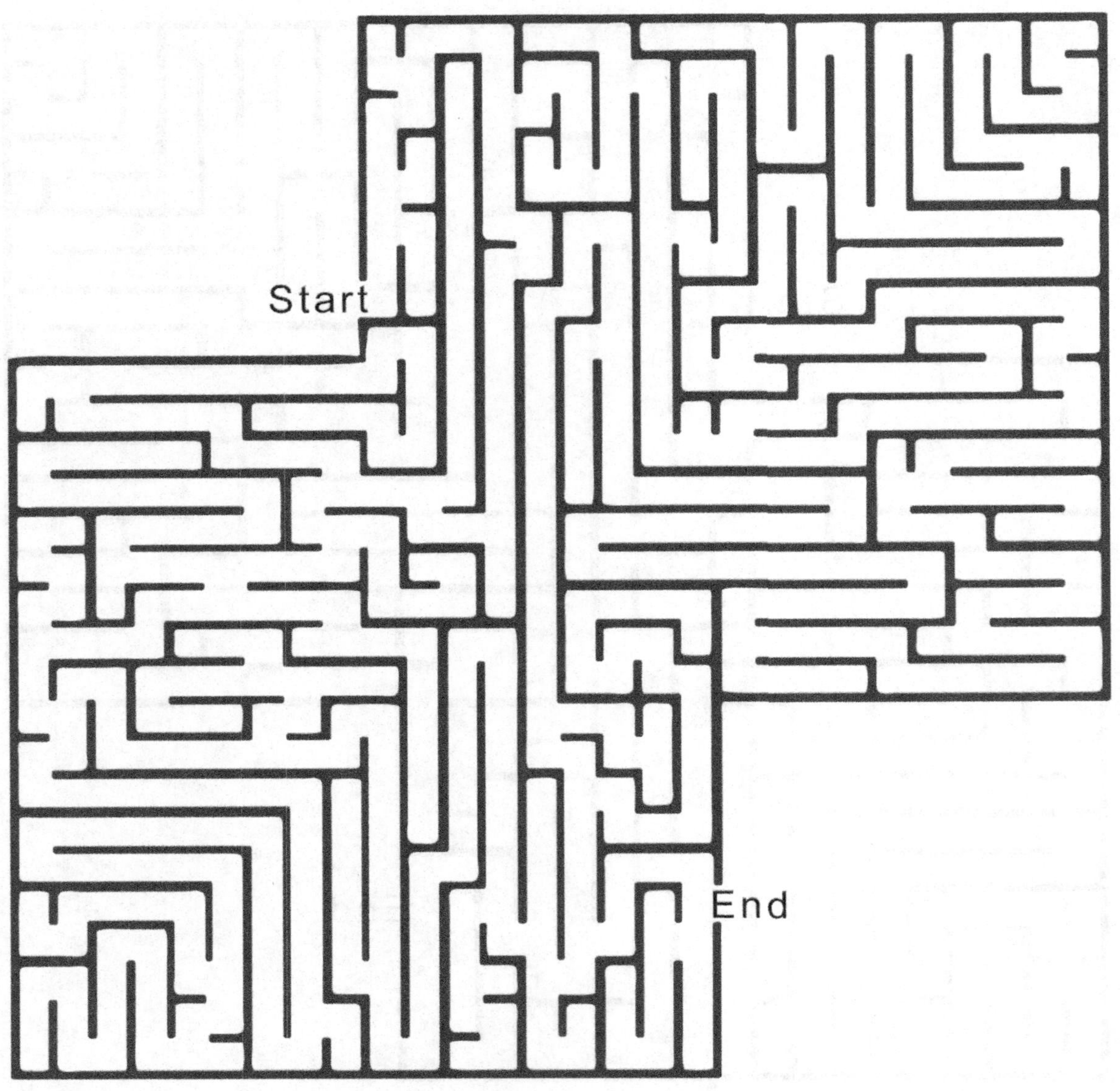

Start time: __________ End time: __________

Total time, maze 2: __________

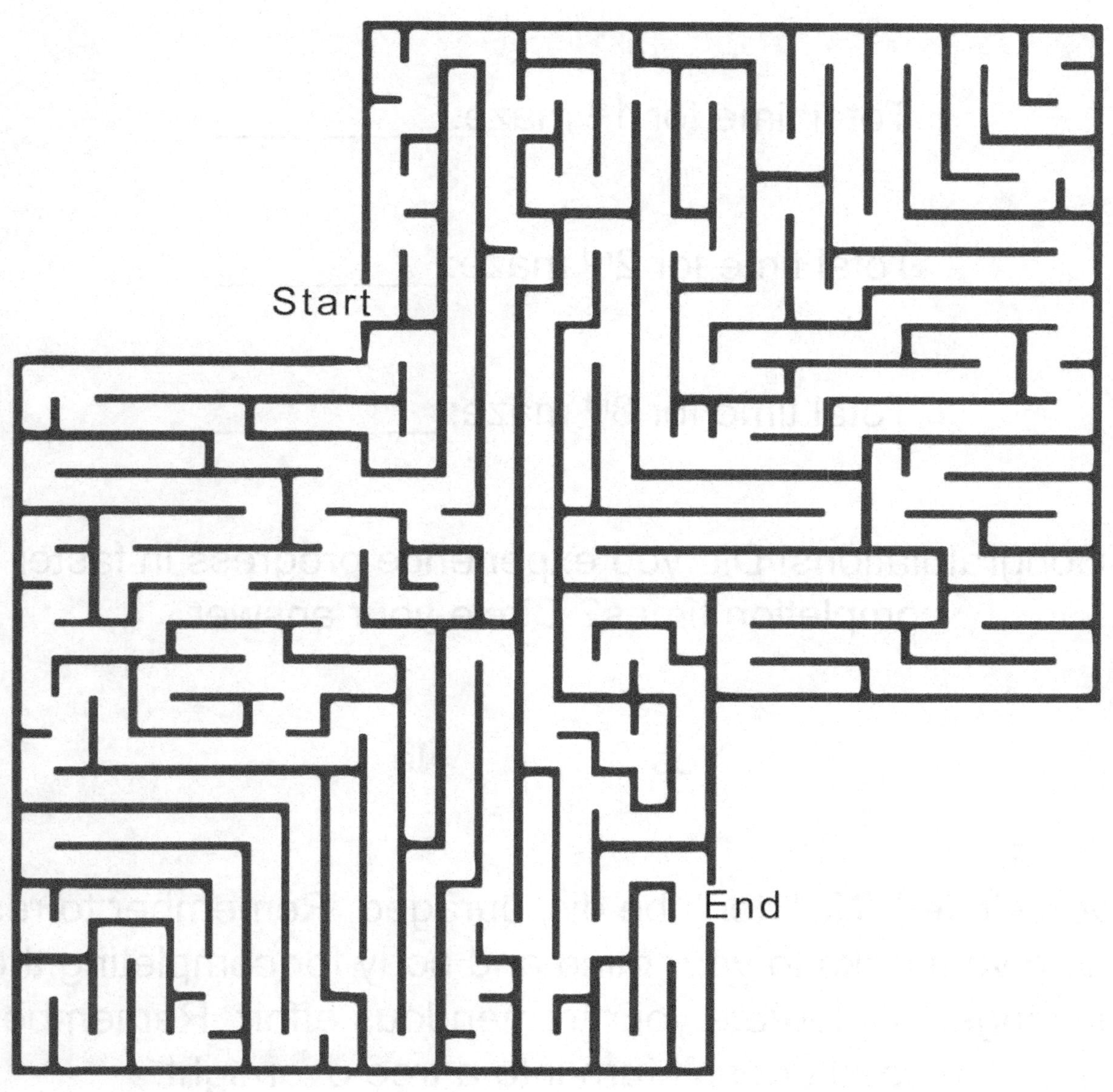

Start time: __________ End time: __________

Total time, maze 3: __________

Total time for 1st maze: __________

Total time for 2nd maze: __________

Total time for 3rd maze: __________

Congratulations! Did you experience progress in faster completion times? Circle your answer.

Yes No

If you circled "No" don't be discouraged. Remember to rest and give thanks to your mind and body for completing the challenges. Celebrate your tremendous effort. Remember, a seed doesn't turn into a tree overnight.

F.E.A.R: has two meanings: 1). Forget Everything And Run or 2). Face Everything And Rise; the choice is yours!

—Zig Ziglar

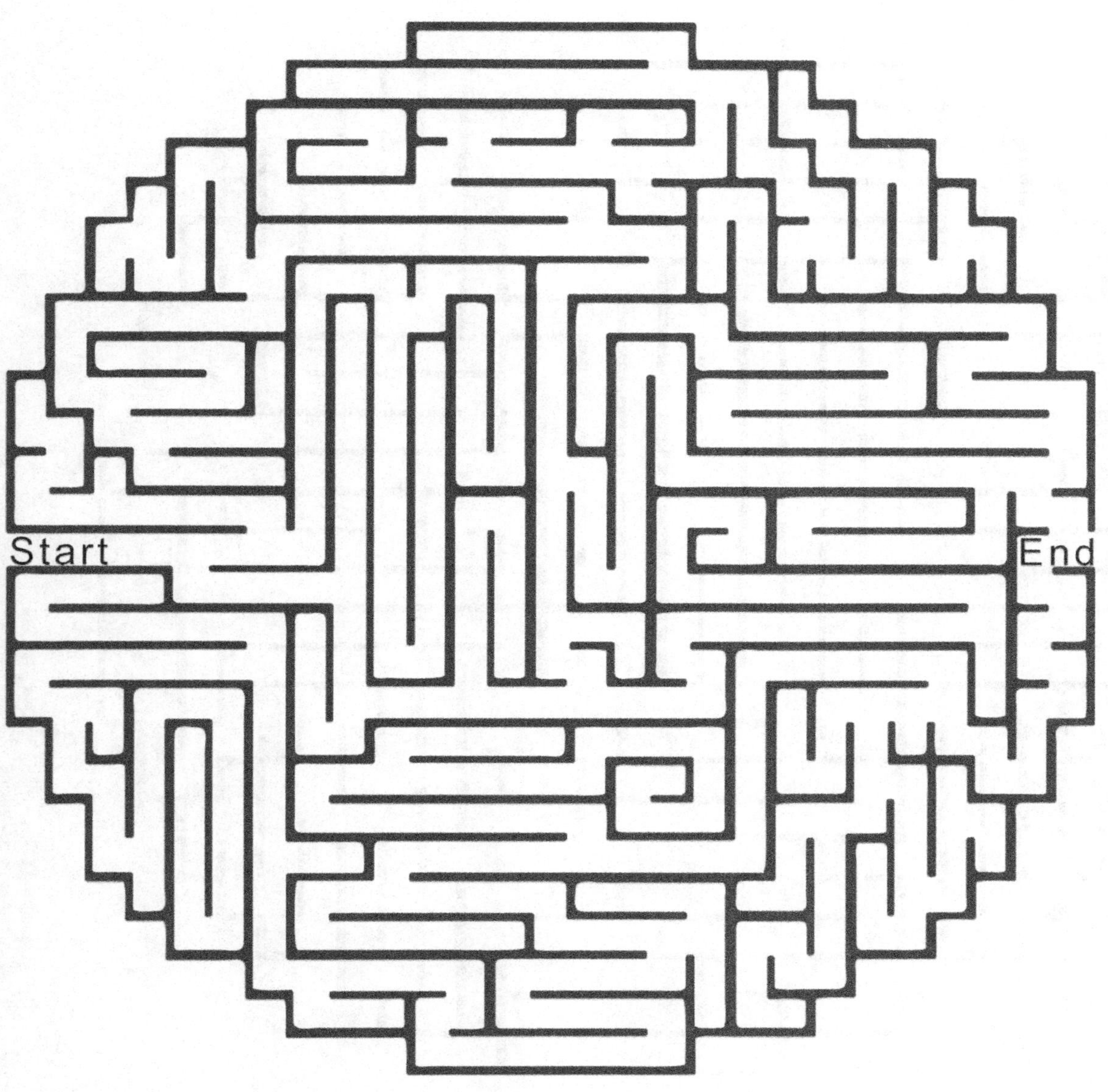

Start time: ___________ End time: ___________

Total time, maze 1: ___________

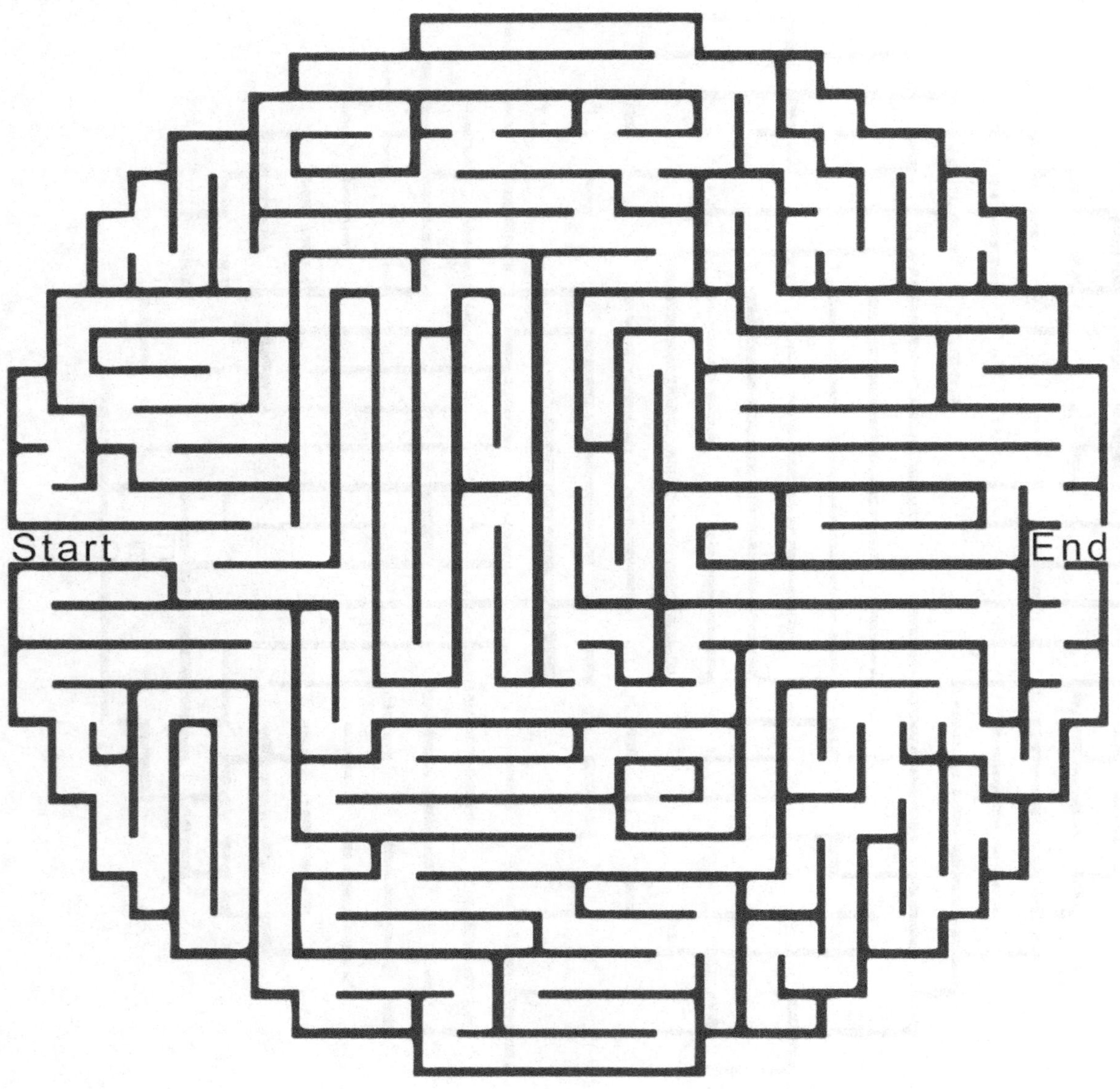

Start time: __________ End time: __________

Total time, maze 2: __________

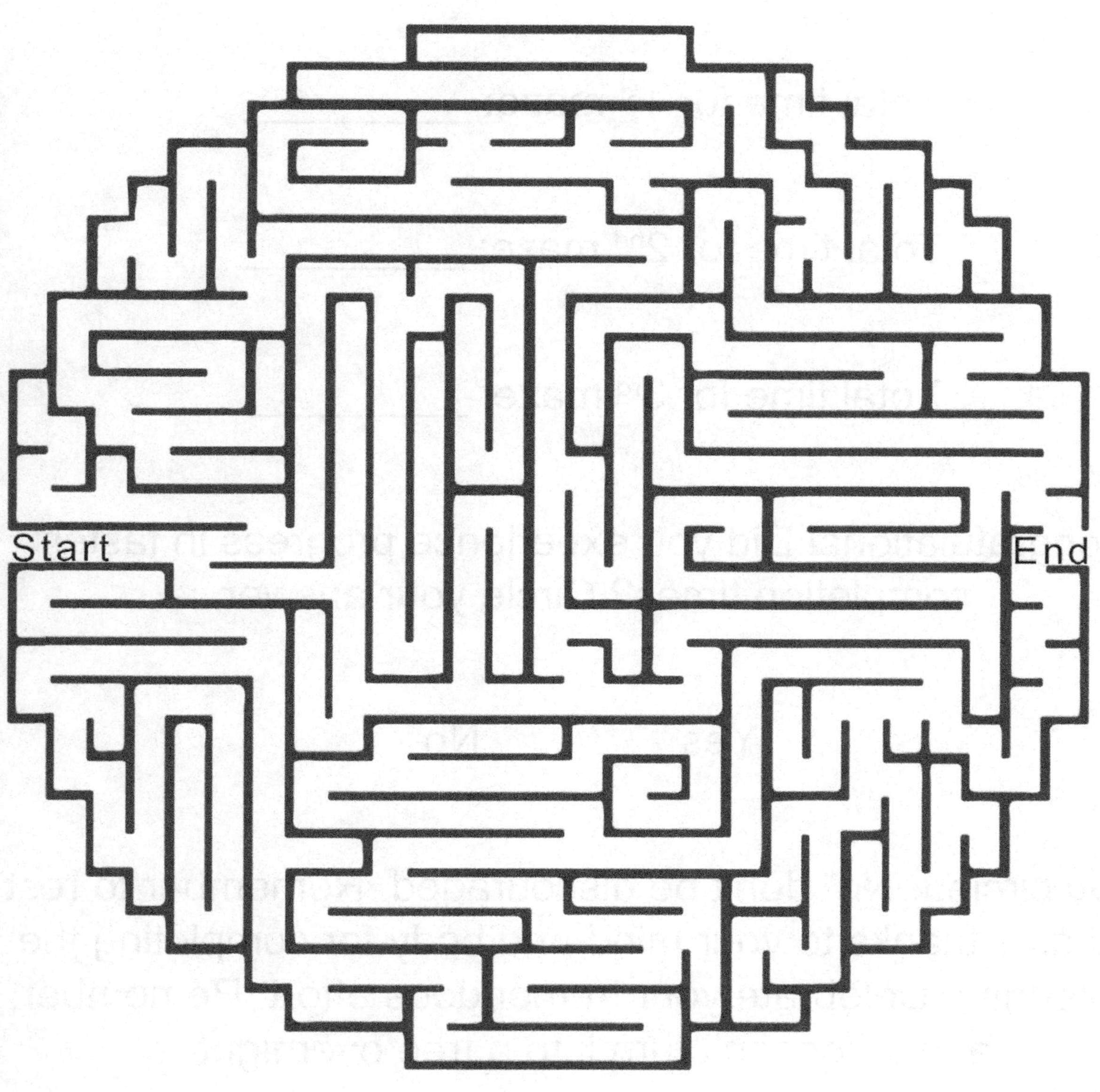

Start time: __________ End time: __________

Total time, maze 3: __________

Total time for 1st maze: __________

Total time for 2nd maze: __________

Total time for 3rd maze: __________

Congratulations! Did you experience progress in faster completion times? Circle your answer.

Yes No

If you circled "No" don't be discouraged. Remember to rest and give thanks to your mind and body for completing the challenges. Celebrate your tremendous effort. Remember, a seed doesn't turn into a tree overnight.

Life is like a camera… Focus on what's important, Capture the good times, Develop from the negatives, and if things don't work out, take another shot.

—Unknown

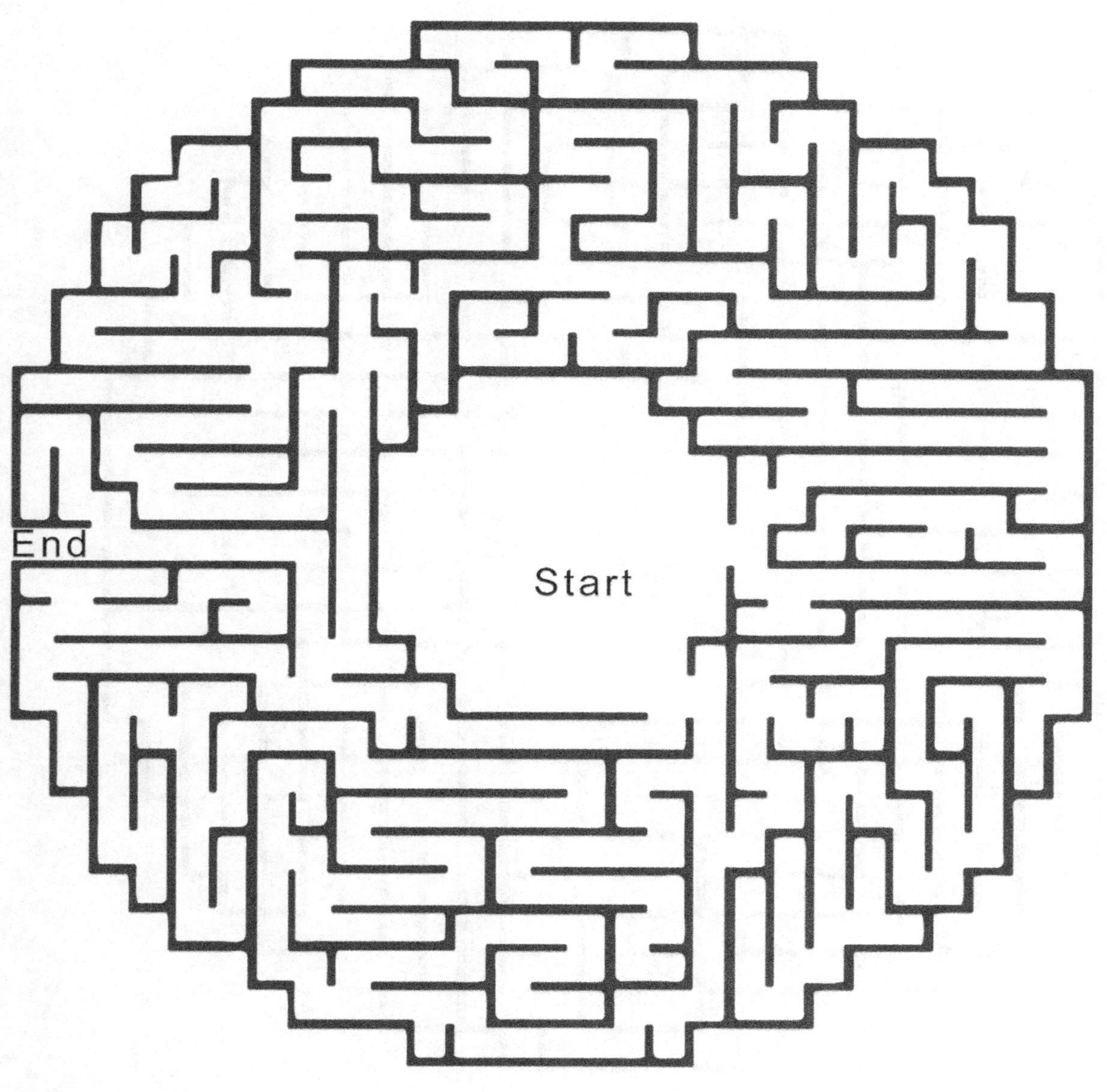

Start time: __________ End time: __________

Total time, maze 1: __________

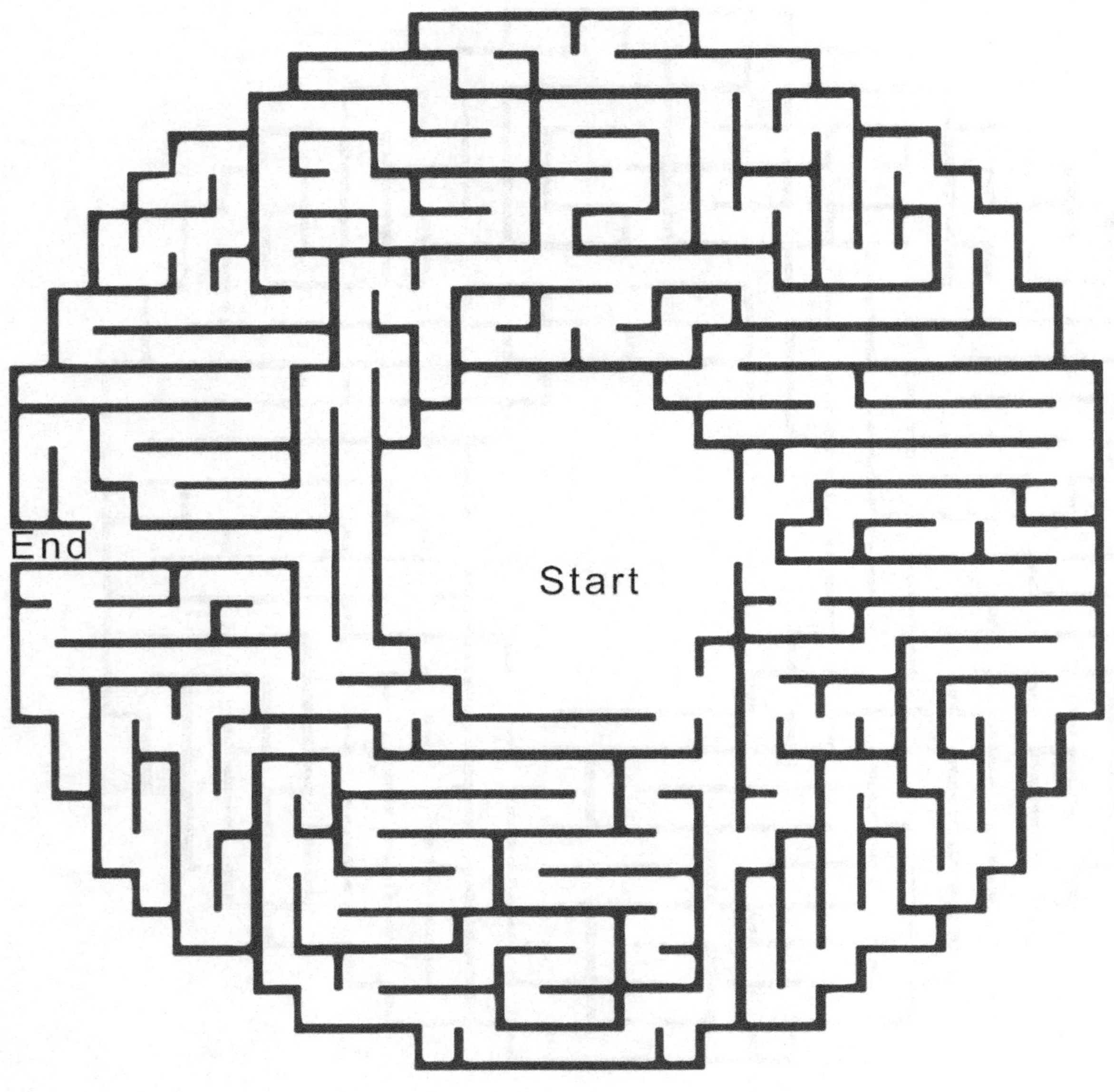

Start time: __________ End time: __________

Total time, maze 2: __________

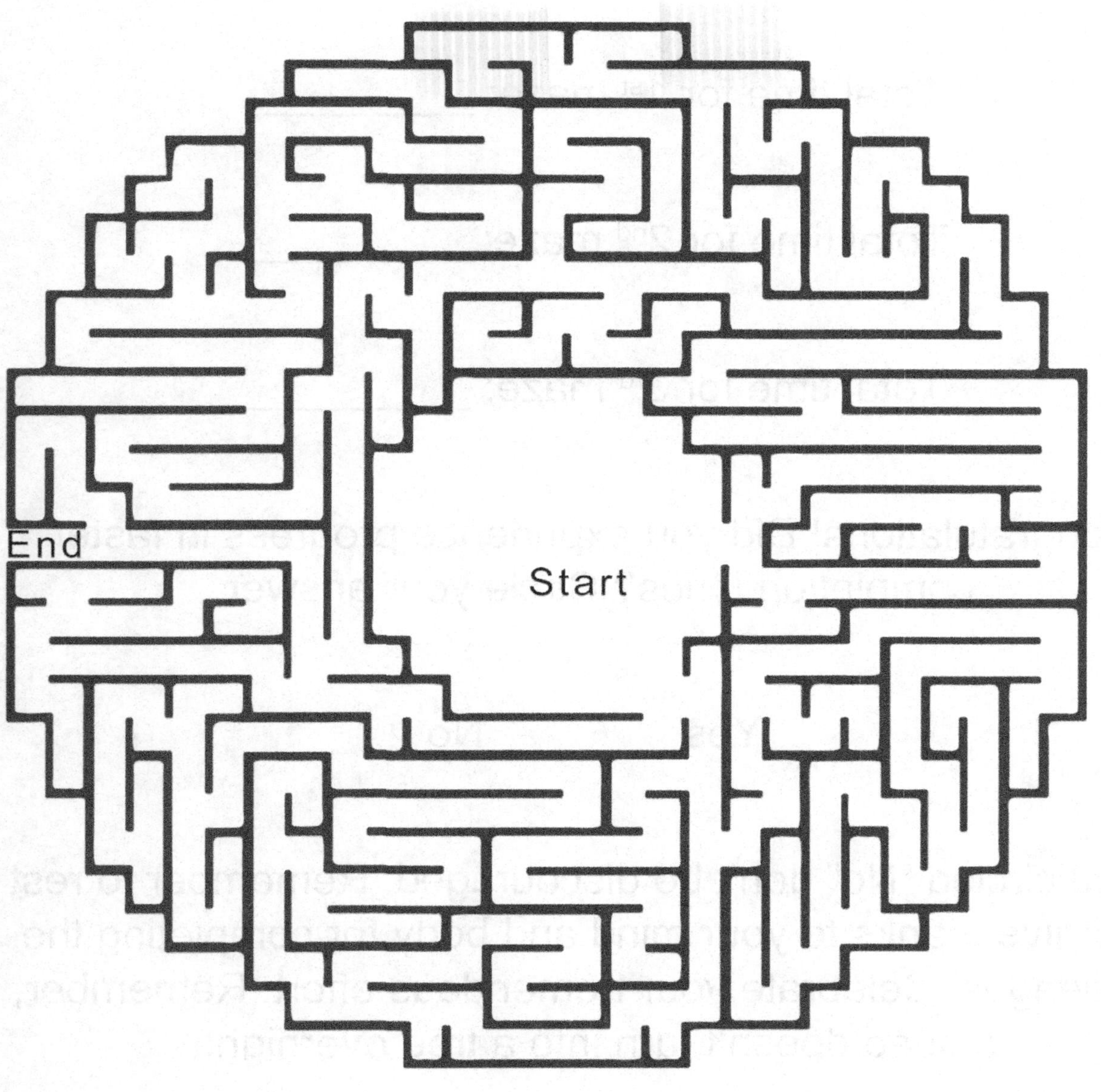

Start time: __________ End time: __________

Total time, maze 3: __________

Total time for 1st maze: __________

Total time for 2nd maze: __________

Total time for 3rd maze: __________

Congratulations! Did you experience progress in faster completion times? Circle your answer.

Yes No

If you circled "No" don't be discouraged. Remember to rest and give thanks to your mind and body for completing the challenges. Celebrate your tremendous effort. Remember, a seed doesn't turn into a tree overnight.

One of the things I learned the hard way was that it doesn't pay to get discouraged. Keeping busy and making optimism a way of life can restore your faith in yourself.

—Lucille Ball

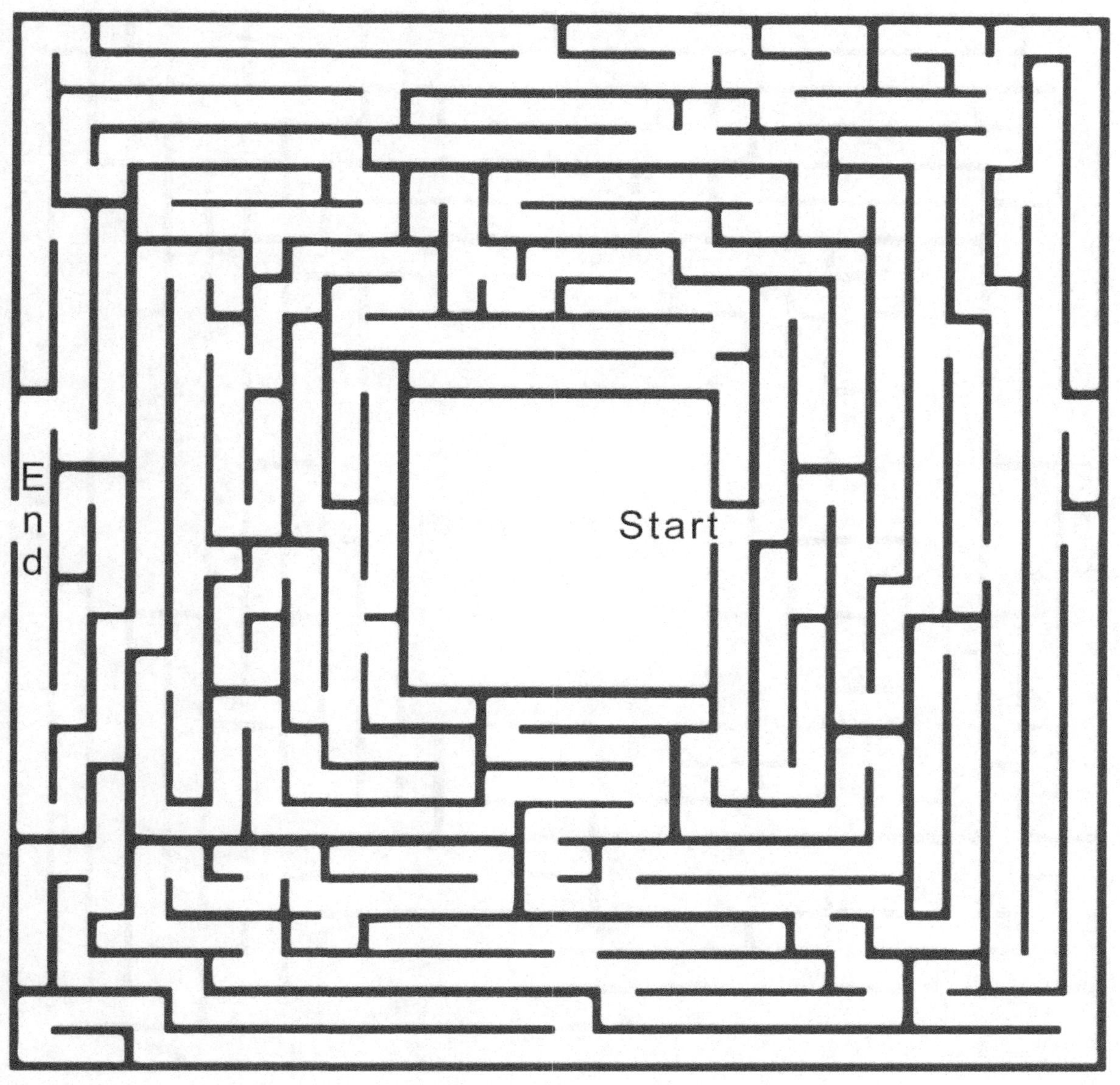

Start time: __________ End time: __________

Total time, maze 1: __________

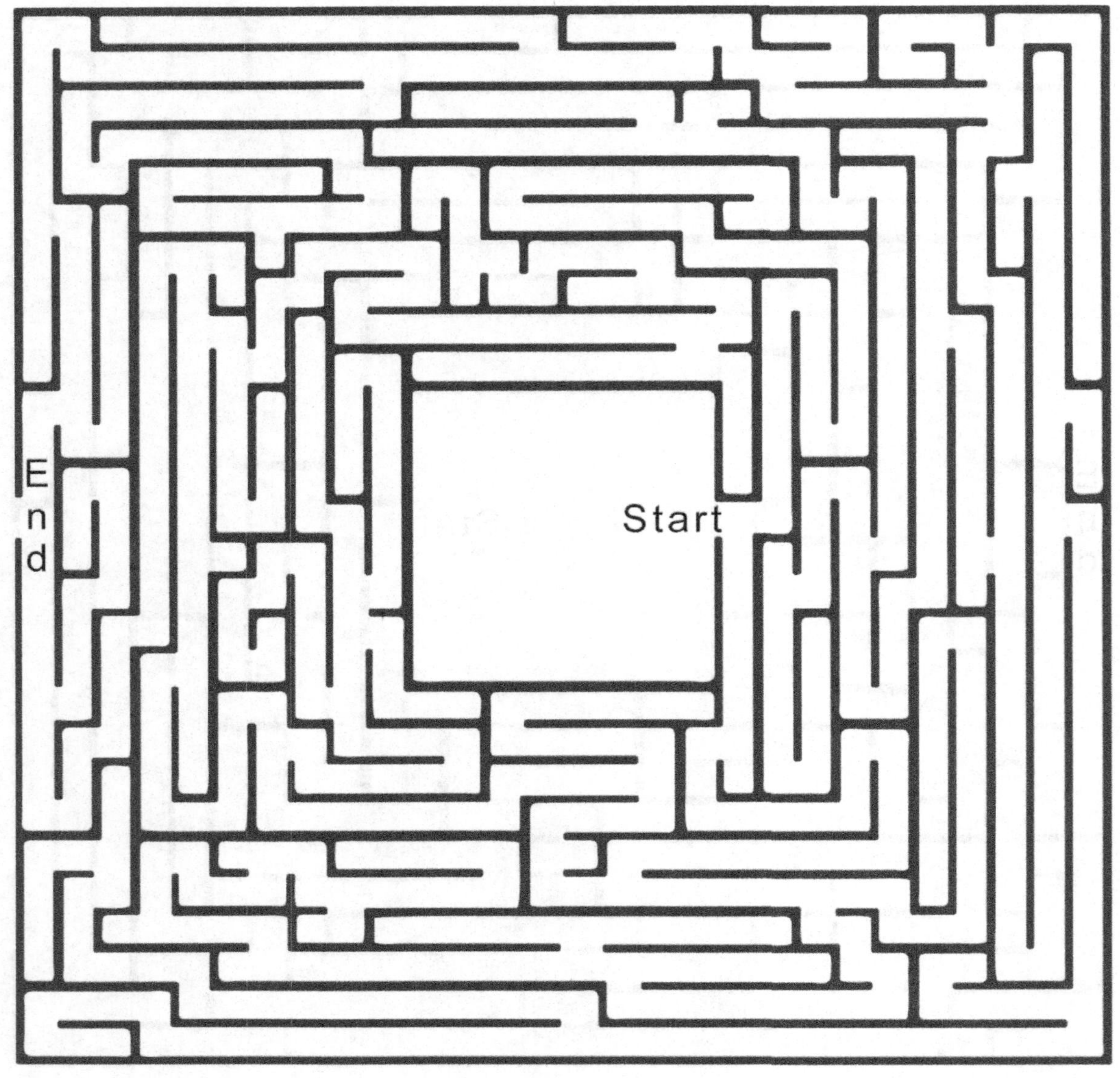

Start time: __________ End time: __________

Total time, maze 2: __________

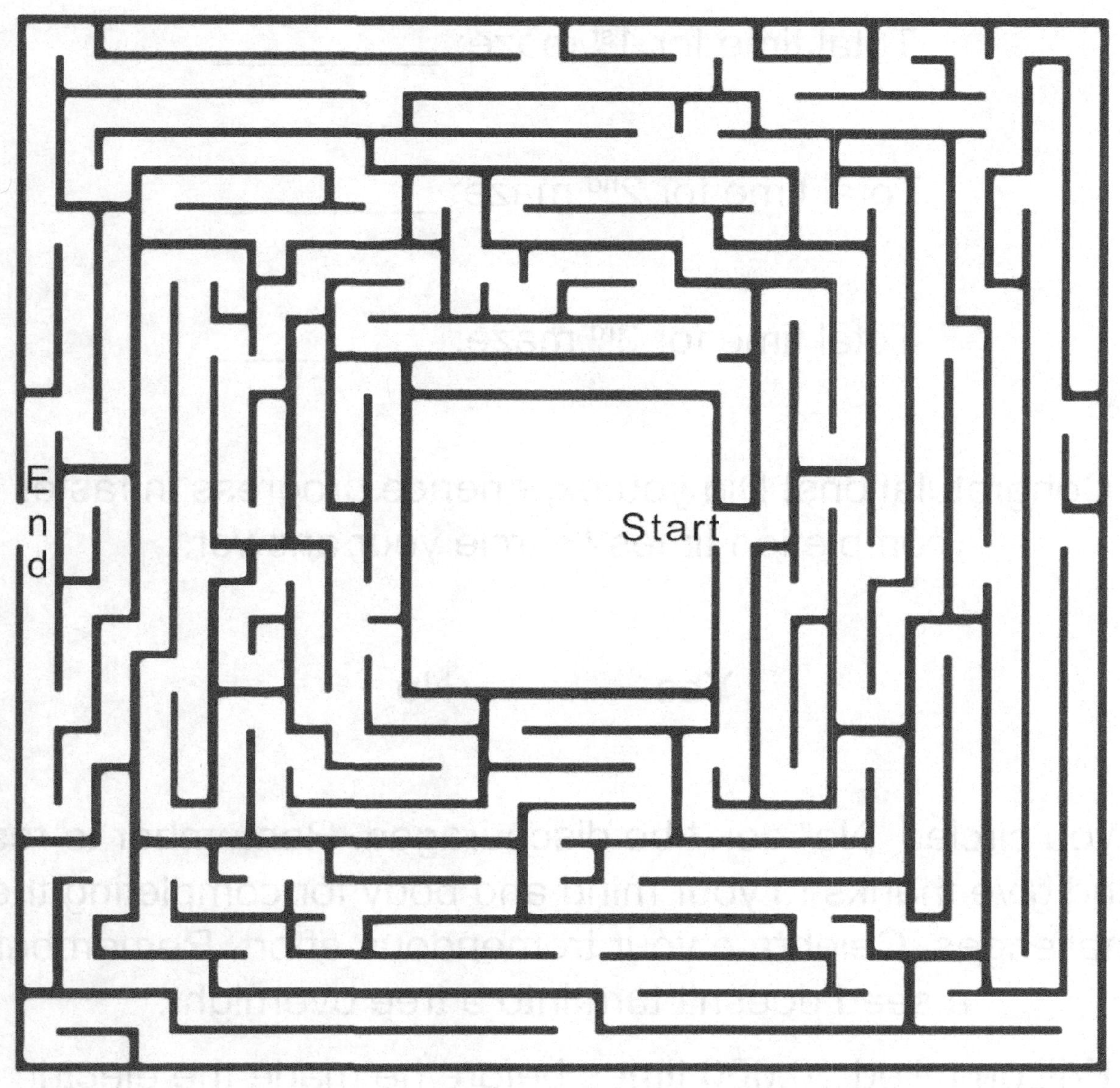

Start time: __________ End time: __________

Total time, maze 3: __________

Total time for 1st maze: __________

Total time for 2nd maze: __________

Total time for 3rd maze: __________

Congratulations! Did you experience progress in faster completion times? Circle your answer.

Yes No

If you circled "No" don't be discouraged. Remember to rest and give thanks to your mind and body for completing the challenges. Celebrate your tremendous effort. Remember, a seed doesn't turn into a tree overnight.

Edison failed 10,000 times before he made the electric light. Do not be discouraged if you fail a few times.

—Napoleon Hill

Your body cannot heal without play.
Your mind cannot heal without laughter.
Your soul cannot heal without joy.

—*Catherine Rippenger*

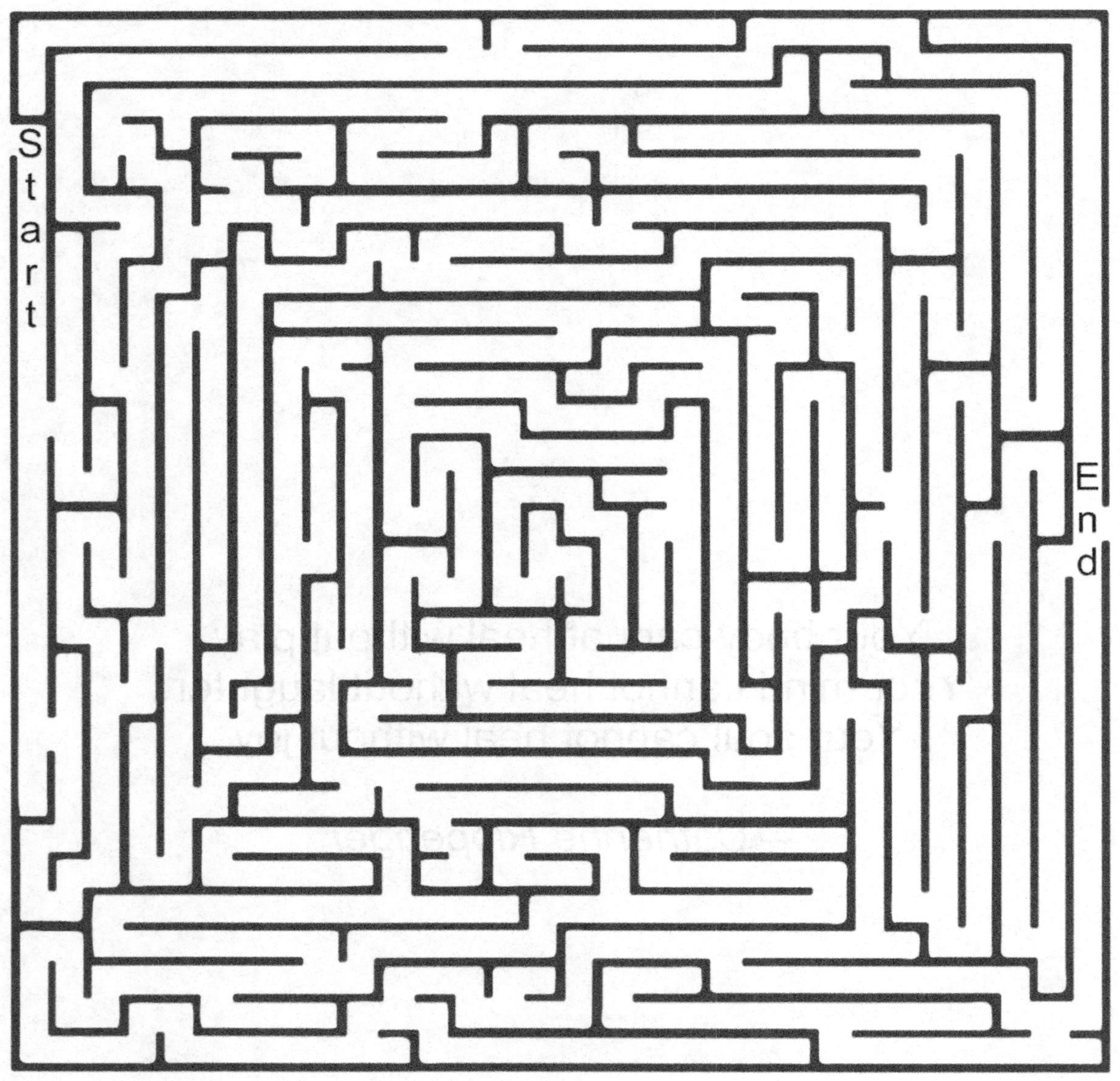

Start time: __________ End time: __________

Total time, maze 1: __________

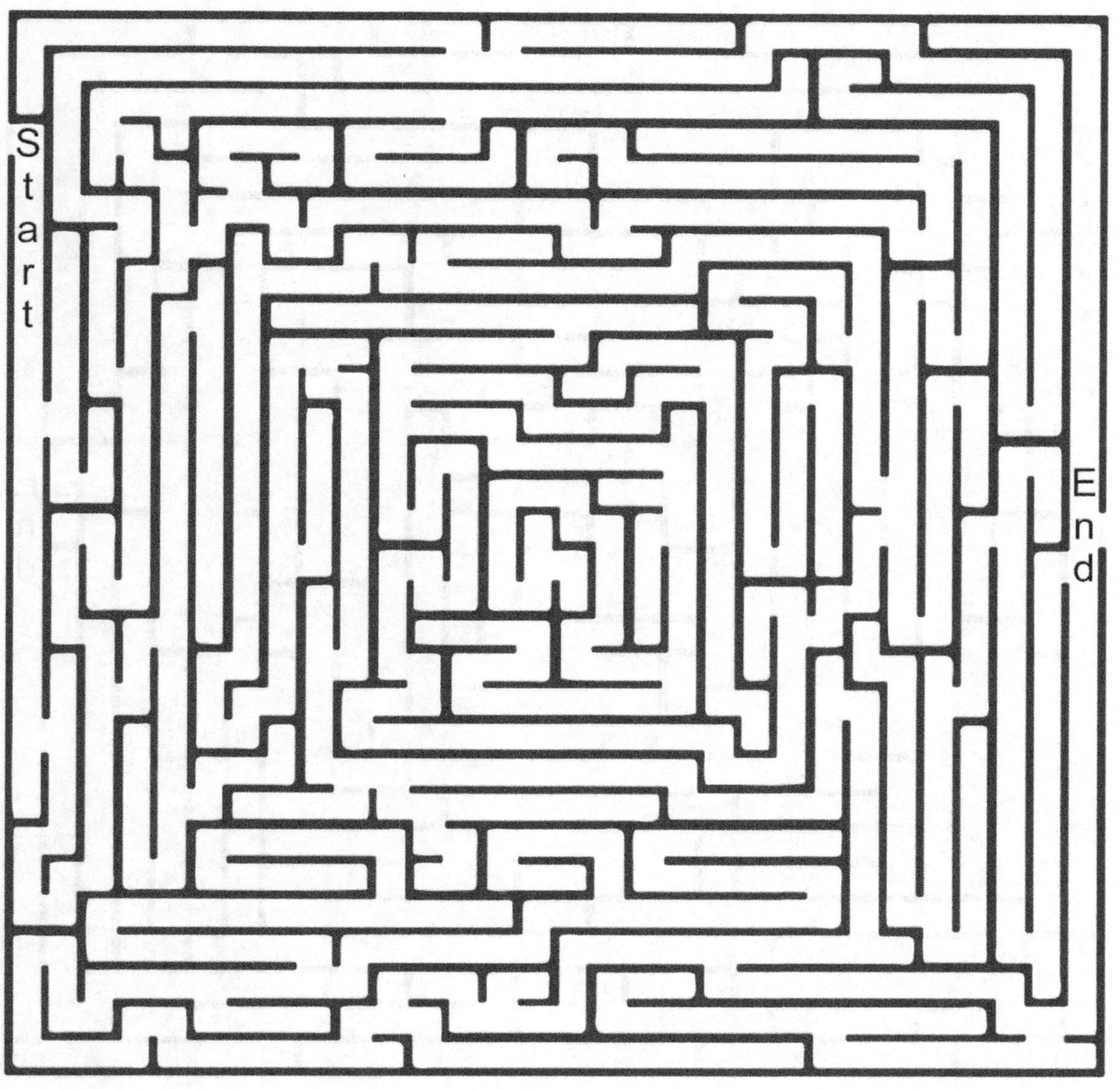

Start time: __________ End time: __________

Total time, maze 2: __________

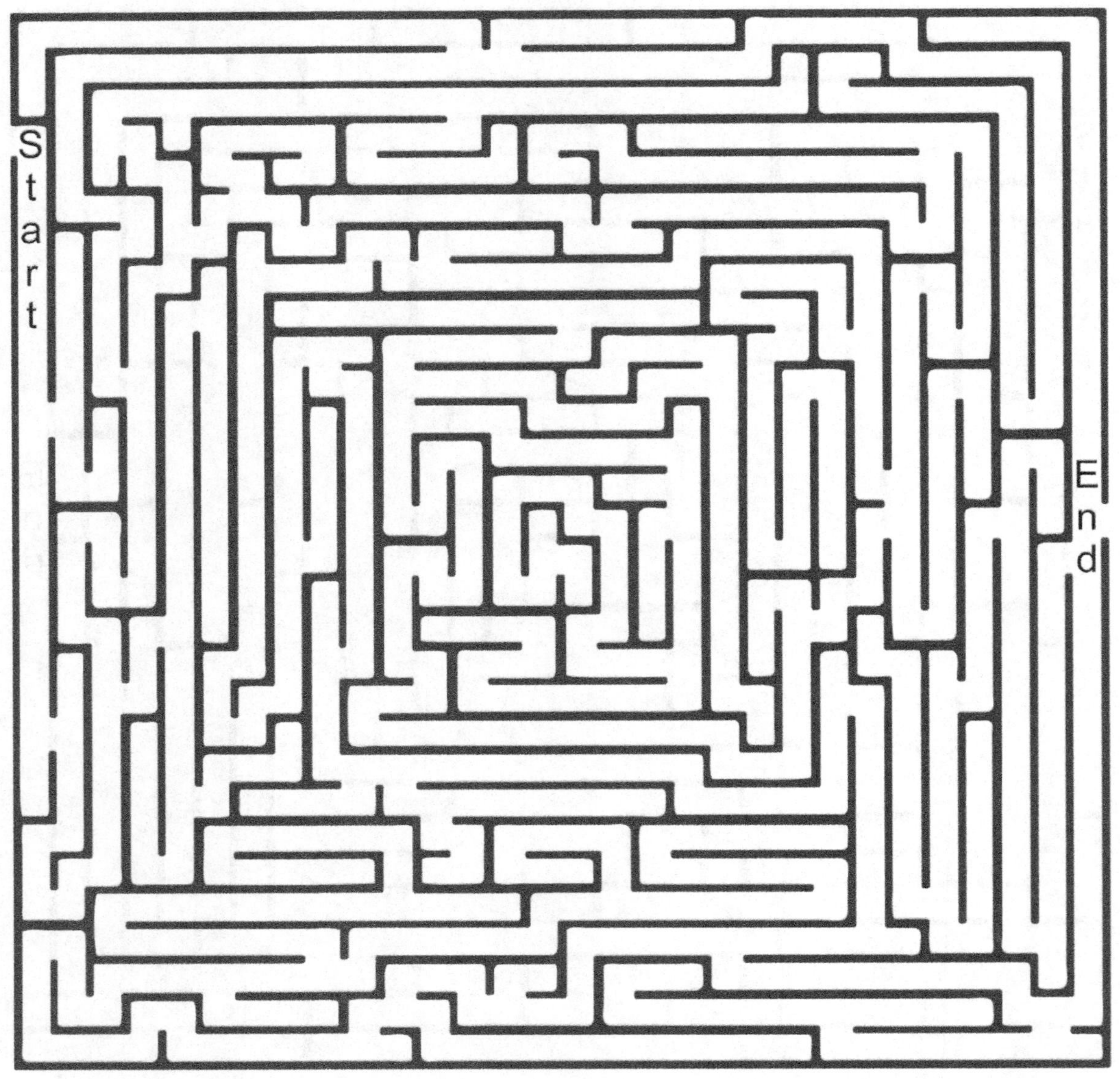

Start time: __________ End time: __________

Total time, maze 3: __________

Total time for 1st maze: __________

Total time for 2nd maze: __________

Total time for 3rd maze: __________

Congratulations! Did you experience progress in faster completion times? Circle your answer.

Yes No

If you circled "No" don't be discouraged. Remember to rest and give thanks to your mind and body for completing the challenges. Celebrate your tremendous effort. Remember, a seed doesn't turn into a tree overnight.

A man can get discouraged many times but he is not a failure until he begins to blame somebody else and stops trying.

—John Burroughs

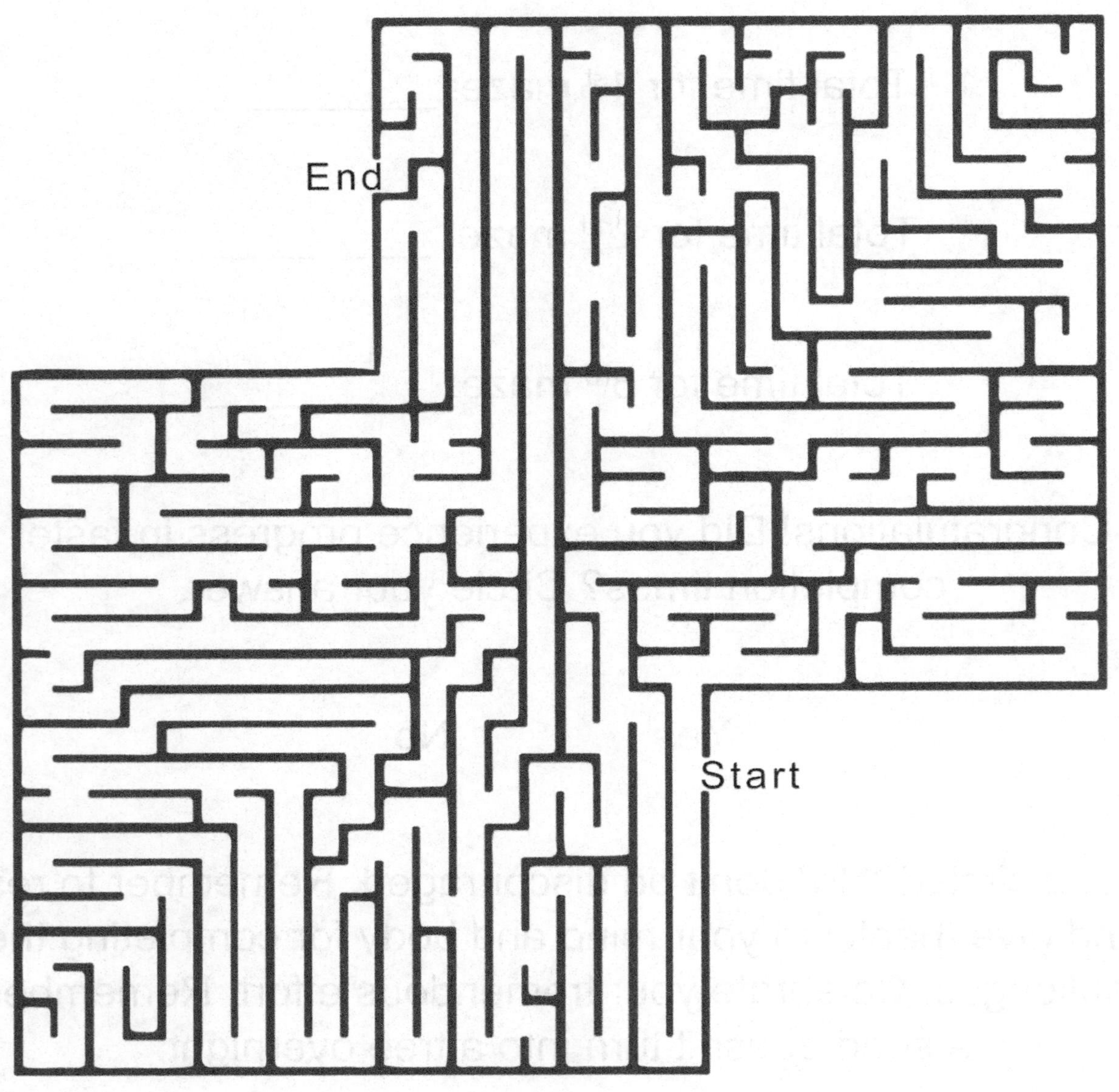

Start time: __________ End time: __________

Total time, maze 1: __________

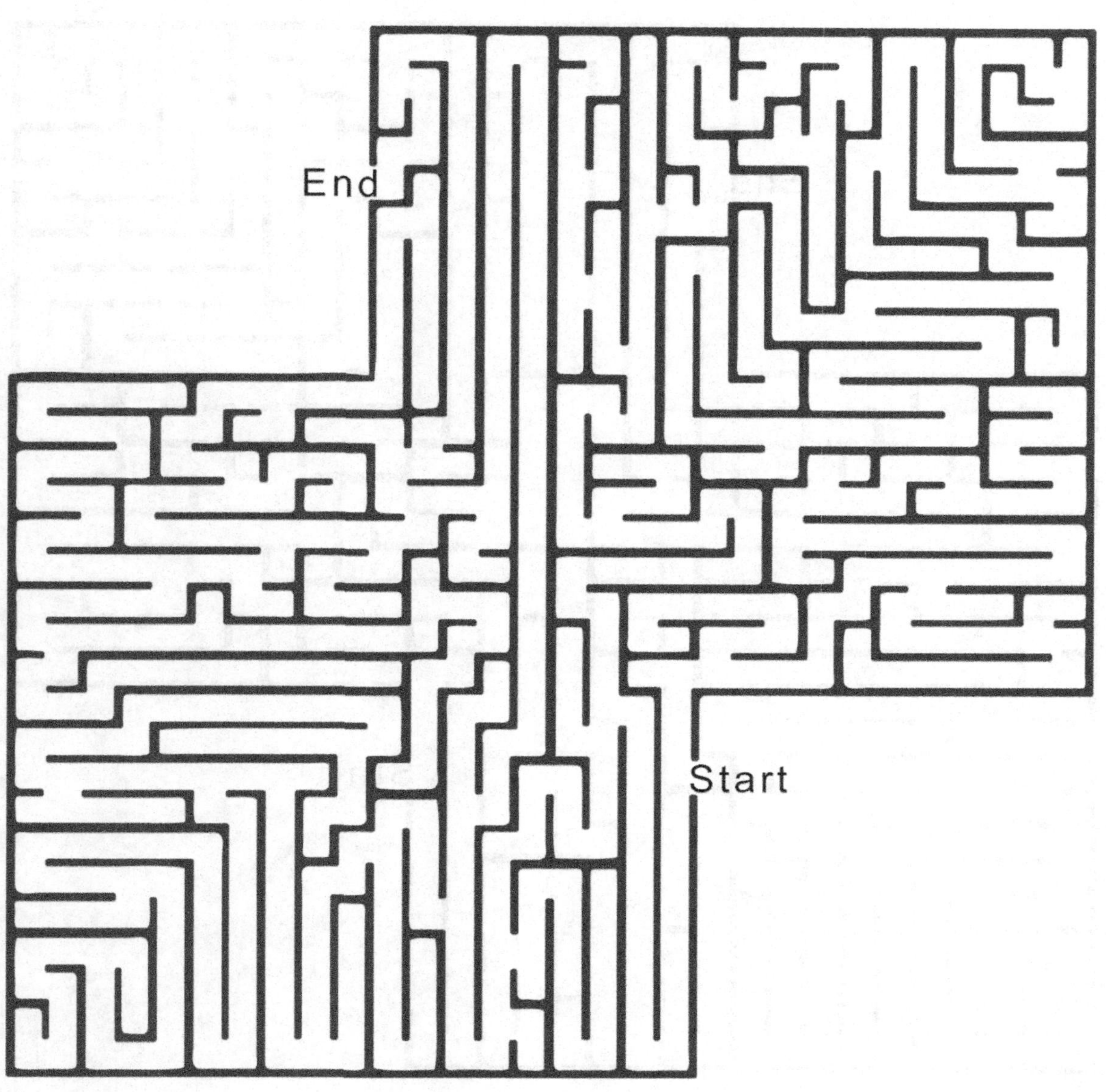

Start time: __________ End time: __________

Total time, maze 2: __________

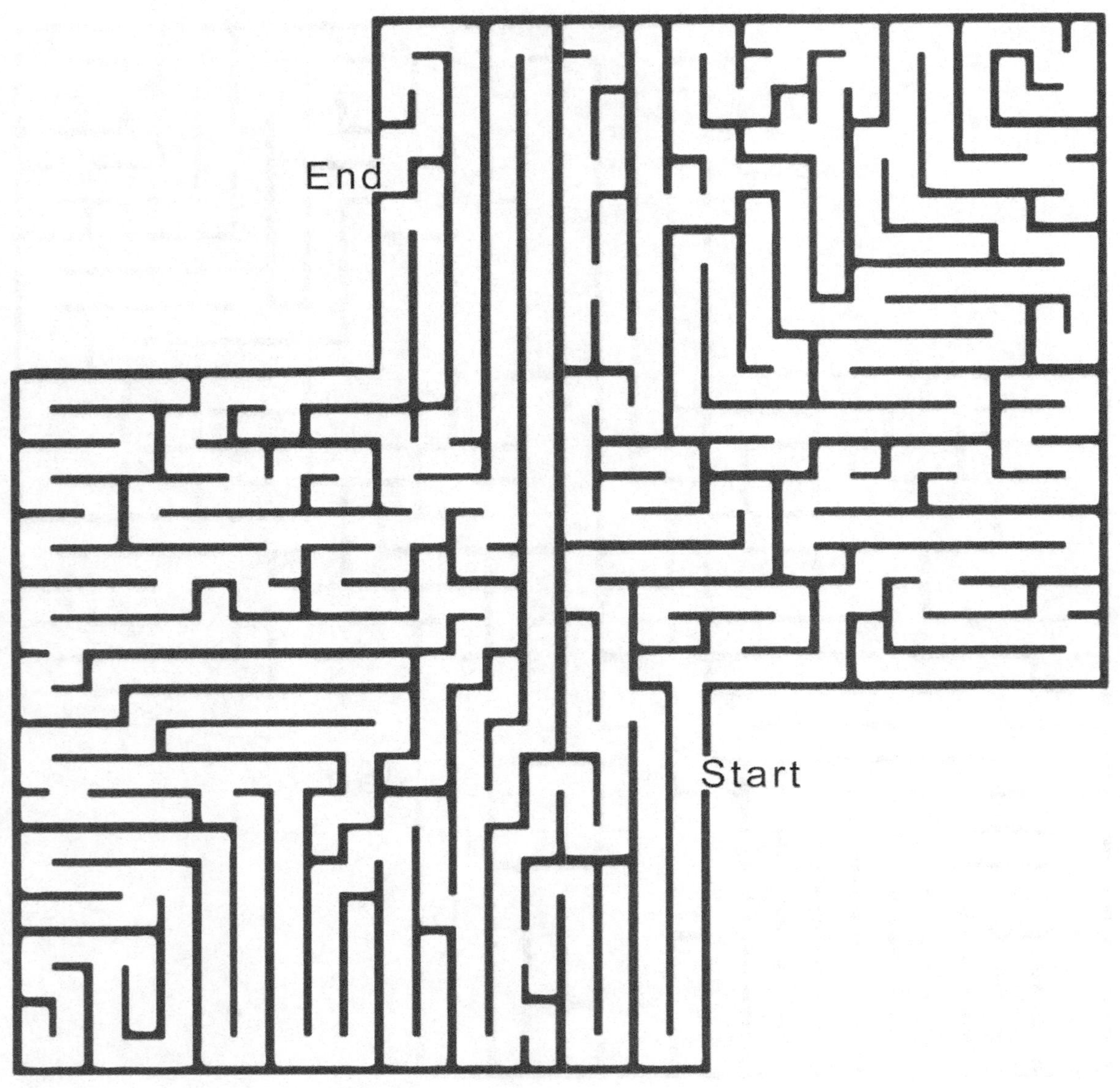

Start time: __________ End time: __________

Total time, maze 3: __________

Total time for 1st maze: __________

Total time for 2nd maze: __________

Total time for 3rd maze: __________

Congratulations! Did you experience progress in faster completion times? Circle your answer.

Yes No

If you circled "No" don't be discouraged. Remember to rest and give thanks to your mind and body for completing the challenges. Celebrate your tremendous effort. Remember, a seed doesn't turn into a tree overnight.

Continuous, unflagging effort, persistence and determination will win. Let not the man be discouraged who has these.

—*James Whitcomb Riley*

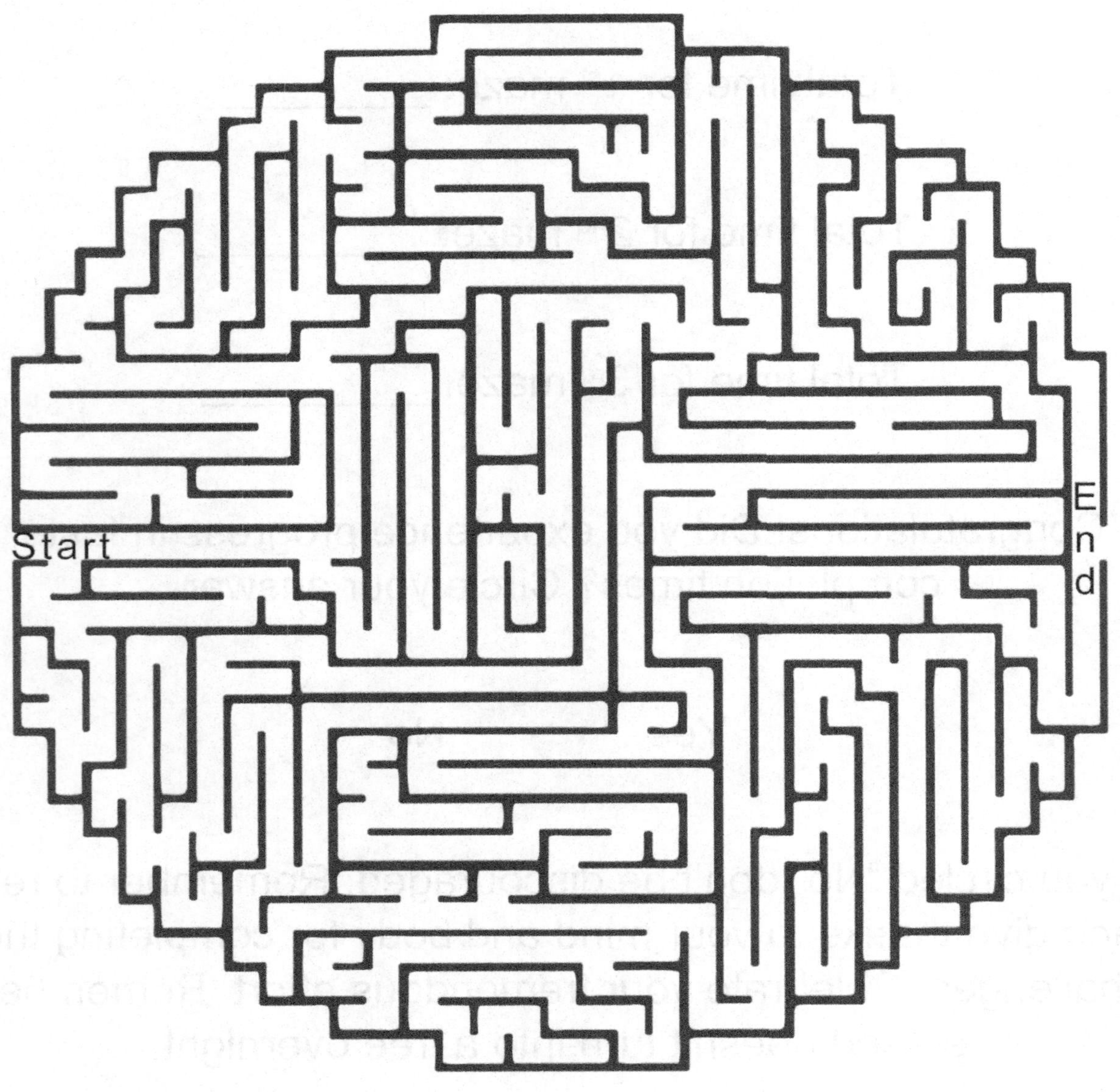

Start time: __________ End time: __________

Total time, maze 1: __________

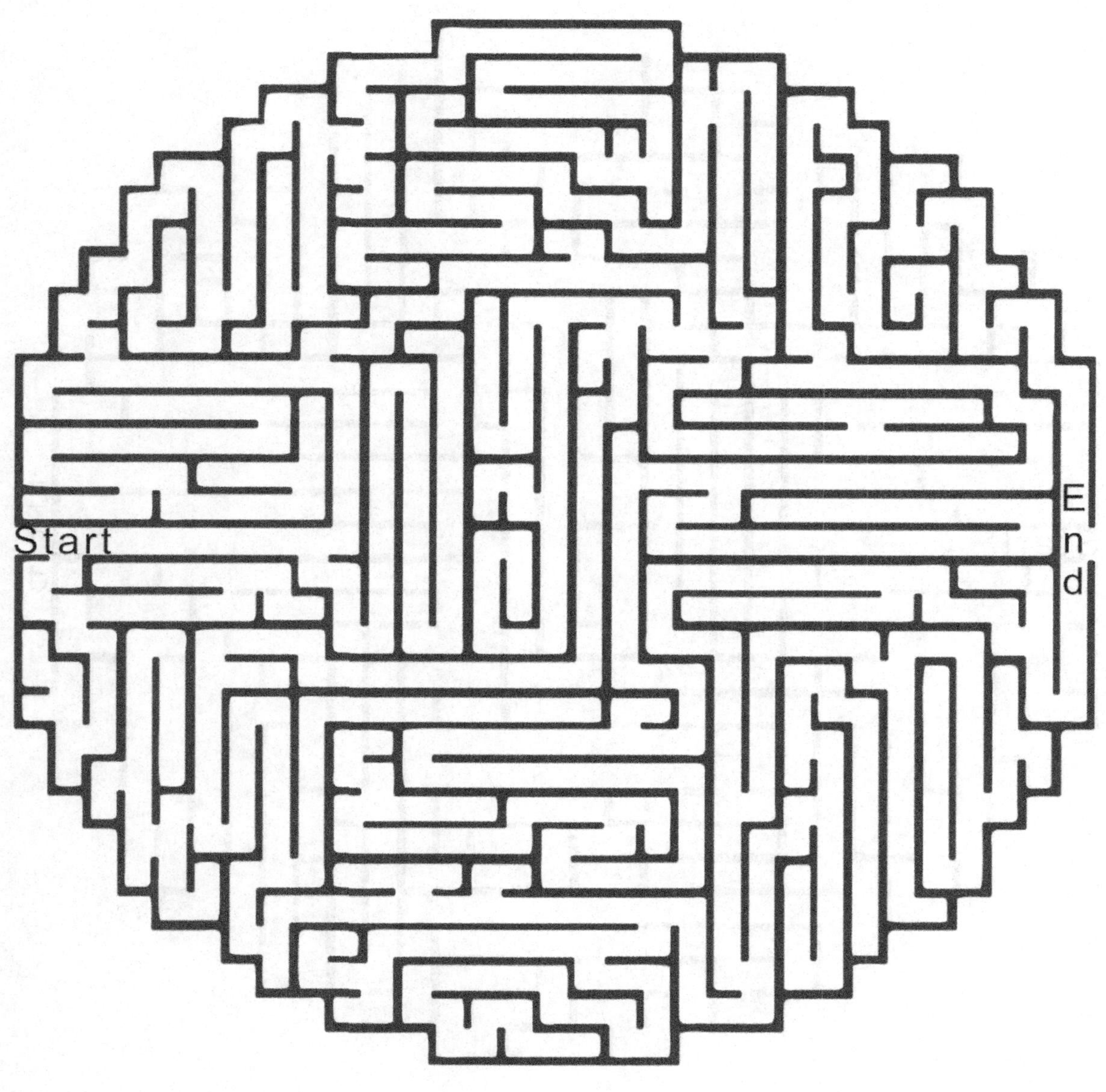

Start time: __________ End time: __________

Total time, maze 2: __________

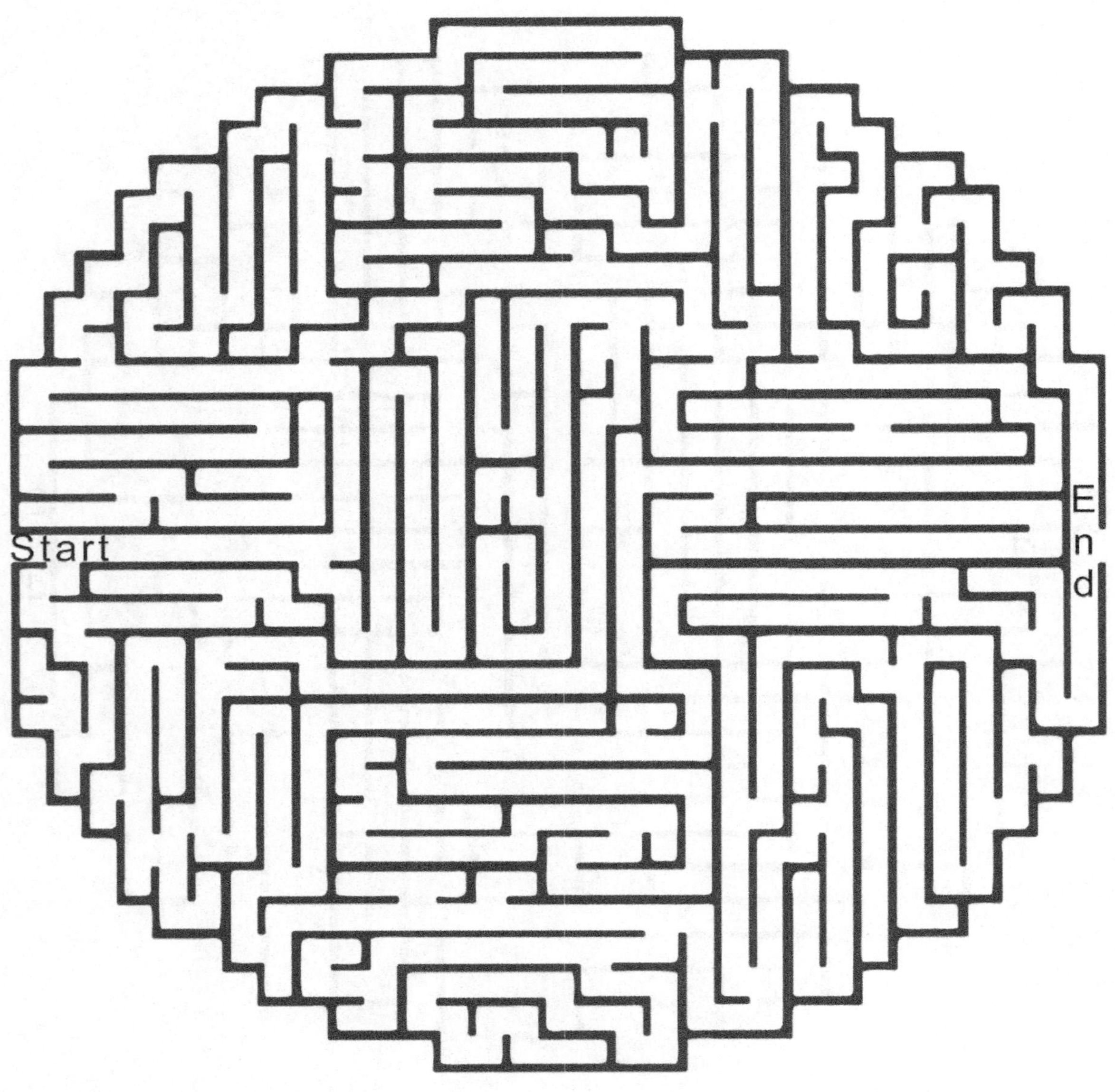

Start time: __________ End time: __________

Total time, maze 3: __________

Total time for 1st maze: __________

Total time for 2nd maze: __________

Total time for 3rd maze: __________

Congratulations! Did you experience progress in faster completion times? Circle your answer.

Yes No

If you circled “No” don’t be discouraged. Remember to rest and give thanks to your mind and body for completing the challenges. Celebrate your tremendous effort. Remember, a seed doesn’t turn into a tree overnight.

What is important is to believe in something so strongly that you're never discouraged.

—*Salma Hayek*

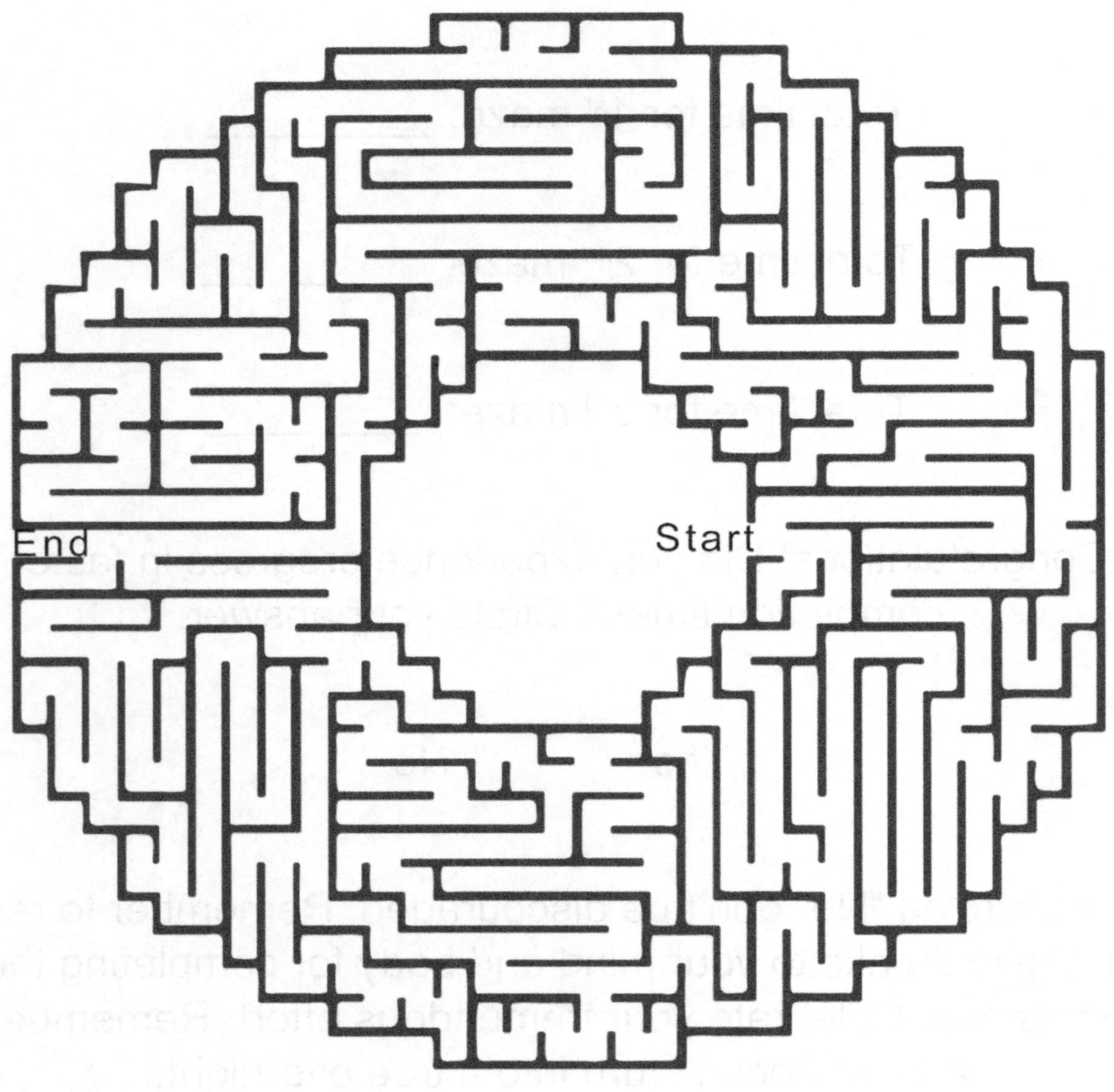

Start time: __________ End time: __________

Total time, maze 1: __________

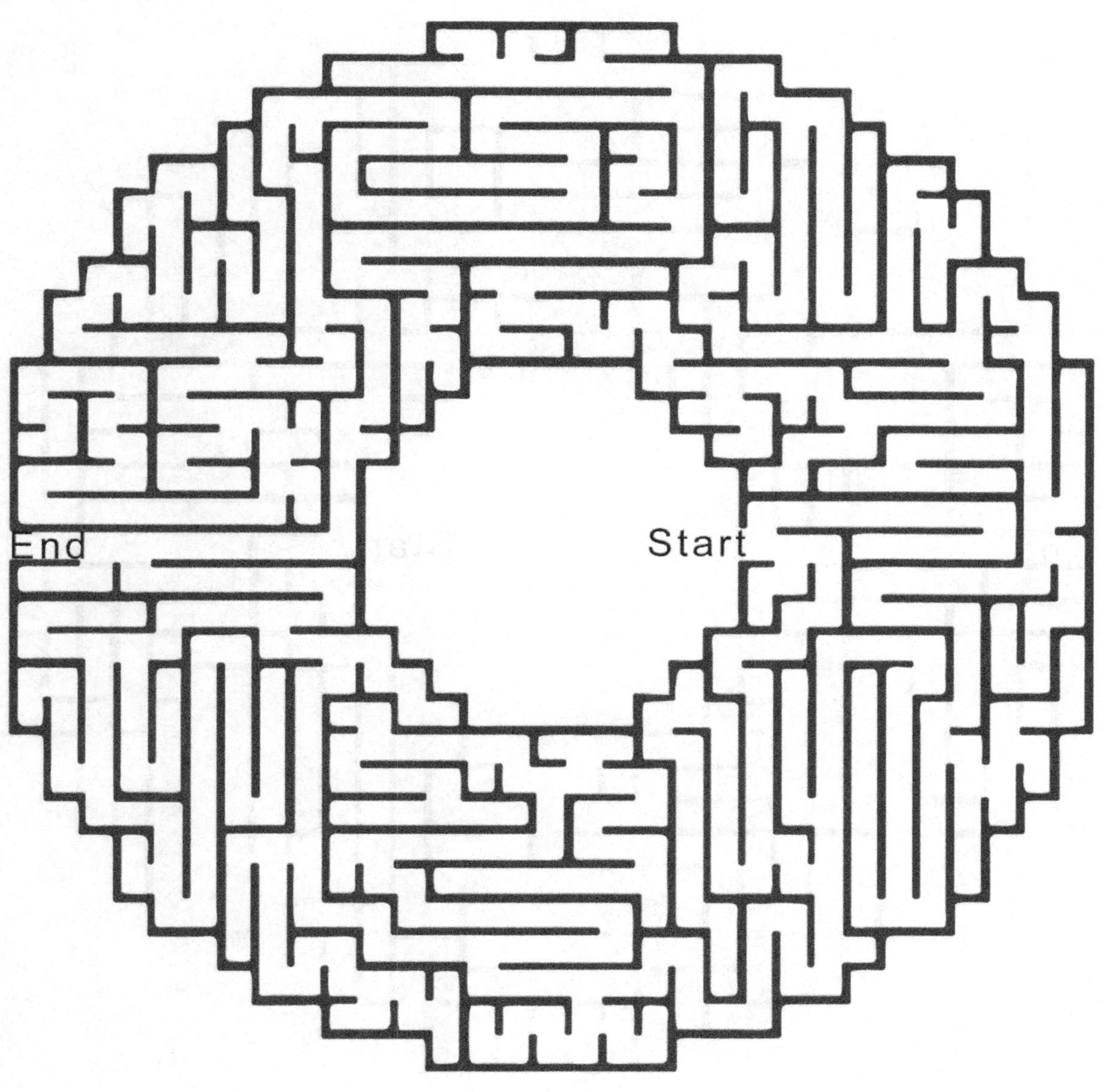

Start time: ____________ End time: ____________

Total time, maze 2: ____________

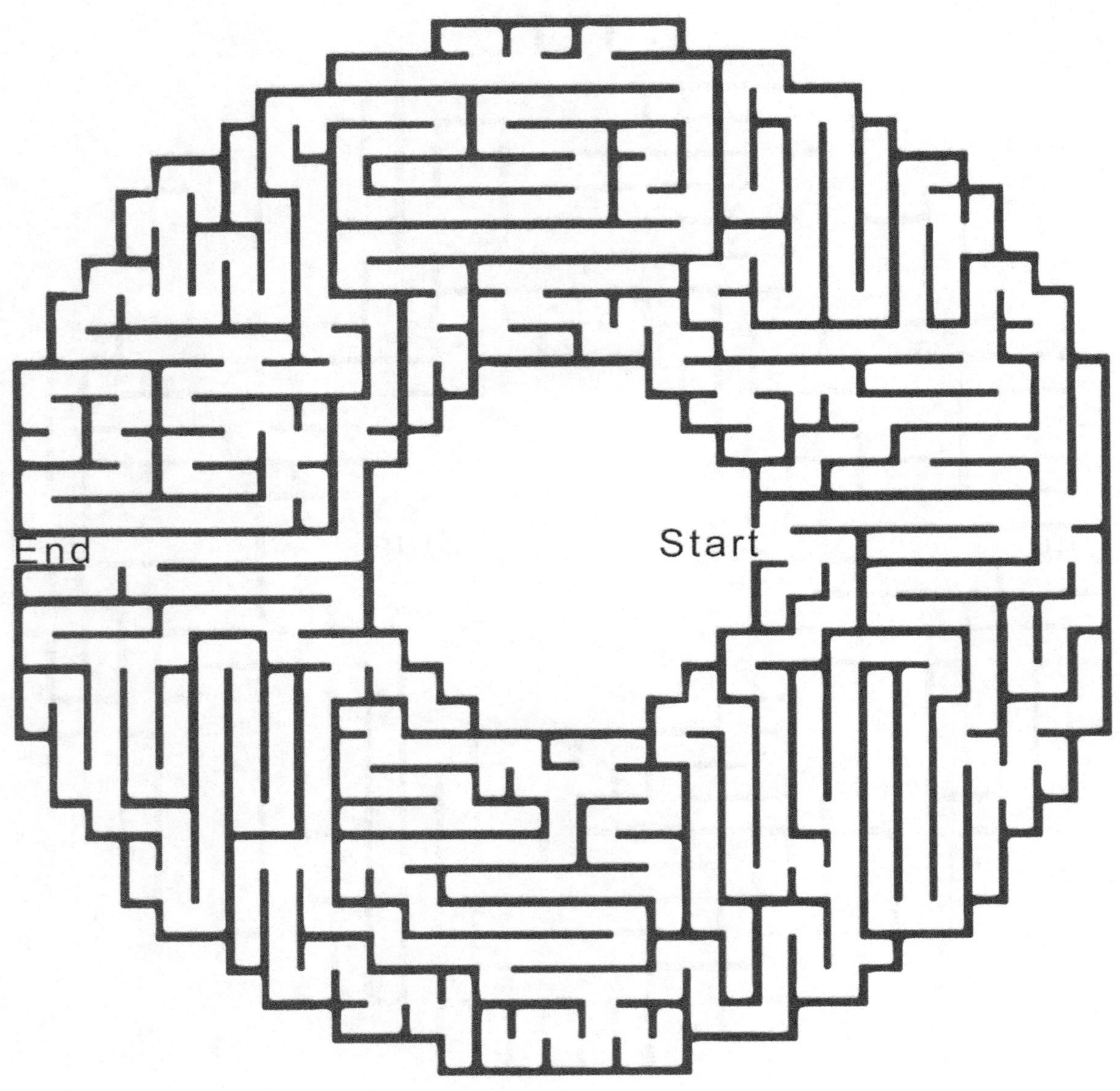

Start time: __________ End time: __________

Total time, maze 3: __________

Total time for 1st maze: __________

Total time for 2nd maze: __________

Total time for 3rd maze: __________

Congratulations! Did you experience progress in faster completion times? Circle your answer.

Yes No

If you circled “No” don’t be discouraged. Remember to rest and give thanks to your mind and body for completing the challenges. Celebrate your tremendous effort. Remember, a seed doesn’t turn into a tree overnight.

Stop beating yourself up. You are a work in progress - which means you get there a little at a time, not all at once.

—Unknown

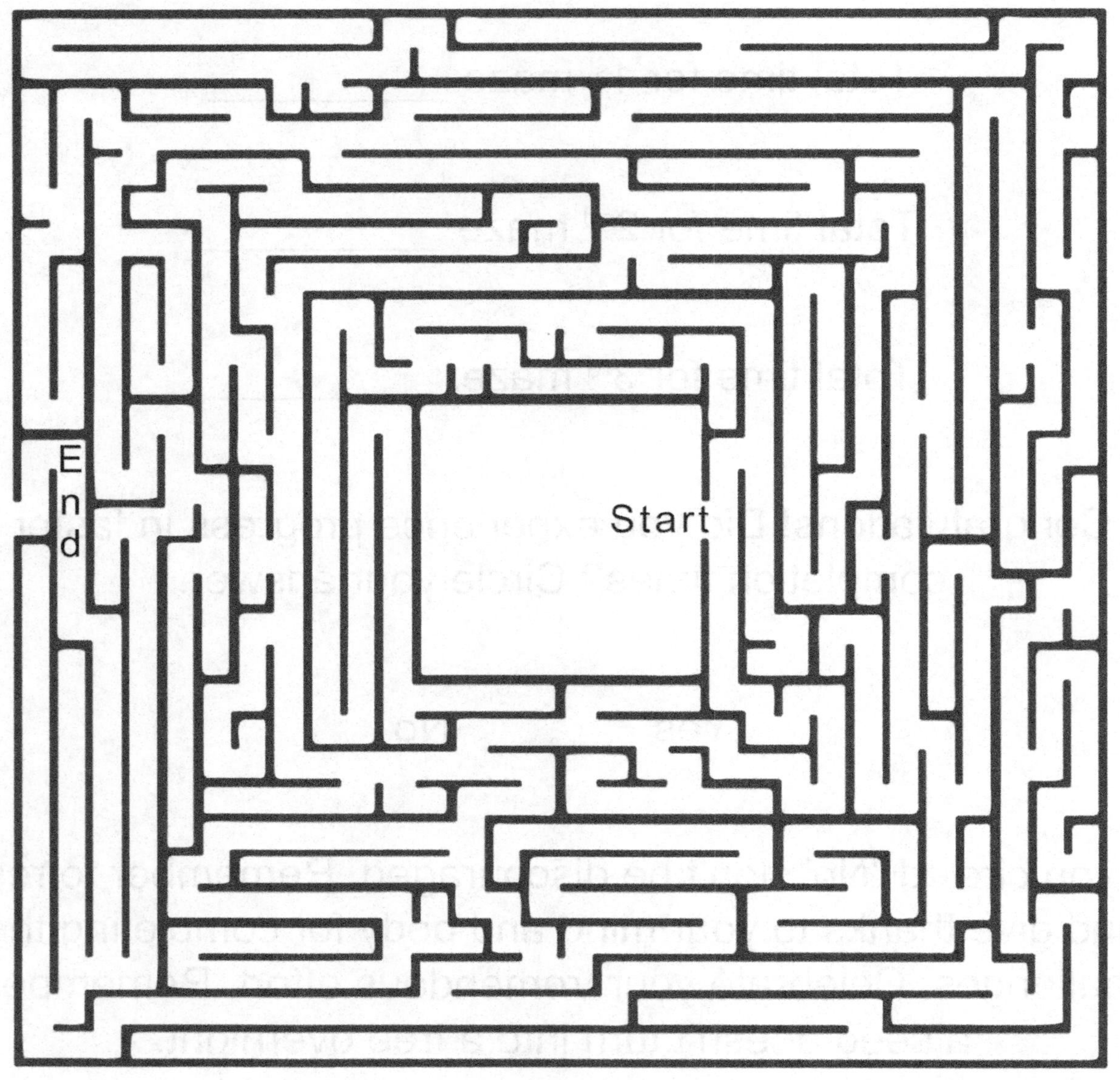

Start time: __________ End time: __________

Total time, maze 1: __________

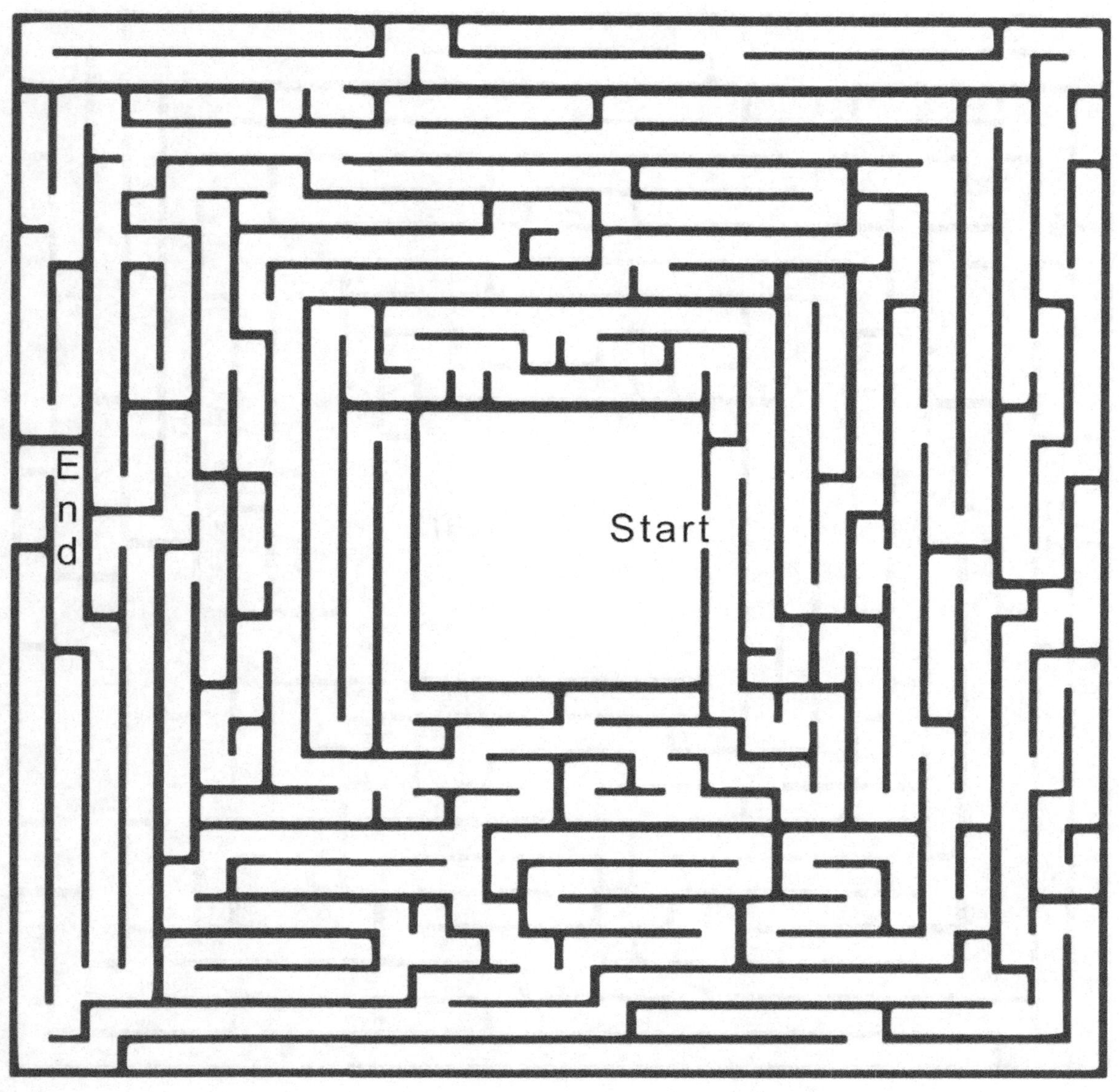

Start time: __________ End time: __________

Total time, maze 2: __________

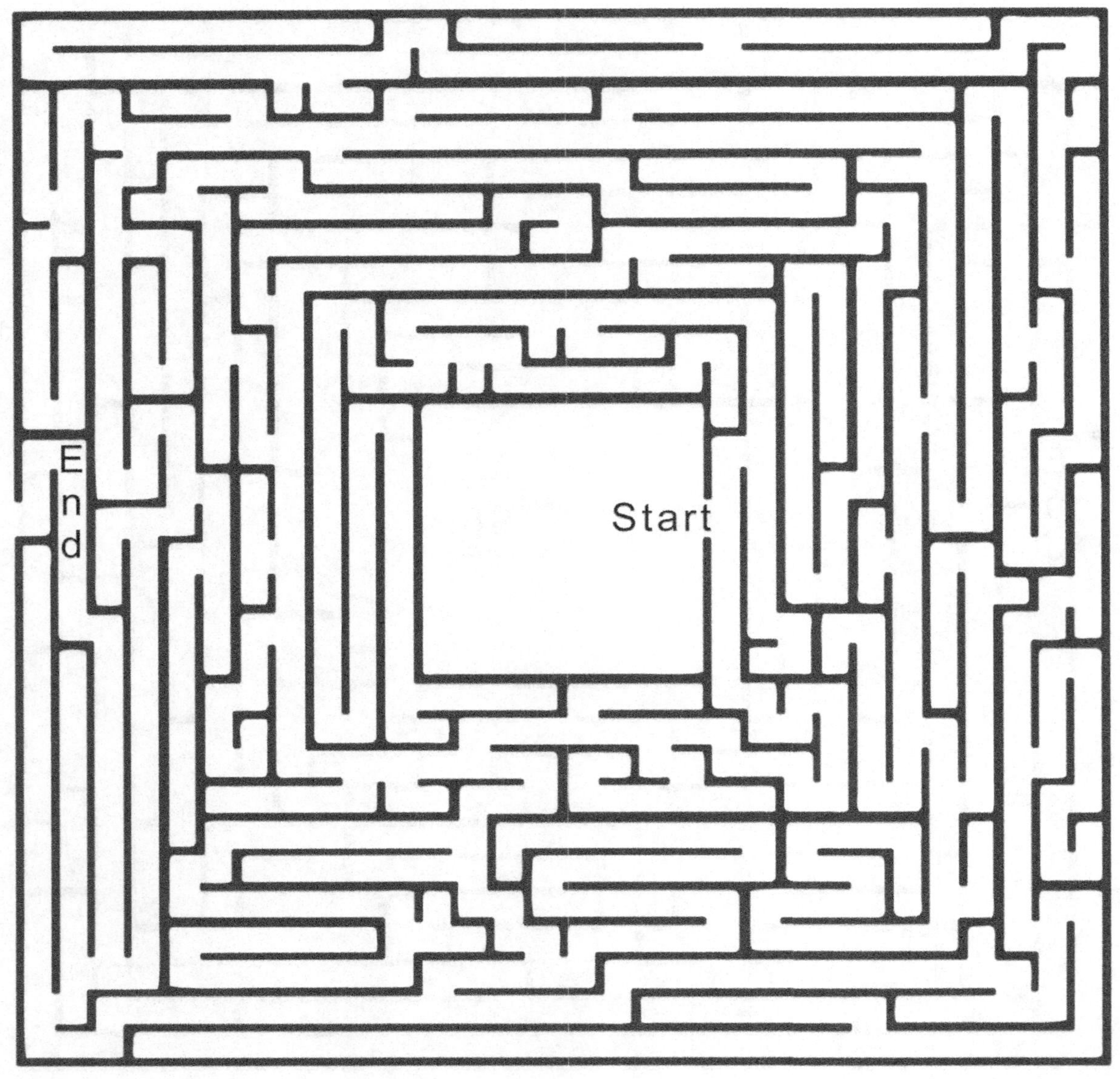

Start time: __________ End time: __________

Total time, maze 3: __________

Total time for 1st maze: __________

Total time for 2nd maze: __________

Total time for 3rd maze: __________

Congratulations! Did you experience progress in faster completion times? Circle your answer.

Yes No

If you circled "No" don't be discouraged. Remember to rest and give thanks to your mind and body for completing the challenges. Celebrate your tremendous effort. Remember, a seed doesn't turn into a tree overnight.

Yesterday I was clever so I wanted to change the world. Today I am wise, so I am changing myself.

—*Rumi*

Your body cannot heal without play.
Your mind cannot heal without laughter.
Your soul cannot heal without joy.

—Catherine Rippenger

Congratulations!

You have completed the Traumatic Brain Injury Workbook, improved your puzzle skills, and are on your way to improved memory and cognitive function. Repeating these exercises can help you realize additional improvements.

Made in the USA
Middletown, DE
28 June 2024